Health Systems Improvement Across the Globe: Success Stories from 60 Countries

T0188262

Health Systems Improvement Across the Globe:
Success Stories from 60 Countries

Series Editor:
Professor Jeffrey Braithwaite, Australian Institute of Health Innovation,
Macquarie University, Australia

Regional Editors:
Professor Jeffrey Braithwaite, Australian Institute of Health Innovation,
Macquarie University, Australia
Professor Russell Mannion, Health Services Management Centre,
University of Birmingham, the United Kingdom
Professor Yukihiro Matsuyama, Canon Institute for Global Studies, Japan
Professor Paul Shekelle, West Los Angeles Veterans Affairs Medical
Center; and the University of California, USA
Professor Stuart Whittaker, School of Public Health and Medicine at the
Faculty of Health Sciences at the University of Cape Town; and School of
Health Systems and Public Health, Faculty of Health Sciences, University of
Pretoria, South Africa
Professor Samir Al-Adawi, Sultan Qaboos University, Oman

Health Systems Improvement Across the Globe: Success Stories from 60 Countries

Edited by
Jeffrey Braithwaite, Russell Mannion, Yukihiro Matsuyama, Paul Shekelle, Stuart Whittaker, and Samir Al-Adawi

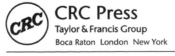

CRC Press
Taylor & Francis Group
Boca Raton London New York

CRC Press is an imprint of the
Taylor & Francis Group, an **informa** business

CRC Press
Taylor & Francis Group
6000 Broken Sound Parkway NW, Suite 300
Boca Raton, FL 33487-2742

First issued in paperback 2019

© 2018 by Jeffrey Braithwaite, Russell Mannion, Yukihiro Matsuyama, Paul Shekelle, Stuart Whittaker, and Samir Al-Adawi.
CRC Press is an imprint of Taylor & Francis Group, an Informa business

No claim to original U.S. Government works

ISBN-13: 978-1-4724-8204-4 (hbk)
ISBN-13: 978-0-367-88174-0 (pbk)

Library of Congress Cataloging-in-Publication Data

Names: Braithwaite, Jeffrey, 1954- editor.
Title: Health systems improvement across the globe : success stories from 60 countries / edited by Jeffrey Braithwaite, Russell Mannion, Yukihiro Matsuyama, Paul Shekelle, Stuart Whittaker and Samir Al-Adawi.
Description: Boca Raton : CRC Press, [2017] | Includes bibliographical references and index.
Identifiers: LCCN 2017000415| ISBN 9781472482044 (hardback : alk. paper) | ISBN 9781315586359 (ebook)
Subjects: | MESH: Delivery of Health Care | Quality Improvement | Health Care Reform | Internationality
Classification: LCC RA441 | NLM W 84.41 | DDC 362.1--dc23
LC record available at https://lccn.loc.gov/2017000415

Visit the Taylor & Francis Web site at
http://www.taylorandfrancis.com

and the CRC Press Web site at
http://www.crcpress.com

Maps have been adapted from
https://mapchart.net/

Contents

Part I   The Americas
Paul Shekelle

Part II Africa
Stuart Whittaker

Part III   Europe
Russell Mannion

Part IV Eastern Mediterranean
Samir Al-Adawi

Part V South-East Asia and the Western Pacific
Yukihiro Matsuyama and Jeffrey Braithwaite

Preface

The world of healthcare is very challenging. Resource-constrained services, creeping bureaucratic requirements, new patient populations with greater needs than ever before, demand in excess of supply, clinician overload, major and minor breaches of patient safety, politicized workplaces, and ideology masquerading as systems planning: everywhere you look, the barriers to the provision of high-quality care are considerable, and often daunting. In the midst of all these problems, where can we turn for help?

One answer is to change the focus and shift from the negatives to the positives. The very countries in which these types of problems reside always contain examples which have risen above the adversity, and provide solutions to problems. These are success stories that overcome difficulties, surmount obstacles, and deliver an accomplishment worthy of study in its own right.

Professor Jeffrey Braithwaite, as health reform series editor, has led a team of internationally renowned scholars to deliver a compendium of work with precisely this focus. Regional experts Professors Russell Mannion (Europe), Yukihiro Matsuyama (South-East Asia), Paul Shekelle (the Americas), Stuart Whittaker (Africa), Samir Al-Adawi (Eastern Mediterranean), and Jeffrey Braithwaite (the Western Pacific) have made a concerted effort to harness the energies, expertise, and analytic ability of 161 authors who have combined to articulate positive messages about healthcare improvement in 60 countries. Rich and poor, northern and southern hemisphere, publicly or privately funded, technologically sophisticated or focused on the basics: the range of health systems examples, and their differing characteristics, is truly impressive.

As you will see, each team of authors presents a single case example, which narrates a story of accomplishment in their home health system. The sheer diversity of case examples is testament to the range of things that can go right in healthcare. They provide plenty of lessons for those who want to improve care in their own system. Collectively, they act as a set of blueprints for what success looks like across many settings, sectors, and initiatives. That every country enrolled in the project, no matter how politically, financially, or logistically challenged, could adduce a shining example of success, is a reminder of what can be done by inspiring people who are determined to provide better services to their patient populations.

In addition to being inspiring, this volume, the second in the Taylor & Francis health reform series, is instructive and practically relevant. It is jam-packed with the expertise of many far-thinking and generous people across the world who take the task of improving the system they work in or on, very seriously indeed.

For those of us whose appetite for reform and improvement can occasionally flag, or in cases when we become reform weary, this book is just the tonic needed. In a word, it's energizing. As the most extensive anthology of health system success stories ever assembled, we commend this book to you.

Clifford F. Hughes

AO, MBBS, DSc, FRACS, FACS, FACC, FIACS(Hon), FAAQHC, FCSANZ, FISQua, AdDipMgt, President, International Society of Quality in Health Care

Wendy Nicklin

RN, BN, MSc(A), CHE, FACHE, FISQua, President-Elect, International Society of Quality in Health Care

Acknowledgments

A book of this magnitude would not be possible without the sustained help of a number of people who willingly provided their expertise and skills to the editorial team. For the care and dedication they applied to their chapters, the authors from the participating countries must be thanked profusely. They told their tales of success from their countries with great aplomb.

To the International Society for Quality in Health Care (ISQua), thank you for once again nominating people to write chapters and helping us bring together the authors. Particularly, we would like to thank Triona Fortune for her kind support and for facilitating the venue for our meeting in Doha, Qatar, in October, 2015.

The job of editing the book was made easier because of the superb expertise of Wendy James, copy editor, and Kristiana Ludlow, administrator and coordinator, who made the job of the regional editors and series editor much easier. In addition, Hsuen P. Ting did the graphs, figures, and statistics; Louise Ellis helped us with the biographies and references; Kate Churacca helped edit the biographies; Jessica Herkes sourced and coordinated the word clouds and map outlines, and worked across a number of whiteboard sessions developing the themes and editing and proofing the documents; and Jackie Mullins and Sue Christian-Hayes are a constant source of support for all the projects we do in the Australian Institute of Health Innovation. On behalf of everyone in the editorial team, our heartfelt thanks.

About the Editors

Series Editor

Jeffrey Braithwaite, BA, MIR (Hons), MBA, DipLR, PhD, FAIM, FCHSM, FFPHRCP (UK), FAcSS (UK), Hon FRACMA, is foundation director, Australian Institute of Health Innovation, director, Centre for Healthcare Resilience and Implementation Science, and professor of health systems research, Faculty of Medicine and Health Sciences, Macquarie University, Sydney, Australia. He has appointments at six other universities internationally, and he is a board member of the International Society for Quality in Health Care (ISQua) and consultant to the World Health Organization.

His research examines the changing nature of health systems, attracting funding of more than AU$102 million (US$76.6 million). He is particularly interested in healthcare as a complex adaptive system, and applying complexity science to healthcare problems. In addition to this, he is very interested in the Anthropocene and the impact of human activity on human and species' health, population, and climate.

Professor Braithwaite has contributed over 600 publications, presented at or chaired international and national conferences, workshops, symposia, and meetings on more than 800 occasions, including 82 keynote addresses. His research appears in journals such as the *British Medical Journal*, *The Lancet*, *Social Science & Medicine*, *BMJ Quality & Safety*, and the *International Journal of Quality in Health Care*. He has received 34 different national and international awards for his teaching and research. Further details are available at his Wikipedia entry: http://en.wikipedia.org/wiki/Jeffrey_Braithwaite

Regional Editors

Russell Mannion, BA (Hons) PG Dip Health Econ, PhD, FRSA, FAcSS, has over 30 years of experience in healthcare research and currently holds the chair in health systems at the University of Birmingham where he is director of research at the Health Services Management Centre. He is also a visiting professor at the Australian Institute for Health Innovation, Macquarie University and is a visiting professor in the Faculty of Medicine,

University of Oslo. He provides expert advice to a range of national and international health agencies, including the World Health Organization, the Organization for Economic Cooperation and Development, the European Health Management Association, and the UK Department of Health. He has published nine books and over 100 peer-reviewed articles in leading scientific journals, including the *British Medical Journal*, the *Milbank Quarterly*, and the *International Journal for Quality in Health Care*. He is an associate editor/ on the editorial board of four international health policy journals and has garnered several international prizes for his research including the Baxter European book award.

Yukihiro Matsuyama, PhD, is research director, the Canon Institute for Global Studies; affiliate professor, Chiba University of Commerce; and visiting professor, the Australian Institute of Health Innovation, the Faculty of Medicine and Health Sciences at Macquarie University. His research examines the sustainability of safety-net systems in Japan, including healthcare, pension, pandemic crisis, and employment through international comparative analyses. He has served as a government committee member, including as advisor to the healthcare working group of the regulatory reform of the Abe administration. He has published many books, including *Healthcare Economics in the United States* (1990), which introduced the theoretical concept of DRG/PPS and managed care into Japan for the first time, *AIDS War: Warning to Japan* (1992), *Health Reform in the United States* (1994), *Breakthrough of Japan's Economy under Half-Population* (2002), *Healthcare Reform and Integrated Healthcare Network*, co-authored with Keiko Kono (2005), *Health Reform and Economic Growth* (2010), and *Depth of Healthcare Reform* (2015).

Paul Shekelle is a staff physician at the West Los Angeles Veterans Affairs Medical Center, and is a professor of medicine at the University of California, Los Angeles (UCLA) School of Medicine. He is widely recognized in the field of guidelines, quality measurement, and evidence-based medicine. In 1996–1997 he spent a year in England as Atlantic Fellow in Public Policy. He is a past chair of the Clinical Guidelines Committee of the American College of Physicians (ACP).

Stuart Whittaker, BSc, MBChB, FFCH (CM), MMed, MD, is the founder and former chief executive officer of the Council for Health Service Accreditation of Southern Africa. He pioneered the concepts of a facilitated accreditation program and graded recognition to assist disadvantaged hospitals in Southern Africa and other developing countries to comply with professional standards and has conducted research and the testing of adverse event monitoring systems for Southern Africa. He has published widely and has presented at numerous international and national conferences.

As a temporary consultant to the World Health Organization, he participated in projects to assess the impact of accreditation on national health systems and choosing quality approaches in health systems. He is a visiting professor at the School of Public Health and Medicine at the Faculty of Health Sciences at the University of Cape Town and extraordinary professor in the School of Health Systems and Public Health, Faculty of Health Sciences, University of Pretoria.

Samir Al-Adawi is a professor of behavioral medicine at the College of Medicine, Sultan Qaboos University. Previously, he was a Fulbright Senior Scholar at the Department of Physical Medicine and Rehabilitation, Harvard Medical School, Boston, Massachusetts, and a research scientist sponsored by Matsumae International Foundation at the Department of Psychosomatic Medicine, Graduate School of Medicine, the University of Tokyo, Japan. His doctorate training was at the Institute of Psychiatry, King's College, United Kingdom. Dr. Al-Adawi has research interests that focus on non-communicable diseases. His research and publications have specifically focused on psychosocial determinants of health and ill health since biological sciences alone in the prevention of and intervention in matters related to disease appear to be an unattainable aspiration in emerging economies such as Oman. Dr. Al-Adawi is a member of the World Health Organization Expert Consultation Group on Feeding and Eating Disorders, reporting to the International Advisory Group for the Revision of International Classification of Diseases (ICD-10) for Mental and Behavioral Disorders.

About the Contributors

Maria Cecilia Acuña, MD, MPH, is an advisor on health systems and services at the Pan American Health Organization/World Health Organization (PAHO/WHO). She was technical coordinator of PAHO's Social Protection in Health Program. In 2010, she was appointed PAHO/WHO Health Systems and Services team leader in Haiti to support the United Nations humanitarian relief efforts and emergency response to the earthquake that devastated that country. She is currently the Health Systems and Services team leader at PAHO-Ecuador and member of WHO Global Patient Safety and Quality Network. She is author and co-author of articles and papers on health policy, health systems reform, access to health, and social protection in health.

William Adu-Krow, MB, ChB, DrPH, is presently the Pan American Health Organization/World Health Organization (PAHO/WHO) representative of Guyana. He was previously the WHO country representative for Papua New Guinea (2010–2014) and Solomon Islands (2008–2010). He is a pro bono adjunct professor at the Center for Population and Family Health of the Mailman School of Public Health at Columbia University, New York. He has worked in Ghana, New York, Washington DC, New Jersey, the Solomon Islands, and Papua New Guinea. His main work has focused on violence against women and the impact of social determinants on global health architecture.

Bruce Agins is medical director of the New York State Department of Health AIDS Institute. He is the principal architect of New York's HIV Quality of Care Program and has over 25 years of HIV-specific QI experience. As a member of the AIDS Institute Executive Team, he has been involved with policy issues and program design focusing on HIV, hepatitis C, and sexually transmitted infections (STIs) for nearly 3 decades. Prior to joining the New York State Department of Health, Dr. Agins directed HIV Centers of Excellence in New York, overseeing inpatient and ambulatory clinics as HIV medical director. He holds academic appointments as full clinical professor in the Division of Epidemiology and Biostatistics in Global Health Sciences, School of Medicine at University of San Francisco and as adjunct professor in the Division of Infectious Diseases and Immunology at New York University School of Medicine.

Emmanuel Aiyenigba, MB, BS, PMP, CPHQ, FISQua, is a physician with a passion for quality and patient safety. He was the inaugural recipient of the Emerging Leader Award and a fellow of the International Society for Quality in Health Care (ISQua). As a certified Lean Six Sigma Black Belt, certified SafeCare assessor, and project management professional, he combines several quality improvement approaches to deliver innovative perspectives to the work of improvement. He was until recently the director of SafeCare programs, Kwara State (PharmAccess Foundation). He currently works as an independent consultant while serving as faculty to the Institute for Healthcare Improvement (IHI) on multiple projects in Africa.

Ahmed Al-Mandhari, MD, DTM&H, PhD, MRCGP (Int.), is a senior consultant in family medicine and public health at Sultan Qaboos University Hospital. He was director general of this hospital, 2010–2013. Currently, he is the director general of the Quality Assurance Centre at the Ministry of Health. He is a World Health Organization (WHO) temporary advisor on patient safety and quality. He is the author of a handbook, *An ABC of Medical Errors Handbook,* as well as chapters in books and many articles on quality in healthcare, patient safety, and health policy.

Yousuf Khalid Al Maslamani is a consultant in general surgery and kidney transplantation. He received his MBBS in 1988 and his fellowship in 1993 from the Royal College of Surgeons, Dublin, Ireland. In 1994, he became a member of the Arab Board of Surgical Specialties. Dr. Al Maslamani did his fellowship in kidney transplantation at the Cleveland Clinic Foundation in 2001. He is head of the kidney transplant section, chairman of the organ transplant committee, and member of the organizing committee, and one of the chairpersons of Gulf Cooperation Council (GCC) Organ Transplantation Congress. He has a range of other international memberships.

Abdullah Al-Raqadi, BSc (computing sciences), MSc (Information Technology), joined the Ministry of Health in 1987. He has extensive experience in health information technology management through working on several national projects within the Ministry of Health. Currently he serves as director general of information technology at the Ministry of Health. He also functions as a chairperson and member in a variety of taskforce teams and committees. He has also presented papers at various conferences at local and international levels.

Khaled Al-Surimi, MSc, PgDip, PhD, is associate professor of health systems and quality management, chairman of the Quality Assurance and Academic Accreditation (QAAA) Unit and former chairman of the Health Systems and Quality Management Department at the College of Public Health and Health Informatics, King Saud ben Abdudlaziz University for Health Sciences, Saudi Arabia. He was previously an assistant professor at the Faculty of Medicine and Health Sciences, Thamar University, Yemen. He is author of books, book chapters, and journal articles, including *Health Care Quality in Developing Countries: Patients' Perception and Quality Policy Development Assessment* and *Total Quality: Concepts, Development, and Tools,* as well as author and co-author of more than 40 articles and conference papers published in international scientific journals and conferences.

Patricia Albisetti holds a bachelor's degree in business administration and a master's degree in health law. She is the general secretary of the Hospital Federation of Vaud (FHV), the umbrella organization for the 12 regional hospitals of the County of Vaud in Switzerland. Her role includes representation and advocacy for its members toward the regional and national authorities, public health agencies, and other partners.

René Amalberti, MD, PhD. After a residency in psychiatry, Professor Amalberti entered the air force in 1977, was appointed to a permanent medical research position in 1982, and became full professor of medicine in 1995. He retired in 2007, dividing his time between the Haute Autorité de Santé (senior advisor, patient safety), a medical insurer, Cie (director risks, MACSF), and a position as volunteer director of a public foundation for safety culture in industry (FONCSI). He has published over 150 papers and authored or co-authored 12 books on human error and system safety (most recently, *Navigating Safety*, Springer, 2013; and *Safer Healthcare*, Springer, 2016).

Hugo Arce, MPH, PhD, is a physician. He was president and chief executive officer of the Technical Institute for Accreditation of Healthcare Organizations, 1994–2010, and president of the Argentine Society for Quality in Health Care; he is director of the Department of Public Health, University Institute of Health Sciences, Barceló Foundation; and president of the International Society of Quality in Health Care (ISQua) International Conference-Buenos Aires 2001 and executive board member in 2002–2003. He is the author of *The Territory of Health Decisions*, *The Quality in the Health Territory*, and *The Health System: Where It Comes From and Where It Goes*, as well as over 170 articles and papers on health policy, hospital management, and quality in healthcare.

Lauren Archer, MPH, works as a technical advisor for health programs at Palladium. Currently, she provides technical support for health systems strengthening and private health sector initiatives in Afghanistan, Zambia, Kenya, and Mali. Previously, she worked at the Center for Advancing Research on Health Systems at Columbia University, where she designed and led research activities focused on the constraints to scale-up in Ghana's primary healthcare system. Early in her career, she served as a community health educator for the US Peace Corps in Nicaragua, with a focus on sexual and reproductive health education.

Toni Ashton, PhD, MA (Hons), BA, is an honorary professor of health economics in the School of Population Health, University of Auckland. Her main research interests are in the funding and organization of health systems and healthcare reform. In addition to numerous articles in referred journals and several book chapters, she has co-edited a book on health policy in New Zealand and co-authored three books on superannuation. Professor

Ashton has been a member of a number of government taskforces on aspects of health policy and has undertaken a range of consultancies, including two for the World Health Organization.

Badar Awladthani, MSc (Information Technology), joined the Ministry of Health in 1998. He has extensive experience in health information technology (IT) management through working on several national projects within the Ministry of Health. Currently, he works as director of the Systems Applications Department in the Directorate General of Information Technology. He is a member in different IT healthcare committees and taskforces.

Luis Azpurua, MD, is the clinical research and education director of Clinica Santa Paula, and also professor of clinical and biomedical engineering in the Universidad Simón Bolívar in Caracas, Venezuela. During his 25 years' journey throughout the healthcare field he has served, among others, as a medical director of the Hospital San Juan de Dios of Caracas. He is co-author of the strategic planning book *De Autoempleados a Empresarios. Como Planificar un Centro de Salud Privado para Potenciar Su Desarrollo.* He is passionate about healthcare quality and patient safety culture.

Natasha Azzopardi-Muscat qualified as a doctor (1995) in public health medicine (2003); she obtained a fellowship (Faculty of Public Health, United Kingdom) (2006) and a PhD from Maastricht University (2016). She previously held various positions in the Ministry of Health of Malta, including chief medical officer. She is a consultant in public health medicine in Malta and is an academic at the University of Malta. Her research centers on EU health policy and in health systems in small states, with several publications on these topics. She is president of the European Public Health Association.

Vasha Elizabeth Bachan, MD, an MPH candidate, is presently the principal investigator/program director of the Ministry of Public Health/Centre for Disease Control and Prevention's Cooperative Agreement. She was previously the director of regional health services for the regional and clinical services of the Ministry of Health (MoH) (2014–2015). She also served as chronic disease coordinator, MoH (2013–2014), regional health officer for region 4, MoH (2012–2014), and district medical officer (sub-region of East Coast Demerara) for region 4, MoH (2011–2012). She also served as a government medical officer working in primary healthcare (2009–2011). Her interest is in public health administration.

G. Ross Baker, PhD, is a professor in the Institute of Health Policy, Management, and Evaluation at the University of Toronto and director of the MSc Program in Quality Improvement and Patient Safety. Professor Baker is co-lead for a large quality improvement-training program in

Ontario—Improving and Driving Excellence Across Sectors (IDEAS). Recent research projects include a review and synthesis of evidence on factors linked to high-performing healthcare systems, an analysis of why progress on patient safety has been slower than expected, and an edited book of case studies on patient engagement strategies (with Maria Judd).

Roland Bal graduated from Health Sciences, University of Maastricht, in science and technology studies (STS). His PhD is from the Law and Public Policy Centre at the University in Leiden, graduating from Twente University. He was previously at the Cultural Sciences Faculty in Maastricht and the Department of Health Policy and Management at Erasmus University. He headed the Research on Information Technology (IT) in Healthcare Practice and Management (Rithm) group before becoming the chair of the Health Care Governance group. He was director of education and currently chairs the advisory board, Health Economics, Policy, and Law master's program, and serves on the advisory board of the Healthcare Management program.

Cynthia Bannerman, MBChB, MPH, FGCPS, is a public health specialist and deputy director of quality assurance for the Ghana Health Service. She has worked in senior management positions for 20 years in the public service and has contributed to the development of national health policies, strategies, protocols, and guidelines. Recently, these have included the ministry's Health Financing Strategy and the Medium-Term Health Development Plan 2014–2017. She has also participated in the annual review of Ghana's health sector program of work (holistic assessment). She co-chaired the Ghana Health Sector Salary Reforms in 2005 and is a champion for healthcare quality and patient safety.

Joshua Bardfield serves as knowledge management director for HEALTHQUAL International. He has extensive public health communications, research, and technical writing experience, with a focus on reproductive health and HIV/AIDS. Over the last several years, Mr Bardfield's work has focused on implementation science and spreading improvement knowledge, with an emphasis on building a sustainable cross-country peer network for improvement among HEALTHQUAL's 15 target countries. He has researched and authored a variety of academic publications focused on women's health, HIV, and quality improvement, and earned his master's degree in public health from Columbia University's Mailman School of Public Health.

Maysa Baroud, MSc, MPH, is a project coordinator at the Education and Youth Policy Research Program at the Issam Fares Institute for Public Policy and International Affairs, American University of Beirut. She is also a researcher at the social innovation lab at the Faculty of Health Sciences, American University of Beirut. Her research focuses on identifying the needs of refugee and host community youth in Lebanon and the Middle East through a participatory action research approach. Maysa holds a master of public health, concentrating in health management and policy, and a master of science in microbiology and immunology.

Apollo Basenero, MBChB, is technical advisor, Quality Management (QM) Program in the Ministry of Health and Social Services Namibia. He is a fellow at the International Society for Quality in Health Care (ISQua) and a fellow at the Arthur Ashe Endowment for the Defeat of AIDS. He has been involved in the development of different QM curricula including consumer involvement in QM curriculum and is part of the team that develops healthcare related guidelines. He has participated in various research projects, authored and co-authored a number of abstracts and has won several professional awards. He serves on various local and international key QM committees.

Roger Bayingana, MD, MPHM, currently works as a consultant in health systems strengthening, research, quality assurance, and accreditation in Rwanda and the region. He has been a principal clinical investigator on many HIV vaccine research studies and also worked as head of training and guidelines for the Ministry of Health HIV research institute. Dr. Bayingana is an author or co-author of several scientific papers mostly on HIV research and programing. He holds a master's degree in research methodologies from the Universite Libre de Bruxelles (ULB) in Belgium and a medical degree from the National University of Rwanda.

Paula Bezzola, MPH, is the chief executive officer (CEO) of EQUAM Foundation (Switzerland), an organization fostering quality in the ambulatory medical sector. From 2006 to 2016, she worked as deputy CEO of the Swiss Patient Safety Foundation, directed the national patient safety improvement program "progress!" (campaign and breakthrough collaboratives), and ran the following working fields: system analyses after incidents, evaluations, developing recommendations, teaching, and consulting in different healthcare system fields. Before 2006, she worked as scientific collaborator at a Swiss cantonal public health state authority (hospital law, introduction of outcome measurements in hospitals).

Mustafa Berktaş, MD, is a clinical microbiology professor. He is managing director of the newly founded Healthcare Quality and Accreditation Institute of Turkey, under Turkish Health Sciences Institute. He lectured in microbiology and fulfilled duties like educational coordinator, director of ethical committee, chief of the Microbiology Department, deputy chief of the Health Sciences Institute, and vice dean of the Medicine Faculty. He was State Hospital's founding chief physician and medical director of a private hospital. He actively engaged with healthcare quality studies at the Ministry of

Health of Turkey. Mr. Berktas has 157 articles published in scientific journals and 141 abstracts presented in conferences both national and international.

Sarah Boucaud, MHA, is a Juris Doctor candidate at Dalhousie University in Halifax, Nova Scotia. She currently works at the Children's Hospital of Eastern Ontario as an administrative resident. She also consults on reports and research projects for Accreditation Canada. She is author of "Patient Safety Incident Reporting: Current Trends and Gaps Within the Canadian Health System," published in *Healthcare Quarterly*.

Denise Boulter has practiced midwifery since 1996 in a variety of settings, including the midwife-led team in the Mater, and is midwifery advisor to the chief nursing officer (CNO) at the Department of Health, Social Services and Public Safety (DHSSPS). Since 2011, she has been midwife consultant within the Public Health Agency in Northern Ireland. This regional role involves being the professional lead on commissioning of maternity services to provide expert professional and public health advice within the Public Health Agency and the Health and Social Care Board; to lead on service development and improvement initiatives, including implementation of the maternity strategy; and be designated responsible officer for serious adverse incidents within maternity.

Mats Brommels is professor and chair of the Department of Learning, Informatics, Management, and Ethics and director of the Medical Management Centre (MMC), Karolinska Institutet. He is a specialist in general internal medicine and holds a qualification in medical administration awarded by the National Board of Health to Finnish medical specialists. His research covers policy analysis in the field of public health services and international comparative studies of public health systems; healthcare utilization studies; and evaluation of medical technologies and professional practice patterns, health services management, quality improvement and patient safety.

Geir Bukholm, MD, PhD, MHA, MPH, is executive director for domain infection control and environmental health at the Norwegian Institute of Public Health, professor at the Norwegian University of Life Sciences, and director of the Scientific Board for the Norwegian Program for Patient Safety. He was department director at the Norwegian Knowledge Centre for the Health Services, when the Norwegian campaign for patient safety was launched and later specialist director for quality in healthcare and patient safety in the Norwegian Ministry of Health and Care Services. He has been the author of several books and more than 100 articles in peer-reviewed journals.

Sandra C. Buttigieg, MD, PhD (Aston), FFPH (UK), MSc (Public Health Medicine), MBA, is associate professor and head of department of health services management, Faculty of Health Sciences, University of Malta, and consultant for public health medicine, Mater Dei Hospital, Malta. She lectures in health services management and public health. She is Honorary Senior Research Fellow at Aston University and at the University of Birmingham, United Kingdom. She has authored and co-authored numerous articles in peer-reviewed management and health journals, and is currently on the editorial advisory board of the *Journal of Health Organization and Management*. She is a member of the research committee of the Health Care Management (HCM) Division, American Academy of Management.

Stephanie Carpenter, MA, has worked with Accreditation Canada as an accreditation product development specialist since 2010. She oversees the Stroke Distinction Accreditation Program and has also worked on a number of other projects, including client- and family-centered care, cancer care, emergency departments, emergency medical services (EMS) and inter-facility transport, and spinal cord injury services.

Edward Chappy, BA, MPA, FACHE, FISQua, is a healthcare quality and accreditation consultant. Previously, he was the chief of part (COP) of the United States Agency for International Development (USAID)-funded Jordan Healthcare Accreditation Project, which established the Health Care Accreditation Council, the national healthcare accreditation agency in Jordan. He has worked in several countries on implanting quality systems in both public and private hospitals, including Eritrea, Indonesia, Pakistan, Turkey, and Saudi Arabia. He has been the chief executive officer (CEO) at private hospitals in Pakistan, Indonesia, and Turkey. He is consulting in Rwanda and Afghanistan, helping to implement quality systems, improve the health facility licensing process, and establish national accreditation agencies.

Patsy Yuen-Kwan Chau, MPhil, is research associate at the JC School of Public Health and Primary Care, the Chinese University of Hong Kong. Her background is in statistics and public health. She has been involved in a wide range of research areas, such as the impacts on mortality and morbidity of air pollution, spatial variation of temperature changes on health, evaluation of hospital accreditation, and evaluation of regulation on sulfur contents of gasoline.

Americo Cicchetti is full professor of healthcare management at the Catholic University, Faculty of Economics, Rome. He is director of the Graduate School of Health Economics and Management at Catholic University of Sacred Heart and chief of research of the Health Technology Assessment Unit and Biomedical Engineering of the Agostino Gemelli University Hospital, Rome, Italy. Among other appointments, he was member of the

Price and Reimbursement Committee of the Italian National Drug Agency (AIFA) from 2009 to 2015 and director of the Health Technology Assessment International (2005–2008). Now he is a member of the executive committee and secretary, and is president of the Italian Society of Health Technology Assessment.

Elisabeth Coll Torres, MD, PhD, is a specialist in preventive medicine and public health. She is medical officer in the Spanish National Transplant Organization (ONT) and associate teacher for the Medical Department of the Alfonso X University. She has extensive experience in training and research, especially in the development of different programs focused on donation and transplantation activity, such as the study of practices in organ donation and end-of-life care, and deceased donation in the EU. During her career, she has participated as an expert in several World Health Organization (WHO) regional consultations and in European Commission working groups. She is the author of articles and chapters of books on donation and transplantation.

Silvia Coretti, MA, MSc, PhD, is postdoctoral research fellow at the Postgraduate School of Health Economics and Management of the Università Cattolica del Sacro Cuore (Rome, Italy). Her PhD dissertation in 2014 was on health-related quality-of-life measures. In that university, she earned a master in health technology assessment in 2010 and, in 2013, she received a master of science at the University of York, United Kingdom. She has collaborated with the Pricing and Reimbursement Office, Italian Agency of Medicines and with the Health Economics Research Unit at the University of Aberdeen. She is interested in health technology assessment and focused on methodological aspects of outcome measures and patients' preferences.

Jacqueline Cumming is professor of health policy and management and director of the Health Services Research Centre at the School of Government at Victoria University of Wellington. She has qualifications in economics, health economics, and public policy; teaches health policy and monitoring and evaluation; and supervises PhD students in health services research. She has led high-profile national evaluations of reforms in health policy and health services. With over 20 years of experience in health services research, she was president of the Health Services Research Association of Australia and New Zealand (2007–2014) and is immediate past president. She has worked with leaders from Counties Manukau District Health Board (DHB) for many years.

Haidee Davis is the general manager for Ko Awatea, having previously held the position of program director for Achieving a Balance for Counties Manukau Health. She has a background in nursing, predominantly working in medicine, oncology, and cardio-respiratory areas as a charge nurse. She developed new models of care for Waikato District Health Board, and led service redesign for the new campus project at Waikato Hospital. Ms. Davis also formed a new program management office, providing standardized project management practices that were repeatable, had reduced costs, and improved project success rates. She has a master in human resources, specializing in clinical leadership and change management.

Ellen Tveter Deilkås, MD, PhD (Organizational Psychology), is a consultant in internal medicine with 20 years of clinical experience. She is a senior scientist at Akershus University Hospital where she conducts research on patient safety culture and improvement. She holds a 20 percent position as a senior advisor for the Norwegian Directorate of Health, specifically responsible for national measurement of medical injury and patient safety culture. The measurements are part of the government's patient safety program. She led the patient safety committee of the Norwegian Medical Association from 2006 to 2016 and works part-time as a consultant with stroke rehabilitation.

Pedro Delgado, MSc, head of Europe and Latin America, Institute for Healthcare Improvement (IHI), has a unique ability to work across cultures, languages, and systems. He has been a driving force in IHI's global strategy. From work on reducing C-sections in Brazil, to improving early years' education in Chile, to improving patient safety in Portugal, and mental health in London, Mr Delgado has led the key senior relationships, and design and implementation of large-scale health system improvement efforts and networks globally. He coaches senior leaders and teams, and lectures extensively worldwide on large-scale change, patient safety, and quality improvement.

Subashnie Devkaran, MScHM, PhD, FACHE, CPHQ, FISQua, BScPT, is a leader in quality, accreditation, and patient experience in the Middle East and Africa region and currently affiliated with Cleveland Clinic Abu Dhabi. She is the vice president of the American College of Healthcare Executives for the Middle East and North Africa Group. In addition, she is an international consultant with Joint Commission International based in Chicago, Illinois. Dr. Devkaran also serves as an associate lecturer with the Royal College of Surgeons in Ireland. She regularly speaks at international conferences and has published several articles on healthcare quality and patient experience. With a passion to reduce the knowledge gap in healthcare quality and patient experience internationally, Dr. Devkaran continues to pursue research in these areas.

Danielle Dorschner, BSc(N), MSc(N), is senior director, programs and client engagement at Accreditation Canada, where she oversees client services, program development, and business development. She is often asked to speak at events and conferences and participate on expert panels regarding accreditation. She also has clinical experience in public health. She has been a certified surveyor with the International Society for Quality in Health Care (ISQua) since 2008. She is also a volunteer on the Canadian Mental Health Association—Champlain East board of directors and was elected as its president in September 2015.

Persephone Doupi, MD, PhD, is a senior researcher at the Welfare Department of the National Institute for Health and Welfare (THL), Finland. Currently, her focus is on injury prevention, safety, and public health informatics. She has over 15 years of experience as key investigator in EU-funded and national projects concerning digital health data and cross-border healthcare services. She has served on multiple national, Nordic, and international expert groups on eHealth, quality, and patient safety and (co)authored several scientific articles, books, and book chapters on medical informatics and eHealth topics.

Adrian Edwards is professor of general practice and co-director of the Division of Population Medicine at Cardiff University, Wales, United Kingdom, and part-time general practitioner in Cwmbran, South Wales, seeing about 60 patients weekly. He holds visiting appointments at Aarhus and Southern Denmark Universities. His main research interests are in risk communication and shared decision-making, communication skills for practitioners, and implementing and evaluating this in routine practice. In 2016, he co-edited *Shared Decision Making in Health Care: Achieving Evidence-based Patient Choice* (Oxford University Press). His current interests include the integration of shared decision-making approaches into healthcare innovations, for example, supporting patients to self-manage long-term conditions through enhanced health literacy.

Carsten Engel, MD, is deputy chief executive at IKAS, the Danish Institute for Quality and Accreditation in Healthcare. His background is in clinical practice as an anesthesiologist, and he has management experience at departmental and hospital level. He has taken a leading part in the development and management of the Danish healthcare accreditation program (DDKM). Through the Accreditation Council of International Society of Quality in Health Care (ISQua), he is engaged in accreditation internationally, and he serves as an ISQua expert.

Jesper Eriksen, MSc Political Science, is special advisor, quality and safety, the Danish Cancer Society. He takes special interest in the interaction between the economic and political organization of the healthcare system and the quality of the healthcare efforts. He works from a policy approach with data-driven quality improvement in cancer treatment and monitors the progress from an organizational, clinical, and user-perceived dimension.

Hong Fung, MBBS (HK), MHP (NSW), FRCS (Edin), FHKAM (Surg), FCSHK, FHKAM (Community Medicine), FHKCCM, FFPHM (UK), FRACMA, FAMS, is professor of practice in health services management at the JC School of Public Health and Primary Care, the Chinese University of Hong Kong (CUHK); he co-directs the master of science in health services management program. He is the executive director of the CUHK Medical Centre and the president of the Hong Kong College of Community Medicine. His expertise is in health leadership, hospital planning, health informatics, and health services management. Previously, he was director of planning and cluster chief executive of New Territories East Cluster in the Hong Kong Hospital Authority.

Ezequiel García-Elorrio, MD, MSc, MBA, PhD, is one of the founders and board members of the Institute for Clinical Effectiveness and Health Policy in Argentina, where he also leads the Department of Health Care Quality and Patient Safety. Elorrio has worked extensively in quality of care and patient safety research, education, and implementation projects in Latin America, sub-Saharan Africa, and South-East Asia. His main interests are related to patient safety, external evaluation, and improvement methods focusing on successful implementation in developing countries. He is an active collaborator of the International Society of Quality in Health Care (ISQua) as associate editor of the society's journal from 2009 and a member of the education committee, as well other activities.

Octavio Gómez-Dantés is senior researcher at the National Institute of Public Health of Mexico. Between 2001 and 2006, he was director general for performance evaluation at the Ministry of Health of Mexico, and, between 2007 and 2008, he worked as director of analysis and evaluation at the CARSO Health Institute. His areas of academic expertise are health policy and global health. Dr. Gómez-Dantés holds a medical degree from the Autonomous Metropolitan University (Mexico), and two master's degrees, one in public health and the other one in health policy and planning, both from the Harvard School of Public Health (Boston, USA).

Jonás Gonseth, MD, MPH, PhD, is a specialist practitioner in preventative medicine and public health by the Ministry of Education of Spain. He is currently serving as a chief executive office of Hospital Dr. Abel Glibert Ponton in Guayaquil and has more than 15 years of experience in different countries as quality and patient safety project manager. He served as associated expert for quality in healthcare in the Pan American Health Organization/World Health Organization (PAHO/WHO) in Washington, DC for the period 2006–2009. He is professor in health service administration at Universidad Católica de Santiago de Guayaquil, Ecuador.

Christine S. Gordon, RN, works at the RM Quality Assurance Unit, Ministry of Health and Social Services (MoHSS), Republic of Namibia.

Jonathon Gray is the director of Ko Awatea, a hub of education, improvement, and innovation that supports health systems and public services and is embedded within the Counties Manukau District Health Board in Aotearoa New Zealand. Professor Gray has more than 30 years of experience in the field of health. Not only is he a doctor with specialist expertise in medical genetics and public health, he also holds various visiting fellowships at organizations in Oxford, Auckland, and through a Health Foundation fellowship, he spent a year studying at the Institute for Healthcare Improvement in Boston (USA). Furthermore, he is the professor of health innovation and improvement at Victoria University in Wellington, New Zealand, with visiting chairs at Auckland University of Technology (AUT) and Cardiff University.

Kenneth Grech, MD, MSc (London), MBA, FFPH (UK), DLSHTM (London), qualified as a medical doctor from the University of Malta, where he lectures. He is a consultant in public health with the Department of Health, Malta. He holds a master's degree in public health from the London School of Hygiene and Tropical Medicine, a master in business administration from the University of Malta, and is a fellow of the Faculty of Public Health Medicine, United Kingdom. He is currently reading for a PhD at University of Warwick on health system performance assessment. He has been chief executive officer of St Luke's Hospital, Malta, and permanent secretary of Malta's Ministry of Health.

Victor Grabois, MD, MPH, MSc, studied undergraduate medicine at the Federal University of Rio de Janeiro and holds an MSc in social medicine from the Institute at Estadual University of Rio de Janeiro. Since 2010, he has been a PhD student at the Public Health National School, Fiocruz. He was formerly the general manager of federal hospitals in Rio de Janeiro and is currently the executive coordinator of the Collaborative Center for Quality of Care and Patient Safety (Proqualis) and official representative of Fundação Oswaldo Cruz at the Implementation Committee of Patient Safety National Program. He has published book chapters and articles on hospital management, clinical judgment, and care management.

Oliver Groene, PhD, MSc, MA, is vice-chairman of the board the population health management company Optimedis AG. Before this, he was senior lecturer/associate professor in health services research at the London School of Hygiene and Tropical Medicine, and he led the Quality of Health Systems and Services Program at the World Health Organization. Dr. Groene has served as principal investigator (PI) or co-PI on various large-scale grants, with total research funding of over five million euros. His research has been cited more than 2000 times, reflected in his h-index of 27. He is deputy editor of the *International Journal for Quality in Health Care.*

Mylai Guerrero, MD, is a physician trained in internal medicine at Hamad Medical Corporation, Doha, Qatar. She then shifted career paths to medical administration in 2014 as a quality and patient safety coordinator in the same organization. She has since facilitated the design, management, and implementation of organization-wide health systems improvements. She is currently completing her master of science in international health management and leadership from the University of Sheffield. She has also trained in lean for healthcare with the University of Tennessee.

The Gulf Health Council for Cooperation Council States was established in 1976. The Council involves in its membership seven countries: the United Arab Emirates, Kingdom of Bahrain, Kingdom of Saudi Arabia, Sultanate of Oman, Qatar, Kuwait, and the Republic of Yemen. The mission of the council includes coordination among member states in the prevention, cure, and rehabilitation fields; dissemination of health knowledge among citizens; assessment of their existing healthcare systems; and the procurement of safe and efficient pharmaceutical products, hospital sundries, and equipment of high quality with appropriate prices through a central group purchase program.

Girdhar Gyani is the director general of the Association of Healthcare Providers, India. The mission of the association is to build capacity in the Indian health system through advocacy and education, with a focus on patient safety and affordability. Prior to this, Dr. Gyani was secretary-general of the Quality Council of India, a peak national body responsible for establishing and operating a national accreditation structure and promoting quality. Dr. Gyani has been instrumental in establishing the national accreditation structure for hospitals (NABH) under the auspices of the International Society for Quality in Health Care (ISQua) accreditation program, bringing patient safety and healthcare quality to the forefront in India.

Gerald Haidinger, MD, is associate professor in epidemiology at the Centre for Public Health, Medical University of Vienna, and was previously interim head of the Department of Epidemiology and adviser to the World Health Organization in HIV/AIDS. In his medical training, he specialized in public health and epidemiology with special research interests in neurology, perinatology, and pediatric allergic diseases. He has participated in numerous national research studies and international projects, including Euro-Peristat and ISAAC as a representative of Austria. He has authored or co-authored more than 160 scientific publications, and has been advisor to Austria's

Ministry of Health, Ministry of Transport and Technology and Statistics Austria for over 10 years.

Ann Hamilton, FRCOG, is a consultant obstetrician and gynecologist and clinical risk director in the South-Eastern Health and Social Care Trust, Northern Ireland. Dr. Hamilton is chair for the regional maternity collaborative and lead obstetrician on the Neonatal Network, Northern Ireland. She completed a Scottish Patient Safety Fellowship Program in 2012. Her main interests include robust and honest investigations when adverse events occur and how lessons can be learned to reduce the risk of recurrence.

Ndapewa Hamunime is senior medical officer, Namibia Ministry of Health and Social Services (MoHSS) and champions the integration of the 3 I's (intensified case finding, infection control, and isoniazid preventive therapy) into the national HIV treatment program. The MoHSS has embraced quality improvement (QI) as an integral component of the government-led strategy for implementation of a national framework for tuberculosis (TB) prevention, care, and treatment.

Qendresa Hasanaj, MSc, is a health services research specialist within the policy and research portfolio at Accreditation Canada. She is responsible for developing provincial and national reports, and supporting collaborative research with partner organizations. She holds a master of science degree in epidemiology from the University of Ottawa, Canada, and has previous experience with population-based health research.

Patricia Hayward is a writer for Ko Awatea, Counties Manukau Health. She has a background in special librarianship, including 7 years as a medical librarian with Counties Manukau Health. She has a master of communication studies from Auckland University of Technology, a bachelor of arts in political studies from the University of Auckland, and a certificate in editing and proofreading. She has edited and contributed to the books *Creating Systems, Population Medicine*, and *Creating Culture*, as well as numerous papers and improvement guides.

Helmut Hildebrandt is founder and director of OptiMedis and founder and managing director of Gesundes Kinzigtal, an integrated care project in the southwest of Germany. After his studies in pharmacy, he worked as a temporary adviser for the World Health Organization. In 1992, he founded Hildebrandt GesundheitsConsult, a strategy and consulting company with a focus on the healthcare market. In 1999–2000, Hildebrandt consulted with the German Ministry of Health regarding integrated care. Mr. Hildebrandt is a board member of the International Foundation for Integrated Care. He was recently awarded an honorary doctorate for his contributions to health services research and policy by the University of Witten-Herdecke in Germany.

Ken Hillman, AO, MBBS, FRCA, FCICM, FRCP, MD, is professor of intensive care at the University of New South Wales, Australia; director, Simpson Centre for Health Services Research; and is an actively practicing clinician in intensive care. He has 165 peer-reviewed publications; 64 chapters in textbooks; co-authored an intensive care textbook; co-edited several textbooks; and written a book—*Vital Signs: Stories from Intensive Care*—and has received over $20 million in grants. He is internationally recognized as a pioneer in the introduction of the medical emergency team (MET) and in 2005 helped establish the first international conference on the MET and has been actively involved since.

Maria M. Hofmarcher-Holzhacker is an economist and health system expert with a research focus on the economics of health and social care, public finance, health and long-term care supply, efficiency, and comparative health and social care research. She is director of HealthSystemIntelligence and research associate at the Department of Health Economics, Medical University of Vienna. She was coordinator of EU FP 7 projects and currently leads work in the area of evaluation of healthcare systems in the context of the EU project BRIDGE Health. Among her many publications, she is the principal author of the publication *Austria: Health System Review*.

Min-Huei Hsu is director of the Department of Information Management, Ministry of Health and Welfare, Taiwan. He has been chief information officer at Taipei Medical University, and a consultant neurosurgeon at Wanfang Hospital, a 746-bed hospital affiliated with Taipei Medical University. He is author and co-author of more than 40 papers and articles in international conferences and scientific journals, focusing on health data, health information technology, e-health, electronic medical record system, hospital information management, and patient safety.

Clifford F. Hughes, AO, MBBS, DSc, FRACS, FACS, FACC, FIACS(Hon), FAAQHC, FCSANZ, FISQua, AdDipMgt, is president of the International Society for Quality in Health Care. He is professor of patient safety and clinical quality at the Australian Institute of Health Innovation at Macquarie University, Sydney, Australia. A former cardiothoracic surgeon and chief executive officer of the Clinical Excellence Commission in New South Wales, Australia, he is a consultant in quality and safety to health services in Australia, New Zealand, the United Kingdome, and the United States. He is passionate about person-based care, better and timely incident management, and the development of clinical leaders. His spare time is devoted to his family and eight grandchildren.

Valentina Iacopino, PhD, is postdoctoral researcher in organization and human resource management at the Faculty of Economics of the Catholic University of Rome. Her research interests and publications focus on the diffusion and adoption processes of innovations in the healthcare context at institutional, organizational, and professional level. In her studies, she also applies social network analysis techniques to understand inter-organizational as well as professional networks' role in the process of adoption and diffusion of medical technologies. She focuses in policy issues and governance of technological innovations both at organizational and institutional level.

Usman Iqbal, PharmD, MBA, PhD, is a senior research fellow at Taipei Medical University (TMU). He has worked at the Aga Khan University Hospital, Pakistan. Dr. Usman is facilitating the International Society for Quality in Health Care (ISQua) fellowship and joint collaborative courses between TMU and the Massachusetts Institute of Technology (MIT)-Harvard (USA). He is also a fellow at Salzburg Global Seminar. Dr. Usman is also working as special assistant for the editor-in-chief of the *International Journal for Quality in Health Care.* He has been an author of multiple peer-reviewed scientific articles, book chapters, and has participated in national and international conferences with a focus on health information technology (IT) and patient safety, healthcare quality and management, and health systems improvement.

Ivan Ivanovic, MD, is a public health specialist and head of Department of Informatics and Biostatistics in the Institute of Public Health (IPH) of Serbia. His main fields of interest and activities in his professional work are coordination of development and the realization of an integrated health information system (IHIS) in the Republic of Serbia; organization and implementation of health statistical research, including responsibility for correctness of data, their timely publishing, accessibility and protection of data; organization and implementation of targeted research projects on health; development and maintenance of databases on a national level; and data analysis and reporting on population health, healthcare system performance, and resources.

Safurah Jaafar, MBChB, MScPH, MBA, FFPH (UK), FAFP (M), MAM(M), is a public health physician currently holding the position as director of the Family Health Development Division with the Ministry of Health, Malaysia. She graduated with an MBCHB from the University of Alexandria in 1981 and completed her master in public health from the National University of Singapore in 1985. In 1993, she secured a master in business administration from Northeastern University in Boston, giving her more extensive capacity for strategic planning and project implementation across health services. She is a fellow in public health with the London Royal College of Physicians.

Wendy James, MA, PhD, works as an editor in the Centre for Healthcare Resilience and Implementation Science at the Australian Institute of Health Innovation, Macquarie University. She has a PhD from the University of New England, and a master's in creative writing from University of Technology Sydney. She is the author of seven works of fiction including *The Mistake* (2012) and *Out of the Silence* (2005), which won the 2006 Ned Kelly Award for Best First Crime Fiction and was shortlisted for the Nita May Dobbie Award for Women's Writing. Her articles and stories have been published widely in journals, newspapers, and magazines. Her latest novel, *The Golden Child*, will be published by HarperCollins in 2017.

Salma Jaouni Araj, since 2012, has been the chief executive officer of the Health Care Accreditation Council (HCAC), Jordan's national arm for quality and patient safety. She was senior advisor to the prime minister of Jordan on public and social policy after serving as founding director and manager of Jordan's National Breast Cancer Program. She has worked with Booz Allen Hamilton, the World Bank, and the United States Agency for International Development (USAID) in the Middle East and North Africa (MENA), consulting and managing public health, poverty, employment, and social services initiatives. She holds an MPA from Harvard Kennedy School, a postgraduate diploma in health systems from the University of London, and a BSc from the American University of Beirut. She is an International Society for Quality in Health Care (ISQua) expert, serves on national boards, and has received several awards for leadership.

Ravichandran Jeganathan is national head of obstetrics and gynecology services and maternal-fetal medicine at the Ministry of Health, Malaysia. He graduated from University Science Malaysia with an MD and a master in obstetrics and gynecology. He is an associate member of the Royal College of Obstetricians and Gynecologists (RCOG). He is the chair of the National Specialist Registry (obstetrics and gynecology) in Malaysia as well as the Confidential Enquiry into Maternal Deaths, Malaysia. He is a life member of the Malaysian Society for Quality and Health and president-elect of the Obstetrical and Gynecological Society of Malaysia. He serves as associate professor of obstetrics and gynecology with Monash Malaysia Medical School and has been a temporary consultant with the World Health Organization (WHO) and the United Nations Population Fund (UNFPA).

Ravindran Jegasothy is dean of the Faculty of Medicine, MAHSA University, Malaysia. He graduated with an MBBS from the University of Malaya and is a fellow of the Royal College of Obstetricians and Gynecologists, London. He has been awarded an MMed (obstetrics and gynecology) from the National University of Singapore, as well as a fellowship from the Academy of Medicine of Malaysia and the Indian Academy of Medical Sciences. He worked in the Ministry of Health,

Malaysia, where he was closely associated with efforts in the reduction of maternal mortality. He is on the International Accreditation Panel of ISQua.

Sara Kaddoura is currently pursuing a master in public administration in environmental science and policy at Columbia University's School of International and Public Affairs. Previously, she was a research assistant in the Faculty of Health Sciences at the American University Beirut (AUB). Her research focused on creating innovative ways to improve health systems mainly in Lebanon and has been working on developing and establishing a Social Innovation Lab for Health and Wellbeing at AUB. She holds a BSc in environmental health with minors in public health and economics. Other projects she has worked on include WASH interventions for Syrian refugees and community/social innovation.

Minna Kaila has been professor in medical management at the University of Helsinki Faculty of Medicine since 2011. She is a pediatrician and public health specialist by training and has special competences in administration and medical education. Previously she has worked in specialized and primary healthcare, and in national clinical practice guideline development and health technology assessment. She has more than 100 original publications. Professor Kaila has been on the boards of Guidelines International Network and the European Health Management Association. She is currently president of the Association for Medical Education in Finland and chair of the Finnish Medical Society Duodecim's delegation.

Ruth Kalda, DrMedSci, is professor of family medicine at the University of Tartu. She is head of the Institute of Family Medicine and Public Health. She is also part-time family doctor and belongs to the board of the Estonian Society of Family Doctors. She belongs to the European Academy of the Teachers in General Practice/Family Medicine (EURACT). She is author and co-author of more than 100 scientific and research articles, among them 45 papers published in international peer-reviewed scientific journals. The main topics of her research interest are the quality of primary healthcare, continuity of care, and care integration.

İbrahim H. Kayral, PhD, has a BSc degree in Economics, and an MBA and a doctorate in BA. He is working for Healthcare Quality and Accreditation Institute of Turkey and coordinating International Society for Quality in Health Care (ISQua) international accreditation programs (IAPs) for the institute, beside establishing accreditation programs. He has different business experiences. After business development consultation for small and medium enterprises (SMEs), Kayral served the Ministry of Health (MoH) of Turkey for years, developing standard sets, training programs, pay-for-performance systems, and strategic plans. He represented MoH in ISQua IAPs.

He is honorary advisor in the Confederation of International Accreditation Commission. Kayral has lots of published books, articles in scientific journals, and presentations in national and international conferences in healthcare.

Edward Kelley is currently director of the Department of Service Delivery and Safety at the World Health Organization (WHO). Prior to this, he served as director of the National Healthcare Reports for the US Department of Health and Human Services in the Agency for Healthcare Research and Quality. He directed the 28-country Health Care Quality Improvement (HCQI) project of the Organization for Economic Cooperation and Development (OECD). Dr. Kelley also previously served as a senior researcher and quality assurance advisor for the United States Agency for International Development (USAID)-sponsored Quality Assurance Project (QAP) and Partnerships for Health Reform Project Plus (PHRPlus). Additionally, he directed the international division of a large U.S.-based hospital consulting firm, the Advisory Board Company. Dr. Kelley's work over 2 decades has focused on strengthening links between health security issues and the quality, safety, and organization of health services, including metrics and measurement in health services and health systems improvement approaches and policies.

Janne Lehmann Knudsen, MD, is a specialist in public health/community medicine. She has a PhD and a master in health management and is director of the Division of Pharmacovigilance and Medical Devices at the Danish Medicines Agency. She has held positions at a research institute, the National Board of Health, and has over 20 years of experience as a leader in quality and safety. She was previously director of quality and safety at the Danish Cancer Society. She has been an associate professor at Copenhagen and Odense Universities. She is a member of national and international committees focusing on quality and safety. She is a board member of the International Society for Quality in Health Care (ISQua) and an ISQua expert. She is author of textbooks, articles, and papers on healthcare issues.

Jorma Komulainen, MD, PhD, adjunct professor, works as the editor-in-chief of the Current Care Guidelines in the Finnish Medical Society Duodecim. He is also a consulting pediatric endocrinologist in South-Carelia Central Hospital. His scientific activities include publications regarding diabetes, pediatric endocrinology, evidence-based medicine, and medical informatics. He is author and co-author of around 20 national Finnish clinical practice guidelines. He is a former member of the Guidelines International Network (G-I-N) board of trustees and a current member of the G-I-N Nordic Steering Group.

Ilkka Kunnamo, MD, PhD, founded Evidence-Based Medicine Guidelines, a comprehensive electronic guideline database published by Duodecim

Medical Publications, Ltd. He serves as the editor-in-chief of the international version, which has been translated into nine languages, and as adjunct professor of general practice at the University of Helsinki. Presently he develops a comprehensive multilingual decision support service (EBMeDS, www.ebmeds.org). He is a member of the GRADE working group, a member of the executive board of DynaMed Plus, EBSCO Health. In 2014, he was elected chair of the World Organization of Family Physicians (WONCA) Working Party on eHealth.

Grace Labadarios is the standards development coordinator at The Council for Health Service Accreditation of Southern Africa, Cape Town, South Africa. She graduated from the University of Stellenbosch in 1992 and was a general practitioner in the United Kingdom until her return to South Africa in 2011. She holds a diploma of the Royal College of Obstetricians and Gynaecologists (DRCOG), a certificate of the Joint Committee on Postgraduate Training for General Practice (JCPTGP), and became a member of the Royal College of General Practitioners (MRCGP) in 2010.

Levette Lamb is regional patient safety advisor with the Northern Ireland Health and Social Care Safety Forum. A nurse by profession, Mrs. Lamb has worked in a range of positions, including service improvement facilitator at the Department of Health Social Services and Public Safety, where she led on a range of multi-professional projects across the region. She has a postgraduate diploma in health and social care management and a master's degree in public administration. She has completed the Patient Safety Executive and Improvement Advisor programs through the Institute of Healthcare Improvement and is a founding member of the Health Foundation Q Programme.

Gavin Lavery is clinical director of the Health and Social Care Safety Forum and a consultant in Critical Care Medicine at Belfast Trust. Dr. Lavery is a graduate of the Advanced Training Programme at Intermountain Healthcare and is a member of the Health Foundation's College of Assessors. He is a standing member (patient safety) on Quality Standards Advisory Committee at the National Institute for Health and Care Excellence (NICE) and a board member at the Centre for Clinical Leadership and Quality in Healthcare at Royal College of Physicians in Ireland. Dr. Lavery has published over 60 peer-reviewed papers and book chapters.

Wui-Chiang Lee is the director of the Department of Medical Affairs and Planning, Taipei Veterans General Hospital, Taiwan. He was the director general of the Department of Medical Affairs, Ministry of Health and Welfare (2013–2014) and chief executive officer of the Joint Commission Taiwan (2011–2013). Dr. Lee has actively participated in many national and international quality improvement and patient safety programs. He has been the president of the Asian Society for Quality in Health Care and also on the board of the International Society for Quality in Health Care since 2013. Dr. Lee received his PhD and MHS from Johns Hopkins University (USA) and an MD from National Yang-Ming University, Taiwan.

Margus Lember, MD, PhD, is professor and head of the Department of Internal Medicine, University of Tartu, and dean of the Faculty of Medicine at the University of Tartu. He was a president of the Estonian Society of Family Doctors and Society of Internal Medicine, and an adviser to the Ministry of Social Affairs in the 1990s, when the Estonian primary care reform was carried out. He is the chairman of the National Practice Guidelines Advisory Board, member of the editorial board of several medical journals, and has been a consultant to the World Bank in healthcare reforms in several countries.

Thomas le Ludec is a hospital director. After several positions as deputy director of French teaching hospitals, he became regional chief executive officer of Marne-La-Vallée Hospitals between 2006 and 2009, and then deputy director of the Haute Autorité de Santé (HAS), the French agency for hospital accreditation, and he worked as head of accreditation certification between 2009 and 2015. He is now chief executive officer of Montpellier Hospital, one of the largest teaching hospitals in France.

Yu-Chuan (Jack) Li, a pioneer of medical informatics research, is dean of the College of Medical Science and Technology and a professor of biomedical informatics at Taipei Medical University (TMU). He has an MD from TMU and a PhD from the University of Utah. He was recognized as one of the "Ten Outstanding Young Persons of the Year" in 2001. He has published 130 scientific papers and three textbooks and is a fellow of the American College of Medical Informatics, the Australian College of Health Informatics, and was president of the Asia-Pacific Association for Medical Informatics. He is editor-in-chief of two international journals—*Computer Methods and Programs in Biomedicine* and the *International Journal for Quality in Health Care.*

Alexander L. Lindenbraten is first deputy director of the National Institute for Research in Public Health (Semashko Institute), and professor of the Health Economics and Management Department at the Higher School of Economics. His main fields of interest include public health economics and health insurance, organizational technology for health management, and assessment of healthcare quality and effectiveness. He is author and co-author of more than 20 books and manuals, and has published more than 270 research and scientific articles.

Kristiana Ludlow, Psych (Hons), is a PhD candidate in health innovation and is employed as a research assistant in the Centre for Healthcare Resilience and Implementation Science at the Australian Institute of Health

Innovation, Macquarie University, Sydney. She has a background in psychology, graduating with first class honors and has fulfilled the requirements for a Master of Research in health innovation at Macquarie University. Her research interests include health systems improvement, patient-centered care, shared decision-making, hearing loss, and aged care.

Melinda Maggard-Gibbons, MD, MSHS, is a professor of surgery at the University of California, Los Angeles (UCLA). She was a fellow in the Robert Wood Johnson Clinical Scholars Program and obtained a master of science in health services. She helped found the Center for Surgical Outcomes and Quality (CSOQ) at UCLA. Her research interests include assessing and improving quality of surgical care, disparities in care, survivorship, and appropriateness of surgical treatment. She has an adjunct appointment at RAND Health and works with the Southern California Evidence-Based Practice Center. Dr. Gibbons serves as the principal investigator (PI) for the Avon Cares for Life Program at Olive View-UCLA Medical Center, providing navigation and support services to underserved breast cancer patients.

Vishwa Mahadeo, MD, MBA, MP, is certified in general surgery, is a registrar in obstetrics and gynecology, and has 27 years of public health experience. He was the regional health officer, region 2 (1994–1995) and, medical superintendent and head of the surgical department of public hospital Suddie (1996–2003). He was medical superintendent and head of the Obstetrics and Gynecology Department of New Amsterdam Regional Hospital (2006–2009), and was regional health officer and chief executive officer of the Pilot Berbice Regional Health Authority in Guyana (2003–2015). Since 2009, he has focused on care of the elderly using a holistic approach.

Geraint Martin, a graduate of the universities of Swansea and Birmingham, has undertaken post graduate study at the University of Aberdeen Medical School and INSEAD; and is chief executive, Counties Manukau District Health Board. His international experience includes developing national policy and leading service provision in primary and secondary care. He was previously director of Health and Social Care Strategy, Wales, and a chief executive in the United Kingdom's National Health Service (NHS). In New Zealand, he has promoted clinical quality, clinical leadership, and improvement methodologies. He was a foundation board member of the New Zealand Health Quality and Safety Commission and leader in residence, Institute for Healthcare Improvement, Boston (USA), 2014.

Rafael Matesanz, MD, PhD, is a nephrologist. He has been founder and director of the Spanish National Transplant Organization (ONT) since September 1989 and is responsible for the "Spanish Model" of organ donation. He was general director of the Spanish National Institute of Health (4 years), president of the Transplant Experts Committee of the Council of

Europe (7 years), president of the Iberoamerican Council of Organ Donation and Transplantation since November 2005, and adviser of the World Health Organization (WHO) in the field of organ donation and transplantation. He is author of more than 500 articles in national and international journals and more than 200 book chapters or monographs about nephrology, organ donation, and clinical management.

Lizo Mazwai is a specialist surgeon who has had a life-long association with Walter Sisulu University in the Eastern Cape where he served as professor of surgery and dean of the Faculty of Health Sciences. He is currently a specialist surgeon in private practice and volunteer consultant responsible for training in surgery at Nelson Mandela Academic Hospital in Mthatha. He is a member of the Eastern Cape Planning Commission, former chair of the South African Medical Research Council board and has served as senior-vice president of the Colleges of Medicine of South Africa.

Feargal McGroarty, FAMLS, has a medical laboratory background and has worked in both medical laboratory and project management roles. His current project has seen the implementation of global standard (GS1) barcoding on hemophilia medication, allowing real-time track and trace of the drug from the manufacturer through to the patient home, including the use of a smartphone app for patients to scan their medication at home, which is the first of its kind. He holds a fellowship in Laboratory Hematology from the Academy of Clinical Science and Laboratory Medicine and a postgraduate diploma in management and employee relations from the National College of Ireland.

Sandra Mesmar is a graduate in public health with a concentration in health management and policy. She is a consultant and project coordinator at the Centre for Research on Population and Health at the American University of Beirut. Her research interests are refugee health, focusing on access to reproductive and chronic care, promoting digital technology with displaced populations, and social innovation during times of conflict.

Lesley Middleton is an independent consultant who works as a research associate with the Health Services Research Centre, Victoria University of Wellington. She has a background in public policy, evaluation, research impact, health services research, and strategy development. She has held previous policy and research roles in the Ministry of Health and the Ministry of Research, Science, and Technology. During her career within government she has overseen the development of new policy directions for research and been a member of senior leadership teams focused on how research is used to solve real-world policy problems.

Jonathan I. Mitchell, MSc, CHE, FISQua, is a healthcare consultant with CADTH, the Canadian Agency for Drugs and Technologies in Health.

From 2011 through 2016, Jonathan was manager of policy and research at Accreditation Canada, where he led the national jurisdictional reporting as well as collaborative research projects with academics and healthcare organizations. Prior, Jonathan led developments to the national and international accreditation programs. From 2005 to 2007, he was a senior analyst at the Canadian Institute for Health Information. Jonathan holds a master of science in business administration from Concordia University's John Molson School of Business in Montreal. He is a certified health executive with the Canadian College of Health Leaders and a fellow of the International Society for Quality in Healthcare.

Jalal Mohammed, MPH, MBA, PGDE(TT), BCom, AFACHSM, is a PhD candidate with the Health Systems Section, School of Population Health, University of Auckland. His PhD research examines the impact of decentralization on access to health services in Fiji. Currently, he is programme leader and lecturer for health administration programmes at the Auckland University of Technology. He has previously held academic positions at the College of Medicine, Nursing, and Health Sciences, Fiji National University, where he was lecturer and program coordinator for health management programs and center coordinator for the Centre for Excellence and Innovation in Learning. His main research interests include access to health services, healthcare reforms, primary healthcare, and online education for health professionals.

Simona Montilla, graduating in chemistry and pharmaceutical technologies at the University of Rome La Sapienza, obtained a doctorate degree in pharmacology, pharmacognosy, and toxicology (in 2003) and master's degrees in drug development (2009) and health technology assessment (HTA) in 2011 from the University of Rome La Cattolica. She is a pharmaceutical policies expert and HTA assessor in the Economic Strategy and Pharmaceutical Policy Department of the Italian Medicines Agency (AIFA). Her expertise is in regulatory science, analysis of pharmaceutical systems, HTA methodology, pricing and reimbursement decision-making processes, pharmaco-epidemiology and rational use of medicines, and evaluation of pharmaceutical innovation. She participates in national and EU projects, co-authoring more than 25 publications.

Ali Mohammad Mosadeghrad, PhD, is an assistant professor of health policy, management and economics at Tehran University of Medical Sciences, Iran. He was the general director for accreditation of healthcare organizations, at the ministry of health. He is an author, speaker, and a professional management consultant and trainer. Mosadeghrad has developed and reviewed hundreds of strategic plans for public and private healthcare organizations. His research interests include global health, strategic management, quality management, organizational health, and organizational change. Mosadeghrad has written extensively on many aspects of healthcare organization and management covering a full spectrum of subjects in strategy formulation, implementation, and evaluation.

Bafana Msibi is a qualified health professional who has more than 15 years of experience in implementing and managing healthcare projects and programs. In addition, he has extensive experience in leading compliance inspection work and health standards development. He holds a degree in health science education and management and is currently studying toward a master's degree in public health (MPH) with the University of Limpopo. He is currently the executive manager for compliance inspections and he is acting as a chief executive officer in the Office of Health Standards Compliance (OHSC). He previously served as the director of compliance inspections and deputy director of women's health at the National Department of Health (NDOH). In addition, he was also the district co-coordinator of maternal child and women's health (MCWH) in the Free State Department of Health in the Thabo Mofutsanyane District.

Wendy Nicklin, RN, MSc(A), CHE, FISQua, is a healthcare consultant. Most recently she was president and chief executive officer of Accreditation Canada (2004 to December 2015). With a nursing background in emergency care, she progressed through a career path that included teaching at Queen's University and senior administrative roles within The Ottawa Hospital. She was a founding member of the Board of the Canadian Patient Safety Institute. Currently, she is president-elect of the International Society for Quality in Healthcare and participates on numerous board committees. She has many publications to her name and is actively engaged in academic and healthcare advisory committees.

José Noronha, MD, DPH, PhD, is senior researcher at the Oswaldo Cruz Foundation of the Brazilian Federal Ministry of Health, where he coordinates the Strategic Foresight of Brazilian Healthcare System Initiative. He is also International Advisor to the Consortium for Brazilian Accreditation of Health Systems and Services, and formerly: national secretary for healthcare of the Brazilian Ministry of Health, president of the Brazilian Association of Public Health, a member of the advisory council and board of the International Society for Quality in Healthcare, and a member of the board of the Joint Commission Resources. He has published book chapters and articles on health policy, healthcare evaluation policies, and quality measures.

Nicola North, PhD, MA (Hons), RN, AFACHSM, a social scientist, is associate professor in health management in the School of Population Health of the Faculty of Medical and Health Sciences, University of Auckland, and is involved in delivering a master of health leadership program. She completed her MA (social science) in 1984 and PhD (social anthropology) in 1996. She has worked previously at Massey University in the Department of Management. Her current research centers on health management and leadership competencies in health systems. She has extensive experience in low-income countries, for example, in community health development in Nepal, evaluations in the Pacific, and a "train the trainers" health management development program in Samoa.

John Øvretveit is director of research and professor of healthcare improvement implementation and evaluation at the Medical Management Centre, the Karolinska Institute, Stockholm, and previously professor of health policy and management at Bergen University Medical School, Norway, and the Nordic School of Public Health, Gothenburg, Sweden. He is a board member for Joint Commission Resources/International, chair of the standards committee, a board member of the Global Implementation Initiative, and chair of the Global Implementation Society. Some of his 300 peer-reviewed scientific papers and books have been translated into nine languages. He was conferred the 2014 Avedis Donabedian international quality award for his work on quality economics.

Charles Pain, LRCP, MRCS, MSc, FFPH (UK), FAFPHM, FCHSM, FISQua, is a public health physician whose 33-year career in medicine has increasingly focused on improving health systems to improve patient care. He was a foundation co-director of the Hamad Health Care Quality Institute in Qatar, and, before that, with the Clinical Excellence Commission in New South Wales (NSW), he led state-wide programs such as the Between the Flags Program, which has had a major impact on hospital mortality. Like many others in his profession around the world, he is trying to build high-reliability healthcare systems that are patient-centered.

José-Artur Paiva is currently the medical director and member of the administration board of Centro Hospitalar São João, Porto, Portugal. Before that, he was director of the Emergency and Intensive Care Management Unit of the same hospital for 9 years. He is a specialist in intensive care medicine and internal medicine and certified in management of healthcare systems by the Portuguese Medical Council. He presided over the National Commission for the Reorganization of Emergency Care and Departments in Portugal in 2012. From 2013 to 2016, he was the director of the National Programme for Prevention and Control of Infection and Antimicrobial Resistance, Directorate General of Health.

Luca Pani is a psychiatrist and expert in pharmacology and molecular biology, Fellow of the National Research Council of Italy, and is currently director general of the Italian Medicines Agency (AIFA), part of the Department of Psychiatry and Behavioral Sciences, University of Miami School of Medicine. His professional trajectory embraced several areas from preclinical study to clinical activity and research and development of CNS drugs. He is an Italian member of CHMP, member of SAWP, participant of WP-CNS, chair of EUMBTC and of ERMS-FG of EMA, and member of the HMA management group. He is the author of over 150 scientific publications, editor and author of several volumes, and has attended more than 1000 events as an invited speaker.

Holger Pfaff is director of the Institute for Medical Sociology, Health Services Research, and Rehabilitation Science (IMVR) of the University of Cologne. Since 2009, he held the professorship in quality development and evaluation in rehabilitation, which is responsible for the teaching fields of medical sociology (Faculty of Medicine) and quality development in rehabilitation (Faculty of Human Sciences). A member of the review board of the German Research Foundation, since January 2016, he is chair of the expert panel of the innovations in healthcare board of the Ministry of Health. This panel makes recommendations on the content of calls for proposals, evaluates applications for funding, and creates recommendations for funding decisions.

Nafiullah Pirzad, MD, is an internal medicine specialist who works as chief executive officer for Afghanistan Private Hospitals Association (APHA). He advises and provides technical assistance to private hospital directors and staff on improving hospital standards and quality at private hospitals. He also coordinates training efforts for private hospitals. Previously, he worked as the minimum required standards (MRS) coordinator at APHA and assisted in the development of the MRS checklist. He has helped the APHA member hospitals to implement MRS and improve basic quality at their hospitals.

Kaja Põlluste, MD, PhD, is senior researcher of internal medicine at the University of Tartu. She has been lecturer of healthcare organization and quality management, and expert and advisor of healthcare quality at the Ministry of Social Affairs of Estonia. Her research is related to the quality of care and the quality of life of people with chronic conditions. She is author and co-author of more than 100 scientific papers and has published 22 articles in international peer-reviewed scientific journals. She is also a co-author of *Quality Policy of Estonian Health Care*.

Martin Powell, BA, PhD, is professor of health and social policy at the Health Services Management Centre, University of Birmingham, United Kingdom. His main research interests are in policy evaluation of the British National Health Service, and he is the author of some 80 articles and 10 books on British social policy. He co-wrote the chapter on England in *Healthcare Reform, Quality, and Safety: Perspectives, Participants, Partnerships, and Prospects in 30 Countries* (Braithwaite, Matsuyama, Mannion, Johnson, Ashgate, 2015).

His most recent book is *Dismantling the NHS?* (edited with Mark Exworthy and Russell Mannion, Policy Press, 2016).

Melissa Ramdeen, BSSW, MBA, has 10 years of experience working in the public health sector of Guyana. She was the focal point for HIV/AIDS in region 6 (2009–2013) and is a trained voluntary counselor and tester. She was the manager of special projects (2012–2015) and assistant hospital administrator (2013–2015) for the Berbice Regional Health Authority. Her main focus has been working with the underprivileged and the elderly as neglected groups.

Ånen Ringard, BA, MSc (Political Science), PhD (Health Policy), is senior advisor for the Association of the Pharmaceutical Industry in Norway (LMI). Before joining LMI, he was a senior scientist at the Health Services Research Unit, Akershus University Hospital. He has been employed by the Ministry of Health and Care Services, and the Norwegian Knowledge Centre for Health Services, where he was lead author of the "Norwegian Health System in Transition" report (commissioned by the World Health Organization [WHO]/The European Observatory of Health Systems and Policies). His research focuses on patient empowerment, hospital choice, priority setting, quality and safety, and health system analysis.

Viviana Rodríguez, MD, MA, graduated from the Medical University of La Plata (UNLP) and is a specialist in internal medicine and infectious diseases. She has an MA in clinical effectiveness from the University of Buenos Aires (UBA). She is chief of the department of infectious diseases at the German Hospital of Buenos Aires where she has coordinated the Patient Safety Committee (2008–2014). Currently, she is a professor and researcher at the Department of Health Care Quality and Patient Safety, Institute for Clinical Effectiveness and Health Policy (IECS). She is also a fellow of the International Society of Quality in Health Care (ISQua) and a certified professional in patient safety by the National Patient Safety Foundation (USA).

Enrique Ruelas, a physician trained in public administration and health administration, was dean, National School of Public Health of Mexico; program director, WK Kellogg Foundation for Latin America; director of institutional development of the Mexican Health Foundation; president and chief executive officer (CEO) of Qualimed; vice minister of health of Mexico; and secretary of the General Health Council. He chaired the Mexican Commission on Accreditation of Health Care Facilities, was founding president of the Mexican Society for Quality in Health Care, president of the International Society for Quality in Health Care (ISQua), and president of the National Academy of Medicine of Mexico. He is a member, board of directors, and senior fellow of the Institute for Healthcare Improvement (IHI).

Hélène Sabourin, RN, BScN, MHA, is senior director of governance, corporate strategy and quality at Accreditation Canada. Prior to holding this position, she was executive director of the Canadian Nurses Foundation. As a registered nurse, she brings over 20 years of progressive senior leadership experience in the not-for-profit sector. Hélène joined the Hospice Care Ottawa board of directors in 2015.

Omarzaman Sayedi, MD, MPH, works with Palladium as deputy chief of party on a United States Agency for International Development (USAID)-funded health sector resiliency project in Afghanistan. He has supported the Afghanistan Ministry of Public Health since 2009 in health policy and health systems strengthening. He has worked in various fields such as health sector governance, health economics, and financing, human resources for health, gender mainstreaming, private sector regulation, public-private partnerships, and quality improvement. He is also a founding member of Afghanistan National Public Health Association (ANPHA).

Richard Selormey, BSc (Med Sci), BDS, is a maxillofacial surgery resident at Komfo Anokye Teaching Hospital, Ghana. He has over 6 years of experience in clinical and administrative roles; as clinical coordinator and infection, prevention, and control (IPC) trainer at the St. Elizabeth District Hospital. He is a Mandela Washington Fellow (public management), an Ashoka change maker scholar (social intrapreneurship), and is currently pursuing a Fellowship of the International Society for Quality in Healthcare. He is also the co-founder and executive director of Oral Health Express-Ghana a nongovernment organization (NGO) that seeks to improve oral health awareness and access to underserved communities.

Syed Shahabuddin is a consultant cardiothoracic surgeon and assistant professor at the Aga Khan University Hospital. He is involved in teaching medical students, nurses, and residents, and in training residents as a residency program coordinator. He is a fellow of the College of Physicians and Surgeons, Pakistan (CPSP). He is interested in outcome research, databases, and quality. He is a member of the Quality Improvement Committee and is involved in monitoring clinical quality indicators to comply with standards of care. He has contributed a number of publications and abstract presentations in national and international meetings.

Amy Showen is a medical student at David Geffen School of Medicine at the University of California, Los Angeles. She is concurrently pursuing her MSc in public health at the London School of Hygiene and Tropical Medicine. She received her BA in human biology from Stanford University.

Paulinus Lingani Ncube Sikosana, MD, MPH, MBA, FRSPH, is a physician, former permanent secretary for health in Zimbabwe, and currently coordinator of health systems and social determinants for health in the World Health Organization country office in Papua New Guinea. He has more than 30 years of experience in public health, health systems development, and health sector reforms. During his career, he has worked in various capacities in Botswana, Ethiopia, Kenya, Lesotho, Malawi, Mozambique, South Africa, and Zambia. He is the author of the book, *Challenges in Reforming the Health Sector in Africa: Reforming Health Systems under Economic Siege—The Zimbabwean Experience* (2010).

Judit Simon, MD, BA, BSc, MSc, DPhil, FFPH, is professor of health economics and head of the Department of Health Economics, Centre for Public Health at the Medical University of Vienna, and visiting professor of cognitive health economics at the University of Oxford. She has a multidisciplinary background specializing in health economics and public health, with primary expertise in economic evaluations, mental health economics, cost-effective clinical guideline development, and health services and systems research. She has been investigator in several applied and methodological research projects funded by, for example, the European Commission, the UK National Institute for Health Research, and the World Health Organization, and authored and co-authored over 60 scientific publications.

Sodzi Sodzi-Tettey is executive director and head of operations for the Africa region for the Institute for Healthcare Improvement. He provides overall strategic and technical leadership while driving new business opportunities. A public health physician, quality improvement advisor, and a fellow of the International Society for Quality in Health Care (ISQua), he has significant district, national, and global experiences facilitating improvement initiatives. He serves on the governing boards of Ghana's National Health Insurance Authority and the University for Health and Allied Sciences. He also writes *Affirmatively Disruptive*, a weekly sociopolitical newspaper column, and is a 2016 Rockefeller Global Fellow for Social Innovation.

Paulo Sousa is currently professor at the National School of Public Health–Universidade Nova de Lisboa, where he coordinates the master in public health and the international course in quality improvement and patient safety (a joint program with the National School of Public Health–Sérgio Arouca, in Brazil). In recent years, he has been involved, and has coordinated, several initiatives and research projects in the area of quality improvement, patient safety, and health outcomes evaluation. He is the author of many chapters in books and articles published in peer-review national and international journals. He is a member of the editorial board of the *Portuguese Journal of Cardiology* and of the *International Journal for Quality in Health Care* (IJQHC).

Anthony Staines currently runs patient safety improvement projects for the Hospital Federation of Vaud (Switzerland), and advises a number of hospitals on patient safety strategies. He holds an MBA from INSEAD Business School (France) and an MPA from IDHEAP School of Public Administration (Switzerland), as well as a PhD in Management from the IFROSS Institute at University of Lyon (France), where he lectures on quality improvement and patient safety. He is the co-author, with John Øvretveit, of a book on improving value in healthcare and serves as deputy editor for the *International Journal for Quality in Health Care*.

David R. Steel, OBE, MA, DPhil, FRCP (Edin), is Honorary Senior Research Fellow at the University of Aberdeen and a senior associate of the Nuffield Trust. He worked for 25 years in National Health Service (NHS) management and was chief executive of NHS Quality Improvement Scotland from its creation in 2003 until 2009. He is author of the *United Kingdom (Scotland): Health System Review*, published in 2012 as part of the European Observatory's *Health Systems in Transition* series. In 2008, he was awarded an OBE for services to healthcare.

Mirjana Živković Šulović is a public health specialist; head of the Department for Analysis, Planning, and Organization of Health Services, Institute of Public Health (IPH) of Serbia; member of the National Committee for Prevention of Child Abuse and Neglect; secretary of the Expert Committee for the Healthcare of Children; and World Health Organization (WHO) National Focal Point (NFP) for equity and social determinants of health. She has a special interest in the development of electronic databases in the field of healthcare. Dr. Šulović has developed and managed a national survey of patient satisfaction. She is author and co-author of more than 10 manuals, books, and papers on health policy and quality in health.

Rosa Suñol, director at Avedis Donabedian Research Institute (FAD), oversees this research and implementation organization that supports quality improvement in health and social care. She holds the Donabedian research chair in quality, Faculty of Medicine, Autonomous University of Barcelona. She has been deputy editor for the *International Journal for Quality in Health Care* since 1991, and has over 30 years of experience in health quality and social care research. She has published articles, books, and participated in EU-funded research projects as leader and partner, and implemented more than 230 internal quality programs (hospitals, primary healthcare [PHC], long-term care, home care, behavioral healthcare, and social services) in Spain and Latin America.

Shamsuzzoha B. Syed, MD, MPH, DPH (Cantab), is the program manager for African Partnerships for Patient Safety (APPS), based at the World Health Organization (WHO) headquarters in Geneva. He assumed responsibility for global partnership development in the newly formed WHO Department of Service Delivery and Safety in 2013. Dr. Syed received his medical degree from St. George's, University of London, and subsequently practiced as an independent general practitioner in the United Kingdom. He received post-graduate public health training at the University of Cambridge. Subsequently, he trained in preventive medicine at Johns Hopkins University. He is US board-certified in public health and preventive medicine and a fellow of the American College of Preventive Medicine. His previous experiences include involvement in a future-focused multi-country health systems research consortium; working at the Pan American Health Organization with seven Caribbean countries on strengthening health systems with a focus on sur-veillance systems; and working as the advisor on family and community health at the WHO Country Office in Trinidad and Tobago with a focus on quality of care.

Reem Talhouk is a doctoral trainee in digital civics at Open Lab, Newcastle University. Her research encompasses the use of technology to build refu-gee community resilience. Her previous work explored the use of technol-ogy in improving access to healthcare by refugees and improving refugee agency within healthcare-provider/refugee relationships. She is a founding member of the Arab Digital Public Health initiative based at the Faculty of Health Sciences, American University of Beirut. She is the author of "Syrian Refugees and Digital Health in Lebanon: Opportunities for Improving Antenatal Health" and co-author of "The Impact of Digital Technology on Health of Populations Affected by Humanitarian Crises: Recent Innovations and Current Gaps."

Andrew Thompson is a social scientist. He holds the chair in public policy and citizenship in the Department of Politics and International Relations at the University of Edinburgh. His main research interests are in two distinct areas: (1) citizenship and public policy (especially health services), in relation to quality improvement, and participatory and deliberative democracy; and (2) European public administration. He is a member of the Participatory and Deliberative Democracy Group of the UK Political Studies Association and the European Consortium for Political Research. He was a regional editor for the *International Journal for Quality in Health Care.*

Claudia Travassos, MD, MPH, PhD, is a senior researcher at the Oswaldo Cruz Foundation, Rio de Janeiro, Brazil. She was a scholar at the Institute of Social Research (ISR), Michigan University (2002), completed her PhD in public administration at the London School of Economics (1992) and before that a master's from the Collaborative Center for Quality of Care and Patient Safety (Proqualis). She is a former member of the Expert Working Group to Advance Measures and Methods for Research on Patient Safety (World Health Organization/Patient Safety), editor emeritus of *Cadernos de Saúde*

Pública (*Reports in Public Health*), and a member of the editorial committee of the *International Journal for Quality in Health Care*.

Leonel Valdivia, MEd, PhD, is professor of global health and director of international relations at the School of Public Health, University of Chile. He currently serves as president of the World Federation of Academic Institutions for Global Health. Before joining the University of Chile, he completed a career in international development in the United States, having worked for the United Nations Population Fund (UNFPA), the Pan American Health Organization/World Health Organization (PAHO/WHO), IPPF, and the United States Agency for International Development (USAID). He started his academic career as a lecturer at the University of Edinburgh, United Kingdom. His research interests focus on the effects of economic globalization on health equity and social justice, particularly in connection with mental and occupational health and non-communicable diseases.

John Van Aerde, MD, PhD, is a neonatologist who fulfilled several leadership roles, including program integration in several Canadian provinces. He holds appointments at the Universities of Alberta and British Columbia, at Royal Roads University, and at the Physician Leadership Institute, helping physicians learn those skills not covered during clinical training. He is the immediate past president of the Canadian Society of Physician Leaders and the editor-in-chief of the *Canadian Journal of Physician Leadership*. From forest regeneration and from living in a self-sustainable house, he discovered models and applications for the Canadian healthcare system as a complex adaptive system.

Pieter Johannes van Maaren is a medical doctor by profession with an MBA in health planning and management. Since March 2014, he is the World Health Organization (WHO) representative in Papua New Guinea. From 2010 to 2014, he was the WHO representative in Cambodia. From 2006 to 2010, he was the regional adviser for Stop Tuberculosis at the WHO's regional office in the Philippines.

Prior to the WHO, he worked with the Royal Tropical Institute in Amsterdam (1999–2001); the National Tuberculosis Program in Egypt (1995–1999); the World Bank in Nepal (1994–1995); and the Ministry of Health of Nepal (1993–1994). From 1983 to 1991, he worked as district medical officer in Botswana and Malawi.

Milena Vasic, DMD, MSc, PhD, is an associate professor, specialist in social medicine and public health and head of department for international cooperation and project management at the Institute of Public Health of Serbia. Dr. Vasic has been assistant director, as well as head of department for research in public health at the Institute of Public Health of Serbia. Dr. Vasic is World Health Organization (WHO) National Focal Point (NFP) for health systems. She has been working as a consultant for the World Bank, World Health Organization, Global Fund, and UNICEF. Her areas of expertise are healthcare planning and financing, monitoring and evaluation, healthcare quality assurance and management, and human resources planning and management.

David Vaughan is a consultant respiratory pediatrician and director of quality and patient safety at the Children's Hospitals Group, Dublin, Ireland. He was previously the executive director for quality and safety in Hamad Medical Corporation, Doha, Qatar. He was previously also director of quality, safety, and leadership in the Royal College of Physicians of Ireland, where he developed and directed a national program of quality improvement for the Irish healthcare system. He also worked in the past as a consultant respiratory pediatrician in the National Children's Hospital, Ireland.

Marcos Vergara, MD, MHA, DPH, is the director of the Institute of Neurosurgery and professor of health policy and management at the School of Public Health, University of Chile. He has over 25 years of experience in healthcare administration at municipal, regional, and national levels. He has directed large hospitals of the Chilean mining sector and has sat on the board of health insurance companies. More recently, he was appointed to the Presidential Commission on Health Financing and the Ministerial Commission for the Design of a Guaranteed Healthcare Plan for Private Insurance Companies. He has been an advisor on health finance to international cooperation agencies, notably the Inter-American Development Bank.

Vasiliy V. Vlassov, MD, DMedSci, is professor of public health at the National Research University Higher School of Economics, Moscow, and president of the Russian Society for Evidence Based Medicine. He serves as a member of the World Health Organization (WHO)-Euro Advisory Committee on Health Research, and as an expert to the Russian Academy of Sciences. He is the author of multiple books including, *Effectiveness of Diagnostic Tests, Reaction of the Organism to External Stimuli, Health Care under Deficit of Resources,* a textbook of epidemiology (all in Russian), as well as more than 200 articles on epidemiology, public health, and evidence-based medicine.

Cordula Wagner, PhD (physiotherapist, sociologist), is executive director of the Netherlands Institute of Health Services Research (NIVEL) in Utrecht and works as a professor of patient safety at VU Medical Center in Amsterdam. She is also head of the patient safety research center "Safety 4 Patients," a collaboration of the Institute for Care and Health Research (EMGO+)/VUmc and NIVEL. For the last 20 years, Professor Wagner has been involved in many projects, including EU research focusing on the implementation of quality systems and the evaluation of national quality programs, for example, quality improvement activities such as guidelines, team-training, and breakthrough projects; the relation between quality systems, care process, and clinical outcomes; and risk management and patient safety.

Eliza Lai-Yi Wong, RN, MPH, PhD, is associate professor at the JC School of Public Health and Primary Care, the Chinese University of Hong Kong. Her research areas include the patient experience of using healthcare, patient-reported outcome measures (PROMs)-EQ5D, acceptability of HPV self-sampling, service delivery from health system approach, and alternative medicine. She is also accredited by the Hong Kong International Arbitration Centre (HKIAC) and the Hong Kong Mediation Accreditation Association Limited (HKMAAL) as a mediator. She runs applied mediation skill workshops for healthcare workers of the Hong Kong Hospital Authority to enhance their communication with patients.

Entela Xoxi, after graduating from the University of Rome La Sapienza in 2001 with highest honors, obtained a PhD in pharmacology, pharmacognosy, and Toxicology (2005), a postgraduate diploma (specialization) in pharmacology (2009), and two master's degrees in drug development (2010) and health technology assessment (2011). Dr. Xoxi is skilled in regulatory science and especially in post-marketing data collection, design, and application of managed entry agreements. Since 2013, she has been coordinating all the activities of the Italian Medicines Agency (AIFA) registries. She is an Italian member of the Commission Expert Group on Safe and Timely Access to Medicines for Patients (STAMP), and provides a regulator and healthcare payer's perspective to national and international events.

Toby Yan, MA, is currently manager of client services at Accreditation Canada, and previously worked as an accreditation specialist and provided guidance to a variety of organizations, including acute care, long-term care, health systems, mental health, and rehabilitation. Along with her knowledge of accreditation, she is an experienced educator, facilitator, and team leader. She frequently presents at conferences and workshops on behalf of Accreditation Canada and has contributed to numerous publications. She has a master's degree in psychology and has worked in private industry and government as well as healthcare.

Nasser Yassin is director of research at the Issam Fares Institute for Public Policy and International Affairs, and professor of policy and planning at the Health Management and Policy Department, American University of Beirut, Lebanon. He holds a PhD from University College London, an MSc from London School of Economics, and an MSc and BSc from the American University of Beirut. His research and practice interests are in development planning and policy-making in countries in transition and in post-conflict situations. He researches and advises on policy and social innovation especially in areas of health, youth, and refugee policies and programs. He is author of more than 25 internationally published articles and reports.

Eng-Kiong Yeoh, FRCP (Edin), FHKCP, FRCP (Lond), FRCP (Glasg), FRACP, FHKAM, FHKCCM, FFPH (UK), FRACMA, is director, JC School of Public Health and Primary Care, the Chinese University of Hong Kong (CUHK), and head of the Division of Health System, Policy and Management at that school. He was head and first chief executive of the Hong Kong Hospital Authority, responsible for the management and transformation of the public hospital system. He was previously secretary for health, welfare, and food for the government of the Hong Kong Special Administrative Region. His research on health systems, services, and policy applies systems thinking to how the complex components of health systems interact to improve health.

Hao Zheng, PhD, MD, MBA, an expert in patient safety, is currently assistant dean and associate professor in public health at Tongji University School of Medicine, Shanghai. Working closely with the China Hospital Association (CHA) since 2014, she has been one of the initiators of the Patient Safety Collaborative of China in 2014—the first nationwide patient safety initiative—and a member of the CHA Steering Committee guiding the development of national patient safety goals and standards. She worked in the World Health Organization Patient Safety Program from 2010 to 2013, leading and coordinating international quality and safety projects worldwide.

Eyal Zimlichman is an internal medicine physician, a healthcare executive, and a researcher focused on assessing and improving healthcare quality and value, patient engagement, and patient safety. He is currently chief medical officer at Sheba Medical Center, Israel's largest hospital. Prior to this, he has held the position of lead researcher at Partners Health Care Clinical Affairs Department in Boston. Dr. Zimlichman is a graduate of the Harvard School of Public Health, Executive Health Care Management Master of Science program and has earned his MD at the Technion Israel Institute of Technology.

Contributors

Maria Cecilia Acuña
Pan American Health
    Organization/World Health
    Organization (PAHO/WHO)
Washington, DC

William Adu-Krow
PAHO/WHO
Washington, DC

Bruce Agins
HEALTHQUAL International
New York State Department of
    Health AIDS Institute
New York, New York

Emmanuel Aiyenigba
Institute for Healthcare
    Improvement (IHI)
Kwara State, Nigeria

Samir Al-Adawi
Behavioral Medicine at College of
    Medicine
Sultan Qaboos University
Muscat, Oman

Patricia Albisetti
Secretary-General of the Hospital
    Federation of Vaud
Prilly, Switzerland

Ahmed Al-Mandhari
Sultan Qaboos University Hospital
Muscat, Oman

Yousuf Khalid Al Maslamani
Hamad General Hospital
Doha, Qatar

Abdullah Al-Raqadi
Ministry of Health
Muscat, Oman

Khaled Al-Surimi
King Saud ben Abudalaziz
    University for Health Sciences
Riyadh, Saudi Arabia, and Thamar
    University
Dhamar, Yemen

René Amalberti
Haute Autorité de Santé (HAS)
Saint-Denis, France

Hugo Arce
University Institute of Health
    Sciences
Barceló Foundation
Buenos Aires, Argentina

Lauren Archer
Palladium
Washington, DC

Toni Ashton
Health Systems Section, School of
    Population Health
University of Auckland
Auckland, New Zealand

Badar Awladthani
Ministry of Health
Muscat, Oman

Luis Azpurua
Clinica Sanitas Santa Paula
Caracas, Venezuela

Natasha Azzopardi-Muscat
University of Malta
Msida, Malta

Vasha Elizabeth Bachan
Ministry of Public Health
Georgetown, Guyana

G. Ross Baker
University of Toronto
Toronto, Canada

Roland Bal
Erasmus University Rotterdam
Rotterdam, Netherlands

Cynthia Bannerman
Ghana Health Service
Accra, Ghana

Joshua Bardfield
HEALTHQUAL International
New York State Department of
   Health AIDS Institute
New York, New York

Maysa Baroud
Issam Fares Institute for Public
   Policy and International Affairs
American University of Beirut
Beirut, Lebanon

Apollo Basenero
Division of Quality Assurance
Ministry of Health and Social
   Services
Windhoek, Republic of Namibia

Roger Bayingana
Health Solutions for Africa
Kigali City, Rwanda

Mustafa Berktaş
Institute of Quality and Accreditation
   in Healthcare of Turkey
Ankara, Turkey

Paula Bezzola
EQUAM Foundation
Patient Safety Foundation
Bern, Switzerland

Sarah Boucaud
Accreditation Canada
Ottawa, Canada

Denise Boulter
Public Health Agency
Belfast, Northern Ireland

Jeffrey Braithwaite
Australian Institute of Health
   Innovation
Macquarie University
Sydney, Australia

Mats Brommels
Medical Management Centre (MMC)
Karolinska Institutet
Solna Municipality, Sweden

Geir Bukholm
Norwegian Institute of Public
   Health
Oslo, Norway

Sandra C. Buttigieg
University of Malta
Msida, Malta

Stephanie Carpenter
Accreditation Canada
Ottawa, Canada

Edward Chappy
Independent Consultant
Wauwatosa, Wisconsin

Patsy Yuen-Kwan Chau
JC School of Public Health and
   Primary Care
The Chinese University of Hong
   Kong
Hong Kong, People's Republic of
   China

Americo Cicchetti
Università Cattolica del Sacro Cuore
Milan, Italy

Elisabeth Coll Torres
Organizacion Nacional de
  Trasplantes
Madrid, Spain

Silvia Coretti
Università Cattolica del Sacro Cuore
Milan, Italy

Jacqueline Cumming
Health Services Resource Centre
Victoria University of Wellington
Wellington, New Zealand

Haidee Davis
Ko Awatea
Counties Manukau Health
Auckland, New Zealand

Ellen Tveter Deilkås
Akershus University Hospital
Lørenskog, Norway

Pedro Delgado
Institute for Healthcare
  Improvement
Cambridge, Massachusetts

Subashnie Devkaran
Cleveland Clinic Abu Dhabi
Abu Dhabi, the United Arab
  Emirates

Danielle Dorschner
Accreditation Canada
Ottawa, Canada

Persephone Doupi
National Institute for Health and
  Welfare–THL
Helsinki, Finland

Adrian Edwards
Cardiff University
Cardiff, Wales

Carsten Engel
IKAS–Danish Institute for Quality
  and Accreditation in Healthcare
Aarhus, Denmark

Jesper Eriksen
Danish Cancer Society
Copenhagen, Denmark

Hong Fung
JC School of Public Health and
  Primary Care
The Chinese University of Hong Kong
Hong Kong, People's Republic of
  China

Ezequiel García-Elorrio
Institute for Clinical Effectiveness
  and Health Policy
Buenos Aires, Argentina

Octavio Gómez-Dantés
National Institute of Public Health
  Mexico
Cuernavaca, Mexico

Jonás Gonseth
Hospital de Especialidades Dr. Abel
  Gilbert Ponton
Guayaquil, Ecuador

Christine S. Gordon
Division of Quality Assurance
Ministry of Health and Social
  Services (MoHSS)
Windhoek, Republic of Namibia

Victor Grabois
Proqualis/Icict/Fiocruz
Rio de Janeiro, Brazil

Jonathon Gray
Ko Awatea
Counties Manukau Health
Auckland, New Zealand

Kenneth Grech
University of Malta
Msida, Malta

Oliver Groene
Optimedis AG
London School of Hygiene and
    Tropical Medicine
London, England

Mylai Guerrero
Hamad Medical Corporation
Doha, Qatar

**The Gulf Health Council for
Cooperation Council States**
Riyadh, Saudi Arabia

Girdhar Gyani
Association of Healthcare Providers
    (INDIA)
New Delhi, India

Gerald Haidinger
Department of Epidemiology
Centre for Public Health
Medical University of Vienna
Vienna, Austria

Ann Hamilton
South Eastern Health and Social
    Care Trust
Belfast, Northern Ireland

Ndapewa Hamunime
Ministry of Health and Social
    Services
Windhoek, Namibia

Qendresa Hasanaj
Accreditation Canada
Ottawa, Canada

Patricia Hayward
Ko Awatea
Counties Manukau Health
Auckland, New Zealand

Helmut Hildebrandt
Optimedis AG
Hamburg, Germany

Ken Hillman
Simpson Centre for Health
Services Research
University of New South Wales
Sydney, Australia

Maria M. Hofmarcher
HS&I Health System Intelligence
    and Medical University Vienna
Vienna, Austria

Min-Huei Hsu
Department of Information
    Management
Ministry of Health and Welfare
Taipei, Taiwan

Clifford F. Hughes
International Society for Quality in
    Health Care (ISQua)
Dublin, Ireland

Valentina Iacopino
Università Cattolica del Sacro Cuore
Milan, Italy

Usman Iqbal
Global Health and Development
    Department
College of Public Heath, and
    International Center for Health
    Information Technology
    (ICHIT)
Taipei Medical University
Taipei, Taiwan

Marcos Vergara Iturriaga
School of Public Health
University of Chile
Santiago, Chile

Ivan Ivanovic
Institute of Public Health of Serbia
Belgrade, Serbia

Safurah Jaafar
Ministry of Health Malaysia
Putrajaya, Malaysia

Wendy James
Australian Institute of Health
  Innovation
Macquarie University
Sydney, Australia

Salma Jaouni Araj
Health Care Accreditation Council
Amman, Jordan

Ravichandran Jeganathan
Ministry of Health Malaysia
Putrajaya, Malaysia

Ravindran Jegasothy
Faculty of Medicine
Mahsa University
Selangor, Malaysia

Sara Kaddoura
School of International and Public
  Affairs (SIPA)
Columbia University
New York, New York

Minna Kaila
Department of Public Health
University of Helsinki
Helsinki, Finland

Ruth Kalda
Department of Family Medicine,
  Institute of Family Medicine and
  Public Health
University of Tartu
Tartu, Estonia

İbrahim H. Kayral
Institute of Quality and
  Accreditation in Healthcare of
  Turkey
Ankara, Turkey

Edward T. Kelley
World Health Organization
Geneva, Switzerland

Janne Lehmann Knudsen
Danish Medicines Agency
Copenhagen, Denmark

Jorma Komulainen
Finnish Medical Society Duodecim
Helsinki, Finland

Ilkka Kunnamo
Duodecim Medical Publications Ltd.
Helsinki, Finland

Grace Labadarios
Council for Health Service
  Accreditation of Southern Africa
Pinelands, South Africa

Levette Lamb
Health and Social Care Safety Forum
Public Health Agency
Belfast, Northern Ireland

Gavin G. Lavery
Health and Social Care Safety Forum
Public Health Agency
Belfast, Northern Ireland

Wui-Chiang Lee
Taipei Veterans General Hospital
  and National Yang-Ming
  University
Taipei, Taiwan

Thomas le Ludec
Centre Hospitalier Universitaire De
  Montpellier
Montpellier, France

Margus Lember
Department of Internal Medicine
Institute of Clinical Medicine
University of Tartu
Tartu, Estonia

Yu-Chuan (Jack) Li
Graduate Institute of Biomedical
  Informatics
College of Medical Science and
  Technology
Taipei Medical University
Taipei, Taiwan

Alexander L. Lindenbraten
National Institute for Research in
  Public Health
Moscow, Russia

Kristiana Ludlow
Australian Institute of Health
  Innovation
Macquarie University
Sydney, Australia

Melinda Maggard-Gibbons
University of California, Los
  Angeles (UCLA) Medical Center
Los Angeles, California

Vishwa Mahadeo
Member of Parliament
Berbice, Guyana

Russell Mannion
Health Services Management Centre
University of Birmingham
Birmingham, England

Geraint Martin
Counties Manukau Health
Auckland, New Zealand

Rafael Matesanz
Organizacion Nacional De Trasplantes
Madrid, Spain

Yukihiro Matsuyama
The Canon Institute of Global Studies
Tokyo, Japan

Lizo Mazwai
The Office of Health Standards
  Compliance
Pretoria, South Africa

Feargal McGroarty
St. James's Hospital
Dublin, Ireland

Sandra Mesmar
American University of Beirut
Beirut, Lebanon

Lesley Middleton
Health Services Research Centre
Victoria University of Wellington
Wellington, New Zealand

Jonathan I. Mitchell
Healthcare Consultant
Ottawa, Canada

Jalal Mohammed
Health Systems Section
School of Population Health
University of Auckland
Auckland, New Zealand

Simona Montilla
Italian Medicines Agency
Roma, Italy

Ali Mohammad Mosadeghrad
School of Public Health, Department
of Health Management and
Economics
Tehran University of Medical
Sciences
Tehran, Iran

Bafana Msibi
The Office of Health Standards
Compliance
Pretoria, South Africa

Wendy Nicklin
International Society for Quality in
Health Care (ISQua)
Dublin, Ireland

José Noronha
Fundação Oswaldo Cruz
Rio de Janeiro, Brazil

Nicola North
Health Systems Section, School of
Population Health
University of Auckland
Auckland, New Zealand

John Øvretveit
Karolinska Institutet
Solna Municipality, Sweden

Charles Pain
Top End Health Service
Darwin, Australia

José-Artur Paiva
Centro Hospitalar Sao Joao and
Faculdade de Medicina da
Universidade do Porto
Porto, Portugal

Luca Pani
Agenzia Italiana del Farmaco
Rome, Italy

Holger Pfaff
University of Cologne
Cologne, Germany

Nafiullah Pirzad
Afghanistan Private Hospitals
Association
Kabul, Afghanistan

Kaja Põlluste
Department of Internal Medicine
Institute of Clinical Medicine
University of Tartu
Tartu, Estonia

Martin Powell
Health Services Management Centre
University of Birmingham
Birmingham, England

Melissa Ramdeen
Former Program Officer of the
Berbice Regional Health
Authority (BRHA)
Berbice, Guyana

Ånen Ringard
Association of the Pharmaceutical
Oslo, Norway

Viviana Rodríguez
Institute for Clinical Effectiveness
and Health Policy
Buenos Aires, Argentina

Enrique Ruelas
Institute for Healthcare
Improvement
Cambridge, Massachusetts

Hélène Sabourin
Accreditation Canada
Ottawa, Canada

Omarzaman Sayedi
Palladium
Kabul, Afghanistan

Richard Selormey
Komfo Anokye Teaching Hospital
Kumasi, Ghana

Syed Shahabuddin
Aga Khan University Hospital
Karachi, Pakistan

Paul Shekelle
West Los Angeles Veterans
   Affairs Medical Center and the
   University of California, Los
   Angeles (UCLA)
Los Angeles, California

Amy Showen
David Geffen School of Medicine at
   the University of California, Los
   Angeles (UCLA)
Los Angeles, California

**Paulinus Lingani Ncube
Sikosana**
World Health Organization
Port Moresby, Papua New Guinea

Judit Simon
Department of Health Economics
Centre for Public Health
Medical University of Vienna
Vienna, Austria

Sodzi Sodzi-Tettey
Institute for Healthcare
   Improvement
Cambridge, Massachusetts

Paulo Sousa
Escola Nacional de Saúde Pública
Universidade Nova de Lisboa
Lisbon, Portugal

Anthony Staines
Hospital Federation of Vaud
Prilly, Switzerland

David Steel
University of Aberdeen
Aberdeen, Scotland

Mirjana Živković Šulović
Institute of Public Health of Serbia
Belgrade, Serbia

Rosa Suñol
Avedis Donabedian Research
   Institute—Universitat Autonoma
   de Barcelona
Bellaterra, Spain

Shamsuzzoha B. Syed
African Partnerships for Patient
   Safety (APPS)
World Health Organization
Geneva, Switzerland

Reem Talhouk
Open Lab
Newcastle University
Newcastle upon Tyne, England

Andrew Thompson
University of Edinburgh
Edinburgh, Scotland

Claudia Travassos
Icict/Fiocruz
Rio de Janeiro, Brazil

Leonel Valdivia
School of Public Health
University of Chile
Santiago, Chile

John Van Aerde
University of British Columbia and
   Alberta
Ladysmith, Canada

Pieter Johannes van Maaren
World Health Organization
Port Moresby, Papua New Guinea

Milena Vasic
Institute of Public Health of Serbia
Belgrade, Serbia

David Vaughan
Hamad Medical Corporation
Doha, Qatar

Vasiliy V. Vlassov
National Research University
   Higher School of Economics
Moscow, Russia

Cordula Wagner
NIVEL
VU University Medical Center
Amsterdam, the Netherlands

Stuart Whittaker
School of Public Health and
   Medicine
Faculty of Health Sciences
University of Cape Town and School
   of Health Systems and Public
   Health
and
Faculty of Health Sciences
University of Pretoria
Pretoria, South Africa

Eliza Lai-Yi Wong
JC School of Public Health and
   Primary Care
The Chinese University of Hong
   Kong
Hong Kong, People's Republic of
   China

Entela Xoxi
Italian Medicines Agency
Rome, Italy

Toby Yan
Accreditation Canada
Ottawa, Canada

Nasser Yassin
American University of Beirut
Beirut, Lebanon

Eng-Kiong Yeoh
JC School of Public Health and
   Primary Care
The Chinese University of Hong
   Kong
Hong Kong, People's Republic of
   China

Hao Zheng
Tongii University School of
   Medicine
Shanghai, China

Eyal Zimlichman
Sheba Medical Center
Ramat Gan, Israel

Introduction

Jeffrey Braithwaite, Russell Mannion, Yukihiro Matsuyama,
Paul Shekelle, Stuart Whittaker, Samir Al-Adawi, Kristiana Ludlow,
and Wendy James

The Book in Context

In this, the second book in the health reform series, now under the Taylor &
Francis banner, we present a series of case studies from authors drawn from
low-, middle-, and high-income countries. The authors were given a specific
assignment by the editors: to choose, from the myriad of things going on in
their health system, one success story. This story didn't necessarily have to
represent the absolute best reform or innovation their country could offer,
but it did have to be in some way instructive. We imagined—or hoped—that
we would receive contributions that ranged quite widely, perhaps dealing
with the eradication of an illness in a low-income country, or the take-up of
a hand hygiene program in a middle-income country, or the effective implementation of a specialized information technology (IT) system in a high-
income country.

As readers will see when they go through the case studies, we got even
more than we banked on. The breadth and extent of case studies is truly
impressive. We provide more details subsequently, but at this point, it's sufficient to highlight that in what follows are success stories ranging from, for
example, Ireland's highly effective National Hemophilia System, China's
efficient self-service encounter system, the innovative use of social media to
coordinate blood donations in Lebanon, the significant reduction of hospital-acquired infections (HAIs) in Portugal, the achievements of community-
based health insurance in Rwanda, and the visionary, if ultimately flawed,
Misión Barrio Adentro in Venezuela.

The first book in this series, *Healthcare Reform, Quality, and Safety: Perspectives,
Participants, Partnerships, and Prospects in 30 Countries* (Braithwaite et al., 2015),
looked at improvement and transformation at the national level in 30 countries, and the relationship of those national reforms to the improvement of
quality of care and safety to patients at macro, meso, and micro levels in each
system. The current book builds on the knowledge assembled in that first
volume. It doubles the number of countries involved (and with 161 authors
to coordinate, this itself was no small task) and changes the focus to one of
achievements rather than challenges. As the authors across this current compendium show, success comes in many guises.

How We Went about Initiating and Compiling This Compendium

As an editorial team, we (Jeffrey Braithwaite, Russell Mannion, Yukihiro Matsuyama, Paul Shekelle, Stuart Whittaker, and Samir Al-Adawi) have, over the decades, contributed substantially to research into how health systems embrace change, reform, and improvement—and have read and digested even more. We know from this experience that most collections like ours tend to identify health system challenges and problems and then try to provide solutions—through presenting research, or ideas, models, or theories about policy enactment or practice improvement. As in most public narratives, good news is often treated as no news—and because the focus is on problems, we rarely hear about success in the level of detail we envisage here.

The approach we took was to begin from a different starting point. In asking, "what does success look like for health systems?" we wanted to acknowledge and celebrate that all health systems, no matter how resource-constrained, politically stressed, or logistically strained, do some things well.

In telling their tales of accomplishment, we sought from our contributors three things. We asked them, first, to briefly provide details of their identified success story and its impact. Next, we wanted an explanation of what they had learned that would help people interested in transferring the knowledge gained from their exemplar to elsewhere in their own health system, or to other health systems. Lastly, we challenged them to write a paragraph or two on the prospects for further success; in other words, what could be done to build on the identified successful initiative either in their own country or in other health systems elsewhere?

Along the way, we were fortunate to secure the services of a research assistant (Kristiana Ludlow) and copy editor (Wendy James) who shouldered much responsibility for the logistics of coordinating and helping shape the chapters. They supported the editorial process, and provided the editors and chapter writers with much additional expertise, and they have joined us as co-authors in this and the final chapter.

In terms of the specific steps taken to develop the book, we initially made contact with chapter writers from the first book in the series (Braithwaite et al., 2015), and asked those who were available to participate in this second book. We were very gratified that from this cohort, 36 authors contributed to this next offering. Because of the expansion of chapters, we also accumulated an additional 125 authors.

We then invited all authors, old and new, to a workshop at a conference run by the International Society for Quality in Health Care (ISQua), held in Doha, Qatar, in October 2015, to discuss the book. There, we provided guidelines to support authors in compiling their contributions. Upon acceptance of their invitation, each group of authors in each country provided us with an outline of their chosen success story. These were discussed leading up to and during the writing period, between October 2015 and August 2016. We then had a short hiatus, while we editors waited patiently for the chapters to emerge. Most contributors kept to their original idea, but some, upon reflection and research, discussed changes to the nature of the success story they wanted to present.

This captures an interesting point we would like to emphasize. Authors in every health system could write several success stories; some could write dozens. In that respect, the book doesn't capture the only, or even the best, success story from the country of origin, assuming there is such a thing. Rather, each story provides a celebrated or effective instance of improvement in that particular health system, one that can serve as a positive example to others. Each case therefore provides insights into what can be done in other countries, for those interested in change and improvement through emulating others' accomplishments.

The World in Context

Leaving aside Taiwan and Hong Kong (because although they are separately reported health systems, they are often reported as part of the Republic of China for data populations), there are 206 states in the world today. According to the United Nations (UN), these 206 include 193 member states, two observer states (the Holy See [The Vatican] and Palestine), and 11 other states, some of which are disputed territories. Whatever number of nations we agree to settle on (and we are not so interested here in the international disputes about what constitutes nationhood), in this book we enrolled 60 countries, or about a third of all the candidate countries in the world.

This is unusual. Most books in this genre focus on developing countries, and often restrict their analyses to Organization for Economic Cooperation and Development (OECD) countries. However, in our quest to represent as many stories of success as we could, it was essential that we cast our net as widely as possible. And although it can be controversial to think about the world in terms of countries, we predicated the book on success stories from health systems.

In Table I.1, we present demographic and socioeconomic data on participating countries' health systems, such as population, median age in years, the proportion living in urban areas, and relevant data on access to drinking water and sanitation. In Table I.2, we present this data by WHO region and World Bank income group. This provides a profile about the contributing countries and their health systems. Tables I.3 and I.4 present data on life expectancy and mortality. Table I.5 provides data on the density of health workforce, health

TABLE I.1

Demographic and Socioeconomic Data by Country

	Population					Gross National Income per Capita (PPP Int.$) 2013b	Gross Domestic Product per Capita[a] (US$) 2015b	Gross Domestic Product per Capita[a] (PPP Int.$) 2015b	Land Area[a] (sq. km) 2015
Country	Total (000s) 2015	Median Age (Years) 2013b	Living in Urban Areas (%) 2013b	Using Improved Drinking Water Sources (%) 2015b	Using Improved Sanitation Facilities (%) 2015b				
Afghanistan	32527	17	26	55	32	2000	590	1934	652860
Argentina[c]	43417	31	92	99	96		13432	20499	2736690
Australia	23969	37	89	100	100	42540	56328	45514	7682300
Austria	8545	43	66	100	100	43840	43439	47824	82531
Bahrain	1377	30	89	100	99	36140	23396	46946	770
Brazil	207848	30	85	98	83	14750	8539	15359	8358140
Canada	35940	40	82	100	100	42610	43249	44310	9093510
Chile	17948	33	89	99	99	21030	13384	22316	743532
China[d]	1400000	37	53	96	76	11850	7925	14239	9388211
Denmark	5669	41	87	100	100	44460	52002	46635	42430
Ecuador	16144	26	63	87	85	10310	6248	11388	248360
Estonia	1313	41	68	100	97	24230	17295	28095	42390
Fiji	892	27	53	96	91	7610	4916	9159	18270
Finland	5504	42	84	100	98	38480	41921	40601	303890
France	64395	41	79	100	99	37580	36248	39678	547557
Germany	80689	46	75	100	99	44540	41219	47268	348540
Ghana	27410	21	53	89	15	3880	1381	4201	227540
Guinea	12609	19	36	77	20	1160	531	1207	245720

(Continued)

TABLE 1.1 (CONTINUED)

Demographic and Socioeconomic Data by Country

| Country | Population | | | | | Gross National Income per Capita (PPP Int.$) 2013b | Gross Domestic Product per Capita[a] (US$) 2015b | Gross Domestic Product per Capita (PPP Int.$) 2015b | Land Area[a] (sq. km) 2015 |
	Total (000s) 2015	Median Age (Years) 2013b	Living in Urban Areas (%) 2013b	Using Improved Drinking Water Sources (%) 2015b	Using Improved Sanitation Facilities (%) 2015b				
Guyana	767	23	28	98	84	6550	4127	7506	196850
Hong Kong[e]	7288	43	95	100	99	54480	42423	56719	1050
India	1300000	26	32	94	40	5350	1582	6089	2973190
Iran	79109	29	72	96	90	15600	5443	17366	1628550
Ireland	4689	35	63	98	90	35090	51290	54654	68890
Israel	8064	30	92	100	100	32140	35330	35432	21640
Italy	59798	44	69	100	100	34100	29847	35896	294140
Japan	126574	46	93	100	100	37630	32477	37322	364560
Jordan	7595	23	83	97	99	11660	4940	10880	88780
Kuwait	3892	29	98	99	100	88170	28985	71312	17820
Lebanon	5851	30	88	99	81	17390	8051	13938	10230
Liberia	4503	19	49	76	17	790	456	836	96320
Malaysia	30331	27	73	98	96	22460	9766	26891	328550
Malta	419	41	95	100	100	28030	22776	29526	320
Mexico	127017	27	79	96	85	16110	9009	17277	1943950
Namibia	2459	21	45	91	34	9590	4696	10414	823290
Netherlands	16925	42	89	100	98	43210	44433	48459	33670
New Zealand	4529	37	86	100		30750	37808	36982	263310

(*Continued*)

TABLE I.1 (CONTINUED)

Demographic and Socioeconomic Data by Country

Country	Population					Gross National Income per Capita (PPP Int.$) 2013b	Gross Domestic Product per Capita (US$) 2015b	Gross Domestic Product per Capita (PPP Int.$) 2015b	Land Area[a] (sq. km) 2015
	Total (000s) 2015	Median Age (Years) 2013b	Living in Urban Areas (%) 2013b	Using Improved Drinking Water Sources (%) 2015b	Using Improved Sanitation Facilities (%) 2015b				
Nigeria	182202	18	46	69	29	5360	2640	5992	910770
Norway	5211	39	80	100	98	66520	74735	61472	365245
Oman	4491	26	77	93	97	52170	15645	38234	309500
Pakistan	188925	23	38	91	64	4920	1429	5042	770880
Papua New Guinea	7619	21	13	40	19	2430	2268	2865	452860
Portugal	10350	42	62	100	100	25360	19223	29214	91600
Qatar	2235	32	99	100	98	123860	74667	143788	11610
Russia	143457	38	74	97	72	23200	9057	24451	16376870
Rwanda	11610	18	27	76	62	1430	697	1759	24670
Saudi Arabia	31540	28	83	97	100	53780	20482	53430	2149690
Serbia	8851	39	55	99	96	12020	5144	13482	87460
Sierra Leone	6453	19	39	63	13	1750	693	1591	72180
South Africa	54490	26	64	93	66	12240	5692	13165	1213090
Spain	46122	41	79	100	100	31850	25832	34527	500210
Sweden	9779	41	86	100	99	44760	50273	46420	407340
Switzerland	8299	42	74	100	100	56580	80215	60535	39516
Taiwan[f]	23381	40	77				22294	46833	36014

(Continued)

TABLE I.1 (CONTINUED)

Demographic and Socioeconomic Data by Country

Country	Total (000s) 2015	Median Age (Years) 2013b	Population Living in Urban Areas (%) 2013b	Using Improved Drinking Water Sources (%) 2015b	Using Improved Sanitation Facilities (%) 2015b	Gross National Income per Capita (PPP Int.$) 2013b	Gross Domestic Product per Capita (US$) 2015b	Gross Domestic Product per Capita (PPP Int.$) 2015b	Land Area[a] (sq. km) 2015
Turkey	78666	29	72	100	95	18760	9130	19618	769630
The United Arab Emirates	9157	30	85	100	98	58090	40438	70238	83600
The United Kingdom	64716	40	82	100	99	35760	43734	41325	241930
The United States of America	321774	37	81	99	100	53960	55837	55837	9147420
Venezuela	31108	27	89	93	94	17890	12265	18309	882050
Yemen	26832	19	34			3820	1408	3792	527970

Source: All data are from World Health Organization (http://apps.who.int/gho/data/node.home) unless stated otherwise. Data accessed in September and October 2016. Table template adapted from World Health Statistics 2015.

[a] Data for land area and GDPs per capita are from the World Bank (http://data.worldbank.org/) unless stated otherwise.

[b] Or nearest year (maximum 2 years prior or 2 years after).

[c] GDP per capita (PPP Int.$) for Argentina is from International Monetary Fund (http://www.imf.org/external/index.htm).

[d] Land area, GNI per capita, and GDPs per capita for China do not include Hong Kong or Macao.

[e] Total population and median age for Hong Kong are from United Nations (https://esa.un.org/unpd/wpp/); % living in urban area, using improved drinking water sources and sanitation facilities are from World Health Organization Western Pacific Region (http://hiip.wpro.who.int/portal/Dataanalytics.aspx).

[f] Total population and median age for Taiwan are from United Nations (https://esa.un.org/unpd/wpp/); % living in urban area is from World Population Prospects 2015; GDP per capita (US$) is from National Statistics Republic of China (Taiwan) (http://eng.stat.gov.tw/); GDP per capita (PPP Int.$) is from International Monetary Fund (http://www.imf.org/external/index.htm); land area is from Ministry of Interior Republic of China (Taiwan) (http://www.moi.gov.tw/english/).

TABLE I.2

Demographic and Socioeconomic Data by WHO Region and World Bank Income

| | | Population | | | Gross National Income per Capita (PPP int.$) 2013 |
		Total (000s) 2013	Median Age (Years) 2013	Living in Urban Areas (%) 2013	
WHO Region	Africa	927371	19	38	3682
	The Americas	966495	32	80	28962
	Eastern Mediterranean	612580	24	51	10968
	Europe	906996	39	71	27369
	South-East Asia	1855068	27	35	5987
	The Western Pacific	1857588	37	56	14238
World Bank Income Group	Low income	848668	21	30	1780
	Lower middle income	2554925	25	39	5953
	Upper middle income	2449819	34	62	13402
	High income	1272686	40	80	40335
Global	Global	7126098	30	53	14233

Source: All data are from World Health Organization (http://apps.who.int/gho/data/node.home) unless stated otherwise. Data accessed in September 2016.
Table template adapted from World Health Statistics 2015.

infrastructure, and technologies. In Tables I.6 and I.7, we present data on health expenditure. We also present several graphs (Figure I.1, life expectancy at birth; Figure I.2, under-five mortality rate; Figure I.3, life expectancy at birth vs. GDP per capita; and Figure I.4, physician density) to provide further information about the range of countries and the types of challenges they face.

What the data show are how wide ranging and diverse the countries (and regions) in the compendium are. On the last metric in Table I.1, land mass, there is a world map (Figure I.5) (Weast, 1981)* the coverage of the book. In summary, the health systems of the countries included provide care to over 69% of the world's 7.4 billion population (some 5.1 billion people) living in over 85.8 million square kilometers of the 148.8 square kilometers of Earth (58%) (Weast, 1981)* and involving five low-income, 22 middle-income, 35 high-income, and

---

* Weast, Robert C. *CRC Handbook of Chemistry and Physics, 61st Edition*. Chemical Rubber Co., 1981, F-202.

TABLE I.3

Life Expectancy and Mortality by Country

Country	Life Expectancy at Birth (Years) 2015a			Life Expectancy at Age 60 (Years) 2015a			Healthy Life Expectancy at Birth (Years) 2015			Neonatal Mortality Rate (per 1000 Live Births) 2015a	Infant Mortality Rate (Probability of Dying by Age 1 per 1000 Live Births) 2015a	Under-Five Mortality Rate (Probability of Dying by Age 5 per 1000 Live Births) 2015a	Adult Mortality Rate (Probability of Dying between 15 and 60 Years of Age per 1000 Population) 2013a			Maternal Mortality Ratio (per 100,000 Live Births) 2015a
	Both Sexes	Male	Female	Both Sexes	Male	Female	Both Sexes	Male	Female	Both Sexes	Both Sexes	Both Sexes	Both Sexes	Male	Female	Female
Afghanistan	61	59	62	16	15	17	52	51	53	35.5	66.3	91.1	242	252	232	396
Argentina	76	73	80	21	19	24	68	65	70	6.3	11.1	12.5	117	151	83	52
Australia	83	81	85	25	24	27	72	71	73	2.2	3.0	3.8	61	78	45	6
Austria	82	79	84	24	22	26	72	70	74	2.1	2.9	3.5	69	91	46	4
Bahrain	77	76	78	20	19	20	67	67	67	1.1	5.3	6.2	64	70	54	15
Brazil	75	71	79	22	20	23	65	63	68	8.9	14.6	16.4	147	197	97	44
Canada	82	80	84	25	23	26	72	71	73	3.2	4.3	4.9	66	81	52	7
Chile	81	77	83	24	22	26	70	69	72	4.9	7.0	8.1	81	107	55	22
China	76	75	78	20	19	21	69	68	69	5.5	9.2	10.7	90	103	76	27
Denmark	81	79	83	23	22	25	71	70	72	2.5	2.9	3.5	80	100	60	6
Ecuador	76	73	79	23	21	24	67	65	69	10.8	18.4	21.6	121	157	85	64
Estonia	78	73	82	22	19	25	69	66	72	1.5	2.3	2.9	129	195	64	9
Fiji	70	67	73	17	15	19	63	61	65	9.6	19.1	22.4	193	239	143	30
Finland	81	78	84	24	22	26	71	69	73	1.3	1.9	2.3	83	114	51	3
France	82	79	85	26	23	28	73	71	74	2.2	3.5	4.3	80	109	52	8
Germany	81	79	83	24	22	25	71	70	73	2.1	3.1	3.7	71	92	50	6
Ghana	62	61	64	16	15	16	55	55	56	28.3	42.8	61.6	241	261	222	319
Guinea	59	58	60	17	16	17	52	51	52	31.3	61.0	93.7	284	301	267	679
Guyana	66	64	69	16	15	17	59	58	60	22.8	32.0	39.4	320	377	256	229
Hong Kong[b]	84	81	87	26	23	28				0.9	1.8	2.6	49	66	34	2
India	68	67	70	18	17	19	60	59	60	27.7	37.9	47.7	201	239	158	174
Iran	76	75	77	20	19	20	67	66	67	9.5	13.4	15.5	119	153	83	25
Ireland	81	79	83	24	23	26	72	70	73	2.3	3.0	3.6	65	82	49	8

(Continued)

TABLE I.3 (CONTINUED)

Life Expectancy and Mortality by Country

Country	Life Expectancy at Birth (Years) 2015a			Life Expectancy at Age 60 (Years) 2015a			Healthy Life Expectancy at Birth (Years) 2015			Neonatal Mortality Rate (per 1000 Live Births) 2015a	Infant Mortality Rate (Probability of Dying by Age 1 per 1000 Live Births) 2015a	Under-Five Mortality Rate (Probability of Dying by Age 5 per 1000 Live Births) 2015a	Adult Mortality Rate (Probability of Dying between 15 and 60 Years of Age per 1000 Population) 2013a			Maternal Mortality Ratio (per 100,000 Live Births) 2015a
	Both Sexes	Male	Female	Both Sexes	Male	Female	Both Sexes	Male	Female	Both Sexes	Both Sexes	Both Sexes	Both Sexes	Male	Female	Female
Israel	83	81	84	25	24	26	73	72	74	2.1	3.2	4.0	56	72	41	5
Italy	83	80	85	25	23	27	73	72	74	2.1	2.9	3.5	54	69	38	4
Japan	84	80	87	26	23	29	75	72	77	0.9	2.0	2.7	62	81	42	5
Jordan	74	73	76	19	18	20	65	64	66	10.6	15.4	17.9	114	131	96	58
Kuwait	75	74	76	18	18	18	66	65	67	3.2	7.3	8.6	52	59	42	4
Lebanon	75	73	76	19	18	20	66	65	67	4.8	7.1	8.3	59	70	46	15
Liberia	61	60	63	16	15	16	53	52	54	24.1	52.8	69.9	259	279	240	725
Malaysia	75	73	77	19	19	20	66	65	68	3.9	6.0	7.0	127	169	86	40
Malta	82	80	84	24	23	26	72	71	73	4.4	5.1	6.4	58	75	41	9
Mexico	77	74	80	22	21	24	67	66	69	7.0	11.3	13.2	132	174	93	38
Namibia	66	63	68	17	16	18	57	56	59	15.9	32.8	45.4	214	255	177	265
Netherlands	82	80	84	24	23	26	72	71	73	2.4	3.2	3.8	61	69	54	7
New Zealand	82	80	83	25	24	26	72	71	72	3.1	4.7	5.7	66	80	52	11
Nigeria	54	53	56	14	14	14	48	47	48	34.3	69.4	108.8	341	357	325	814
Norway	82	80	84	24	23	26	72	71	73	1.5	2.0	2.6	61	73	47	5
Oman	77	75	79	21	20	22	67	66	68	5.2	9.9	11.6	100	116	73	17
Pakistan	66	65	67	18	18	18	58	57	58	45.5	65.8	81.1	173	189	155	178
Papua New Guinea	63	61	65	15	13	17	56	55	58	24.5	44.5	57.3	282	319	243	215
Portugal	81	78	84	24	22	26	71	69	73	2.0	3.0	3.6	80	111	48	10
Qatar	78	77	80	21	21	22	68	67	68	3.8	6.8	8.0	67	72	50	13
Russia	70	65	76	19	15	21	63	59	68	5.0	8.2	9.6	232	339	126	25
Rwanda	66	61	71	18	16	20	57	52	61	18.7	31.1	41.7	220	246	196	290
Saudi Arabia	75	73	76	19	18	20	64	64	65	7.9	12.5	14.5	80	89	67	12

(Continued)

TABLE I.3 (CONTINUED)

Life Expectancy and Mortality by Country

Country	Life Expectancy at Birth (Years) 2015a			Life Expectancy at Age 60 (Years) 2015a			Healthy Life Expectancy at Birth (Years) 2015			Neonatal Mortality Rate (per 1000 Live Births) 2015a	Infant Mortality Rate (Probability of Dying by Age 1 per 1000 Live Births) 2015a	Under-Five Mortality Rate (Probability of Dying by Age 5 per 1000 Live Births) 2015a	Adult Mortality Rate (Probability of Dying between 15 and 60 Years of Age per 1000 Population) 2013a			Maternal Mortality Ratio (per 100,000 Live Births) 2015a
	Both Sexes	Male	Female	Both Sexes	Male	Female	Both Sexes	Male	Female	Both Sexes	Both Sexes	Both Sexes	Both Sexes	Male	Female	Female
Serbia	76	73	78	20	18	21	68	66	70	4.2	5.9	6.7	128	172	84	17
Sierra Leone	50	49	51	13	13	13	44	44	45	34.9	87.1	120.4	433	444	423	1360
South Africa	63	59	66	17	14	19	54	52	57	11.0	33.6	40.5	378	441	320	138
Spain	83	80	85	25	23	27	72	71	74	2.8	3.5	4.1	63	86	40	5
Sweden	82	81	84	25	24	26	72	71	73	1.6	2.4	3.0	56	69	43	4
Switzerland	83	81	85	26	24	27	73	72	74	2.7	3.4	3.9	53	66	40	5
Taiwan[c]	79	76	82	23	22	25				2.3	4.2	5.3	98	137	58	9
Turkey	76	73	79	21	19	23	66	65	68	7.1	11.6	13.5	109	147	73	16
The United Arab Emirates	77	76	79	20	20	21	68	68	69	3.5	5.9	6.8	76	84	59	6
The United Kingdom	81	79	83	24	23	25	71	70	73	2.4	3.5	4.2	72	88	55	9
The United States of America	79	77	82	24	22	25	69	68	70	3.6	5.6	6.5	102	128	76	14
Venezuela	74	70	78	21	19	23	65	62	68	8.9	12.9	14.9	145	198	88	95
Yemen	66	64	67	16	16	17	58	57	58	22.1	33.8	41.9	232	255	211	385

Source: All data are from World Health Organization (http://apps.who.int/gho/data/node.home) unless stated otherwise. Data accessed in September 2016. Table template adapted from World Health Statistics 2015.

a Or nearest year (maximum 3 years prior). Life expectancies, infant, under-five, and adult mortality rate for Hong Kong and Taiwan are from period 2010-2015.

b Life expectancies, infant, under-five, and adult mortality rate for Hong Kong are from United Nations (https://esa.un.org/unpd/wpp/); neonatal mortality rate is from World Health Organization Western Pacific Region (http://hiip.wpro.who.int/portal/Dataanalytics.aspx); maternal mortality rate is from Health Facts of Hong Kong 2016 Edition.

c Life expectancies, infant, under-five and adult mortality rate for Taiwan are from United Nations (https://esa.un.org/unpd/wpp/); neonatal and maternal mortality rate are from Health Promotion Administration (http://www.hpa.gov.tw/English/index.aspx).

TABLE I.4

Life Expectancy and Mortality by WHO Region and World Bank Income Group

		Life Expectancy at Birth (Years) 2015			Life Expectancy at Age 60 (Years) 2015			Healthy Life Expectancy at Birth (Years) 2015			Neonatal Mortality Rate (per 1000 Live Births) 2015	Infant Mortality Rate (Probability of Dying by Age 1 per 1000 Live Births) 2015	Under-Five Mortality Rate (Probability of Dying by Age 5 per 1000 Live Births) 2015	Adult Mortality Rate (Probability of Dying between 15 and 60 Years of Age per 1000 Population) 2013			Maternal Mortality Ratio (per 100,000 Live Births) 2015
		Both Sexes	Male	Female	Both Sexes	Male	Female	Both Sexes	Male	Female	Both Sexes	Both Sexes	Both Sexes	Both Sexes	Male	Female	Female
WHO Region	Africa	60	58	62	17	16	17	52	51	54	28.0	55.4	81.3	306	332	281	542
	The Americas	77	74	80	23	21	24	67	65	69	7.7	12.5	14.7	122	157	87	52
	Eastern Mediterranean	69	67	70	18	17	19	60	59	61	26.6	40.5	52.0	159	181	135	166
	Europe	77	73	80	22	20	24	68	66	71	6.0	9.8	11.3	128	178	79	16
	South-East Asia	69	67	71	18	17	19	61	60	62	24.3	34.0	42.5	184	219	146	164
	The Western Pacific	77	75	79	21	19	22	69	67	70	6.7	11.3	13.5	95	114	76	41
World Bank Income Group	Low income										26.9	53.1	76.1	241	264	219	
	Lower middle income										25.8	40.0	52.8	199	236	160	
	Upper middle income										8.9	15.2	19.1	115	139	89	
	High income										3.7	5.8	6.8	101	135	66	
Global	Global	71	69	74	20	19	22	63	62	65	19.2	32.0	43.0	152	182	121	216

Source: All data are from World Health Organization (http://apps.who.int/gho/data/node.home) unless stated otherwise. Data accessed in September 2016.

Table template adapted from World Health Statistics 2015.

TABLE I.5

Health Systems Data by Country

Country	Density of Health Workforce (per 10,000 Population)					Density of Health Infrastructure and Technologies				
	Physicians 2007–2015	Nursing and Midwifery Personnel 2007–2015	Dentistry Personnel 2007–2015	Pharmaceutical Personnel 2007–2015	Psychiatrists 2011–2014	Hospitals (per 100 000 Population) 2013a	Psychiatric Beds (per 100 000 Population) 2014	Computed Tomography Units (per Million Population) 2013a	Radiotherapy Units (per Million Population) 2013a	Mammography Units (per Million Females Aged 50–69 Years) 2014a
Afghanistan	2.7	5.0	<0.05	0.5	<0.05	0.4	0.6	0.2	0.0	0.0
Argentina	38.6				0.9		343.3		2.8	
Australia	32.7	106.5	5.4	10.2	2.0		101.3		4.0	
Austria			2.4	1.5	0.5		16.8	28.5	5.4	
Bahrain	9.2	23.7	12.2	7.2	0.3		13.0		1.7	
Brazil	18.9	76.0	12.6	10.3						
Canada	20.7	92.9			1.3	2.3		13.8	8.1	32.2
Chile	10.2	1.4	<0.05	<0.05	0.5	1.0	21.5	12.6	0.9	
China	14.9	16.6		2.7	0.2		16.8		1.1	
Denmark	34.9	167.9	7.9		1.0	1.0	104.7	23.8	9.6	138.4
Ecuador	17.2	21.6	2.8	0.6	0.1	0.3	9.3	1.6	0.1	
Estonia	32.4	63.8	8.9	6.3	1.4	1.9	54.8	15.5	2.3	
Fiji	4.3	22.4	2.0	0.9	<0.05	0.0	4.6	3.4	0.0	28.8
Finland	29.1	108.6	7.3	11.1	1.8	1.4	210.6	20.1	7.4	223.2
France	31.9	3.3	6.6	10.9	1.4		89.6		7.5	
Germany	38.9		8.1	6.2	1.5		86.1		6.4	
Ghana	1.0	9.3	0.1	0.7	<0.05	1.4	6.0	0.2	0.1	
Guinea					<0.05	0.4	1.4	0.0	0.0	0.0
Guyana	2.1	5.3	0.6	1.2	<0.05	3.4	27.4	3.8	1.3	70.0
Hong Kong[b]	18.8	75.2	3.8	3.4		0.7				
India	7.0	17.1	1.0	5.0	<0.05		2.1		0.4	
Iran				5.4	0.2		16.4		0.9	
Ireland	26.7			11.7	0.6			4.5	3.9	23.2
Israel	33.4	49.6	7.0		1.2	0.6	87.9	7.5	3.4	112.3
Italy	37.6			7.8	1.1	2.1	44.5		6.4	

(Continued)

TABLE I.5 (CONTINUED)

Health Systems Data by Country

Country	Density of Health Workforce (per 10,000 Population)					Density of Health Infrastructure and Technologies				
	Physicians 2007–2015	Nursing and Midwifery Personnel 2007–2015	Dentistry Personnel 2007–2015	Pharmaceutical Personnel 2007–2015	Psychiatrists 2011–2014	Hospitals (per 100 000 Population) 2013a	Psychiatric Beds (per 100 000 Population) 2014	Computed Tomography Units (per Million Population) 2013a	Radiotherapy Units (per Million Population) 2013a	Mammography Units (per Million Females Aged 50–69 Years) 2014a
Japan	23.0	114.9	7.9	21.5	1.0	1.9	284.7	101.2	7.2	227.3
Jordan	25.6	40.5	9.0	21.4	0.1		7.5	5.5	0.8	129.1
Kuwait	17.9	45.5	3.5	3.0	0.3		17.2		1.2	
Lebanon	32.0	27.2	14.7	15.7	0.1	3.1	0.8	25.1	1.9	370.2
Liberia	0.1	2.7	<0.05	0.8	<0.05	0.4	1.8		0.0	
Malaysia	12.0	32.8	3.6	4.3	0.1	0.5	14.0	6.4	1.4	86.7
Malta	34.9	74.9	4.7	11.2	0.3	0.9		9.3	4.7	99.7
Mexico	21.0	25.3	1.2		0.1	3.5	3.4	3.7	0.5	74.5
Namibia	3.7	27.8	0.4	1.8	<0.05	1.9	12.0	4.8	0.4	42.3
Netherlands		1.6		2.1	2.0	0.8	89.2	12.2	7.2	
New Zealand	27.4	108.7	4.6	10.1	1.0		77.0	15.8	6.2	227.9
Nigeria	4.1	16.1	0.2	1.1	<0.05		1.5		0.1	
Norway	42.8	172.7	8.8	6.8	3.0		84.5		8.1	
Oman	24.3	53.8	2.8	18.8	0.2	1.3	5.9	6.9	0.6	149.8
Pakistan	8.3	5.7	0.6		<0.05	0.5	5.6	0.3	0.1	1.6
Papua New Guinea	0.6	5.7	0.2	0.5	<0.05	1.6	1.3	0.4	0.1	8.5
Portugal	41.0	61.1	7.6	10.2	0.4		21.7	27.4	4.1	272.0
Qatar	77.4	118.7			0.3		3.5	8.3	0.9	225.1
Russia					1.1		102.8		2.3	
Rwanda	0.6	6.9	0.1	0.1	<0.05		2.9			
Saudi Arabia	24.9	48.7		5.4	0.2	1.0	19.8	3.8	0.1	40.6
Serbia	21.1		2.3	2.1	0.7	1.1	58.9	13.7	1.5	84.6
Sierra Leone	0.2	1.7	<0.05	0.2	<0.05		6.4	0.3	0.0	

(Continued)

TABLE I.5 (CONTINUED)

Health Systems Data by Country

Country	Density of Health Workforce (per 10,000 Population)					Density of Health Infrastructure and Technologies				
	Physicians 2007–2015	Nursing and Midwifery Personnel 2007–2015	Dentistry Personnel 2007–2015	Pharmaceutical Personnel 2007–2015	Psychiatrists 2011–2014	Hospitals (per 100 000 Population) 2013a	Psychiatric Beds (per 100 000 Population) 2014	Computed Tomography Units (per Million Population) 2013a	Radiotherapy Units (per Million Population) 2013a	Mammography Units (per Million Females Aged 50–69 Years) 2014a
South Africa	7.8	51.1	2.0	4.1	<0.05	0.7	22.7	1.0	0.6	7.8
Spain	49.5	56.7	8.2	14.2	0.8	1.6	38.7	13.9	4.2	
Sweden	39.3	7.4	8.1	7.7	1.8		72.5		6.9	
Switzerland	40.5	3.2	5.4	5.6	4.1		31.8		9.8	
Taiwan[c]	18.7	53.9	5.8	6.8		2.1				
Turkey	17.1	24.0	2.9	3.5	0.2	1.5	9.3	14.5	2.0	230.4
The United Arab Emirates	25.3	31.6	4.3	5.9	<0.05		1.2		0.6	
The United Kingdom	28.1	88.0	5.4	8.1	1.5		136.3		5.0	
The United States of America	24.5			3.8	1.2		50.2		12.4	
Venezuela									2.5	
Yemen	2.0	6.8	0.4	0.9	<0.05	3.0		3.6	0.1	17.6

Source: All data are from World Health Organization (http://apps.who.int/gho/data/node.home) unless stated otherwise. Data accessed in September 2016.

Table template adapted from World Health Statistics 2015.

[a] Or nearest year (maximum 4 years prior or 2 years after).

[b] Health workforce and hospital density for Hong Kong are derived from Health Facts of Hong Kong 2016 Edition. Dentistry personnel includes dentists and dental hygienists; pharmaceutical personnel include pharmacists only.

[c] Health workforce, hospital, and psychiatric beds density for Taiwan are derived from Ministry of Health and Welfare, Taiwan (http://www.mohw.gov.tw/en/Ministry/Index.aspx). Dentistry personnel includes dentists, dental technicians, and technologists; pharmaceutical personnel include pharmacists and pharmacist assistants.

TABLE I.6

Health Expenditure by Country

Country	Total Expenditure on Health as % of Gross Domestic Product 2014a	Health Expenditure Ratios							Per Capita Health Expenditures			
		General Government Expenditure on Health as % of Total Government Expenditure 2014a	Private Expenditure on Health as % of Total Expenditure on Health 2014a	General Government Expenditure on Health as % of Total Expenditure on Health 2014a	External Resources for Health as % of Total Expenditure on Health 2014a	Social Security Expenditure on Health as % of General Government Expenditure on Health 2014a	Out-of-Pocket Expenditure as % of Private Expenditure on Health 2014	Private Prepaid Plans as % of Private Expenditure on Health 2014a	Per Capita Total Expenditure on Health at Average Exchange Rate (US$) 2014	Per Capita Total Expenditure on Health (PPP int. $) 2014	Per Capita Government Expenditure on Health at Average Exchange Rate (US$) 2014	Per Capita Government Expenditure on Health (PPP int. $) 2014
Afghanistan	8.2	12.0	64.2	35.8	23.0	0.0	99.6	0.0	56.57	166.52	20.28	59.69
Argentina	4.8	6.9	44.6	55.4	0.8	82.8	68.9	21.7	605.19	1137.24	335.44	630.34
Australia	9.4	17.3	33.0	67.0		0.0	57.1	25.4	6031.11	4357.26	4043.18	2921.05
Austria	11.2	16.3	22.1	77.9	0.0	56.0	73.0	20.8	5580.49	5038.88	4345.19	3923.47
Bahrain	5.0	10.5	36.7	63.3	0.0	1.3	63.5	25.9	1242.84	2272.90	786.14	1437.67
Brazil	8.3	6.8	54.0	46.0	0.1	0.0	47.2	49.7	947.43	1318.17	436.19	606.87
Canada	10.4	18.8	29.1	70.9		2.0	46.8	43.4	5291.75	4640.95	3753.46	3291.84
Chile	7.8	15.9	50.5	49.5	0.0	9.0	62.4	37.6	1137.36	1749.36	562.60	865.33
China	5.5	10.4	44.2	55.8	0.0	67.6	72.3	10.2	419.73	730.52	234.16	407.53
Denmark	10.8	16.8	15.2	84.8	0.0	0.0	87.7	11.9	6463.24	4782.06	5478.52	4053.47
Ecuador	9.2	10.2	50.8	49.2	0.3	50.2	95.3	2.8	579.19	1039.76	285.02	511.66
Estonia	6.4	13.5	21.2	78.8	1.4	78.0	97.8	1.1	1248.28	1668.31	983.94	1315.03
Fiji	4.5	9.2	34.2	65.8	9.9	0.0	67.3	21.2	204.01	364.05	134.26	239.58
Finland	9.7	12.4	24.7	75.3	0.0	17.6	73.8	8.1	4612.29	3701.14	3473.46	2787.28
France	11.5	15.7	21.8	78.2		94.7	29.1	61.0	4958.99	4508.13	3878.19	3525.60
Germany	11.3	19.6	23.0	77.0		89.2	57.3	38.8	5410.63	5182.11	4165.49	3989.56
Ghana	3.6	6.8	40.2	59.8	15.4	32.5	66.8	2.0	57.89	145.37	34.65	87.00
Guinea	5.6	9.0	51.5	48.5	12.6	3.4	88.0	1.1	30.46	68.46	14.77	33.18
Guyana	5.2	9.4	40.6	59.4	7.3	4.1	92.3	0.2	221.78	378.79	131.85	225.18

(Continued)

TABLE 1.6 (CONTINUED)

Health Expenditure by Country

Country	Total Expenditure on Health as % of Gross Domestic Product 2014a	General Government Expenditure on Health as % of Total Government Expenditure 2014a	Private Expenditure on Health as % of Total Expenditure on Health 2014a	General Government Expenditure on Health as % of Total Expenditure on Health 2014a	External Resources for Health as % of Total Expenditure on Health 2014a	Social Security Expenditure on Health as % of General Government Expenditure on Health 2014a	Out-of-Pocket Expenditure as % of Private Expenditure on Health 2014	Private Prepaid Plans as % of Private Expenditure on Health 2014a	Per Capita Total Expenditure on Health at Average Exchange Rate (US$) 2014	Per Capita Total Expenditure on Health (PPP int. $) 2014	Per Capita Government Expenditure on Health at Average Exchange Rate (US$) 2014	Per Capita Government Expenditure on Health (PPP int. $) 2014
Hong Kong^b	5.4	13.3	52.4	47.6								
India	4.7	5.0	70.0	30.0	1.0	5.7	89.2	2.5	74.99	267.41	22.53	80.32
Iran	6.9	17.5	58.8	41.2	0.0	31.3	81.3	6.7	350.74	1081.67	144.51	445.66
Ireland	7.8	13.4	33.9	66.1		0.2	52.0	41.2	4239.15	3801.06	2800.33	2510.94
Israel	7.8	11.6	39.1	60.9		74.9	68.9	26.4	2910.29	2599.13	1771.04	1581.69
Italy	9.2	13.7	24.4	75.6		0.4	86.9	3.7	3257.75	3238.89	2463.29	2449.03
Japan	10.2	20.3	16.4	83.6		87.3	84.8	14.8	3702.95	3726.68	3095.25	3115.08
Jordan	7.5	13.7	30.3	69.7	6.0	8.7	68.8	22.8	358.91	797.59	250.08	555.75
Kuwait	3.0	5.8	14.1	85.9	0.0	0.0	90.5	9.5	1385.78	2319.60	1190.85	1993.32
Lebanon	6.4	10.7	52.4	47.6	1.0	52.5	69.5	29.6	568.71	987.39	270.75	470.08
Liberia	10.0	11.9	68.5	31.5	49.1	0.0	44.8	5.4	46.27	98.29	14.57	30.94
Malaysia	4.2	6.4	44.8	55.2	0.0	1.1	78.8	15.9	455.83	1040.23	251.50	573.95
Malta	9.7	15.6	30.8	69.2	0.0	2.7	93.6	5.7	2470.60	3071.63	1708.76	2124.46
Mexico	6.3	11.6	48.2	51.8	0.4	56.5	91.2	8.8	677.19	1121.99	350.57	580.83
Namibia	8.9	13.9	40.0	60.0	8.0	2.5	17.9	61.2	499.02	869.30	299.41	521.57
Netherlands	10.9	20.9	13.0	87.0	0.0	93.0	40.2	45.8	5693.86	5201.70	4953.91	4525.71

(Continued)

TABLE I.6 (CONTINUED)

Health Expenditure by Country

Country	Total Expenditure on Health as % of Gross Domestic Product 2014a	General Government Expenditure on Health as % of Total Government Expenditure 2014a	Private Expenditure on Health as % of Total Expenditure on Health 2014a	General Government Expenditure on Health as % of Total Expenditure on Health 2014a	External Resources for Health as % of Total Expenditure on Health 2014a	Social Security Expenditure on Health as % of General Government Expenditure on Health 2014a	Out-of-Pocket Expenditure as % of Private Expenditure on Health 2014	Private Prepaid Plans as % of Private Expenditure on Health 2014a	Per Capita Total Expenditure on Health at Average Exchange Rate (US$) 2014	Per Capita Total Expenditure on Health (PPP int. $) 2014	Per Capita Government Expenditure on Health at Average Exchange Rate (US$) 2014	Per Capita Government Expenditure on Health (PPP int. $) 2014
New Zealand	11.0	23.4	17.7	82.3		8.6	62.6	24.5	4896.35	4018.31	4032.04	3308.99
Nigeria	3.7	8.2	74.9	25.1	6.7	0.0	95.7	3.1	117.52	216.87	29.55	54.53
Norway	9.7	18.2	14.5	85.5	0.0	12.0	93.8	21.5	9522.22	6346.62	8140.77	5425.87
Oman	3.6	6.8	10.2	89.8	0.0	0.0	56.5		675.04	1441.97	605.96	1294.40
Pakistan	2.6	4.7	64.8	35.2	8.0	2.9	86.8	0.9	36.15	128.99	12.71	45.34
Papua New Guinea	4.3	9.5	18.7	81.3	21.1	0.0	55.9	5.5	92.36	109.49	75.07	88.99
Portugal	9.5	11.9	35.2	64.8		1.7	76.3	14.4	2096.82	2689.94	1359.07	1743.51
Qatar	2.2	5.8	14.3	85.7	0.0	0.0	48.1	51.0	2106.36	3071.19	1806.19	2633.52
Russia	7.1	9.5	47.8	52.2		53.1	95.9	3.5	892.85	1835.71	466.09	958.29
Rwanda	7.5	9.9	61.9	38.1	46.2	25.5	45.4	7.8	52.48	125.07	20.00	47.65
Saudi Arabia	4.7	8.2	25.5	74.5	0.0		56.2	22.3	1147.45	2465.98	855.13	1837.76
Serbia	10.4	13.9	38.1	61.9	0.2	93.6	96.0	0.8	632.92	1312.22	391.67	812.04
Sierra Leone	11.1	10.8	83.0	17.0	17.1	0.0	73.4	0.2	85.91	223.74	14.59	38.01
South Africa	8.8	14.2	51.8	48.2	1.8	2.4	12.5	82.8	570.21	1148.37	275.04	553.92
Spain	9.0	14.5	29.1	70.9		6.9	82.4	15.1	2658.27	2965.82	1884.07	2102.04
Sweden	11.9	19.0	16.0	84.0	0.0	0.0	88.1	3.4	6807.72	5218.86	5720.55	4385.43
Switzerland	11.7	22.7	34.0	66.0	0.0	71.5	78.8	21.8	9673.52	6468.50	6384.53	4269.21

(Continued)

TABLE I.6 (CONTINUED)

Health Expenditure by Country

Country	Health Expenditure Ratios								Per Capita Health Expenditures			
	Total Expenditure on Health as % of Gross Domestic Product 2014a	General Government Expenditure on Health as % of Total Government Expenditure 2014a	Private Expenditure on Health as % of Total Expenditure on Health 2014a	General Government Expenditure on Health as % of Total Expenditure on Health 2014a	External Resources for Health as % of Total Expenditure on Health 2014a	Social Security Expenditure on Health as % of General Government Expenditure on Health 2014a	Out-of-Pocket Expenditure as % of Private Expenditure on Health 2014	Private Prepaid Plans as % of Private Expenditure on Health 2014a	Per Capita Total Expenditure on Health at Average Exchange Rate (US$) 2014	Per Capita Total Expenditure on Health (PPP int. $) 2014	Per Capita Government Expenditure on Health at Average Exchange Rate (US$) 2014	Per Capita Government Expenditure on Health (PPP int. $) 2014
Taiwan[c]	6.2		40.6	59.4		88.5	85.7		1324	2697	827	1686
Turkey	5.4	10.5	22.6	77.4	0.0	70.0	78.7		567.63	1036.47	439.62	802.72
The United Arab Emirates	3.6	8.7	27.7	72.3	0.0	0.0	64.4	26.0	1610.80	2405.37	1165.29	1740.10
The United Kingdom	9.1	16.5	16.9	83.1			57.7	20.4	3934.82	3376.87	3271.52	2807.62
The United States of America	17.1	21.3	51.7	48.3		88.3	21.4	64.2	9402.54	9402.54	4541.17	4541.17
Venezuela	5.3	5.8	70.7	29.3	0.0	32.0	91.1	3.4	873.38	922.99	256.33	270.88
Yemen	5.6	3.9	77.4	22.6	6.4	0.0	98.7	1.3	79.94	202.16	18.04	45.61

Source: All data are from World Health Organization (http://apps.who.int/gho/data/node.home) unless stated otherwise. Data accessed in September 2016.

Table template adapted from World Health Statistics 2015. Health expenditure ratios for Hong Kong are from 2012/2013.

[a] Or nearest year (maximum 4 years prior).

[b] Health expenditure ratios for Hong Kong are from Health Facts of Hong Kong 2016 Edition.

[c] Data for Taiwan are from Ministry of Health and Welfare, Taiwan (http://www.mohw.gov.tw/en/Ministry/Index.aspx).

TABLE I.7

Health Expenditure by WHO Region and World Bank Income Group

		Health Expenditure Ratios								Per Capita Health Expenditures			
		Total Expenditure on Health as % of Gross Domestic Product 2014	General Government Expenditure on Health as % of Total Government Expenditure 2014	Private Expenditure on Health as % of Total Expenditure on Health 2014	General Government Expenditure on Health as % of Total Expenditure on Health 2014	External Resources for Health as % of Total Expenditure on Health 2014	Social Security Expenditure on Health as % of General Government Expenditure on Health 2014	Out-of-Pocket Expenditure as % of Private Expenditure on Health 2014	Private Prepaid Plans as % of Private Expenditure on Health 2014	Per Capita Total Expenditure on Health at Average Exchange Rate (US$) 2014	Per Capita Total Expenditure on Health (PPP int. $) 2014	Per Capita Government Expenditure on Health at Average Exchange Rate (US$) 2014	Per Capita Government Expenditure on Health (PPP int. $) 2014
WHO Region	Africa	5.5	10.0	52.2	47.8	9.6	10.5	60.0	28.5	108.0	228.0	51.6	111.4
	The Americas	14.2	18.1	50.2	49.8	0.0	74.8	27.3	59.7	3730.2	3958.8	1858.3	1983.3
	Eastern Mediterranean	4.8	7.9	43.2	56.8	1.2	8.8	81.3	9.6	242.6	597.5	137.9	317.5
	Europe	9.5	15.5	24.6	75.4	0.0	50.7	69.4	22.4	2425.9	2580.0	1828.1	1884.2
	South-East Asia	4.3	7.1	59.3	40.7	1.5	7.8	85.9	3.5	83.5	275.9	34.0	107.0
	The Western Pacific	7.1	14.3	33.6	66.4	0.1	67.3	74.3	12.7	745.9	1007.4	495.3	635.1
World Bank Income Group	Low income	5.9	10.5	58.8	41.2	28.3	5.2	65.5	3.4	36.5	92.1	15.0	37.9
	Lower middle income	4.5	6.7	63.8	36.2	3.3	15.0	87.5	3.6	89.3	267.6	32.3	95.4
	Upper middle income	6.1	10.2	43.8	56.2	0.2	48.9	68.4	20.6	486.9	869.1	273.5	494.6
	High income	12.0	17.6	38.1	61.9	0.0	65.1	37.6	50.2	4538.7	4608.3	2810.9	2825.3
Global		9.9	15.5	39.9	60.1	0.2	61.7	45.5	42.5	1058.3	1273.1	636.3	738.9

Source: All data are from World Health Organization (http://apps.who.int/gho/data/node.home) unless stated otherwise. Data accessed in September 2016.

Table template adapted from World Health Statistics 2015.

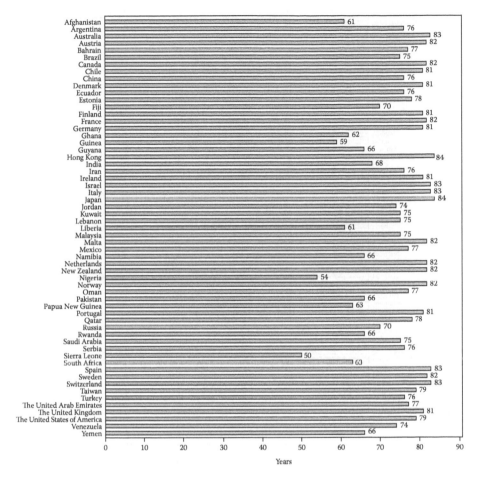

FIGURE I.1

Life expectancy at birth, 2015 (or nearest year). (From World Health Organization [http://apps.who. int/gho/data/node.home] unless stated otherwise; data for Hong Kong is derived from Health Facts of Hong Kong 2016 Edition; data for Taiwan is derived from Ministry of Health and Welfare, Taiwan [http://www.mohw.gov.tw/en/Ministry/Index.aspx]; data accessed in September 2016.)

one currently unclassified health system. We would have liked more representation from Africa, and South-East Asia, but, overall, representation is wide, as you will see, and stories are most instructive.

Structure of the Book

There are many ways we could have presented the countries in the chapters that follow: by income status, by type of health system (e.g., mainly privately

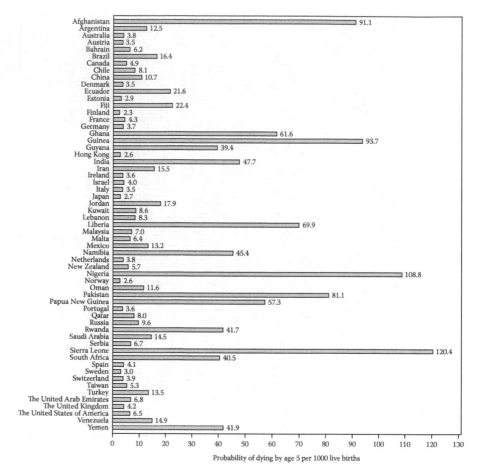

FIGURE I.2

Under-five mortality rate 2015 (or nearest year). Data from Hong Kong and Taiwan are from 2010 to 2015. (From World Health Organization [http://apps.who.int/gho/data/node.home] unless stated otherwise; data for Hong Kong and Taiwan are from United Nations [http://esa.un.org/unpd/wpp/]; data accessed in September 2016.)

operated or publicly funded), or by categorizing the success stories into themes. As editors, we thought long and hard about this, especially as the chapters were rolling in and we were engaging with the authors and their work, providing editorial feedback and support.

We eventually decided to structure the book in alignment with WHO regions (http://www.who.int/about/regions/en/). This was also the way we assigned responsibilities among the editors. Table I.8 shows the regions, the countries involved, and the editors responsible for each region.

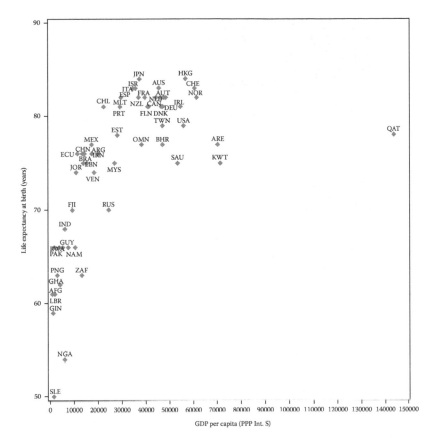

FIGURE I.3

Life expectancy at birth 2015 (or nearest year, maximum 2 years prior) versus GDP per capita 2015 (or nearest year, maximum 2 years prior). Life expectancy for Hong Kong and Taiwan are from 2010 to 2015. (From World Health Organization for life expectancy [http://apps.who.int/gho/data/node.home] and from World Bank for GDP per capita [http://data.worldbank.org/] unless stated otherwise; life expectancy data for Hong Kong and Taiwan are from United Nations [http://esa.un.org/unpd/wpp/]; GDP per capita data for China do not include Hong Kong or Macao; GPD per capita data for Taiwan is from International Monetary Fund [http://www.imf.org/external/index/htm]; data accessed in September and October 2016.)

Our Readership

If you are a reader of this book, it's likely that you will be someone who is not merely interested in learning, in a detached way, about your own health system. It's likely that you will be a healthcare policymaker, or a bureaucrat, manager, clinician, patient, patient advocate or delegate, researcher, or someone from the media who specializes in health and medicine. You might be interested in your own country and its success story, or you might

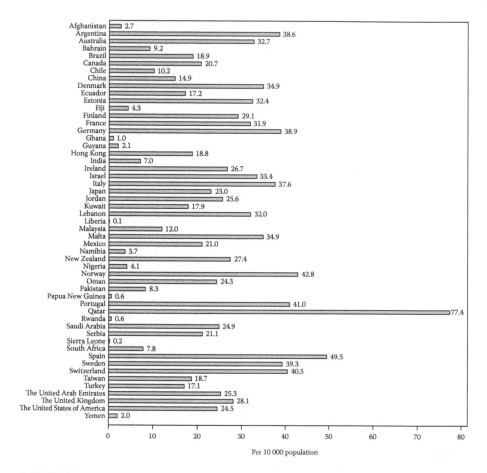

FIGURE I.4
Physician density, 2007–2015. (From World Health Organization [http://apps.who.int/gho/data/node.home] unless stated otherwise; data for Hong Kong is derived from Health Facts of Hong Kong 2016 edition; data for Taiwan is derived from Ministry of Health and Welfare, Taiwan [http://www.mohw.gov.tw/en/Ministry/Index.aspx]; data accessed in September 2016.)

be interested more broadly in what the blueprint for success is among different types of change or improvement efforts. You might want to find out how you can emulate specific programs that have proved valuable in other countries, or to discover systems that might be successfully translated into entirely new contexts. You could be interested in international health reform. You might be looking for new ways of tackling a particular public health or health systems problem, searching for fresh perspectives on possible solutions, or learning from those who have traveled further down the same road.

Or you might simply be interested in immersing yourself in the fascinating world of healthcare, and in learning about how stakeholders have gone

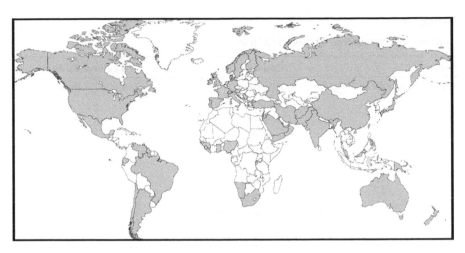

FIGURE I.5
Coverage of the health systems in the book. (Adapted from https://mapchart.net/.)

about trying to improve their part of that world. Whatever your position, there is something here, we believe, for everyone.

In fact, we suggest there's no other book like it. Most books dealing with health reform and improvement, whether concerned with macro, meso, or micro levels of complex health systems, tend to look at how the system is governed, or how care is delivered, or target specific conditions, or present patients' perspectives on how (or how not) to engage with the system. This book presents all these elements, but from the vantage point of a unique mix of authors.

In short, we think there is a very wide audience for what follows. Whatever your interest, we invite you to sample the work of our writers and their success stories. It's a gold mine of narratives about what constitutes success from many different stances, across many different countries, representing many different themes—and providing a panoramic vision of global healthcare reform.

It remains for us to say one final thing. There's much to read, and it will be a challenging task to absorb all that we and our authors have to say. So, you might want to sample the offerings by theme (in which case, be guided by Table D.1 in the Discussion and Conclusion, which collates the topics covered in the book), or by income group (see Table I.1), or by region (see Table I.8). But for the real aficionado of health systems reform, you have everything to gain and much to learn by partaking of the whole. However you approach it, we think the effort will be repaid many times over. It was a great pleasure to envision, edit, and assemble this book—and we hope this pleasure will be shared by you, our readers.

TABLE I.8

Regions, Countries, and Regional Editors

Region	Countries	Regional Editor
Part I: The Americas	Argentina	Professor Paul Shekelle
	Brazil	
	Canada	
	Chile	
	Colombia	
	Ecuador	
	Guyana	
	Mexico	
	The United States of America	
	Venezuela	
Part II: Africa	Ghana	Professor Stuart Whittaker
	Namibia	
	Nigeria	
	South Africa	
	Rwanda	
	West Africa (Guinea, Liberia, Sierra Leone)	
Part III: Europe	Austria	Professor Russell Mannion
	Denmark	
	England	
	Estonia	
	Finland	
	France	
	Germany	
	Israel	
	Italy	
	Malta	
	Netherlands	
	Northern Ireland	
	Norway	
	Portugal	
	Russia	
	Scotland	
	Serbia	
	Spain	
	Sweden	
	Switzerland	
	Turkey	
	Wales	

(Continued)

TABLE I.8 (CONTINUED)

Regions, Countries, and Regional Editors

Region	Countries	Regional Editor
Part IV: Eastern Mediterranean	Afghanistan	Professor Samir Al-Adawi
	Iran	
	Jordan	
	Lebanon	
	Oman	
	Pakistan	
	Qatar	
	The Gulf States (Bahrain, Kuwait, Oman, Qatar, Saudi Arabia, and the United Arab Emirates)	
	The United Arab Emirates	
	Yemen	
Part V: South-East Asia and the Western Pacific	Australia	Professor Yukihiro Matsuyama and Professor Jeffrey Braithwaite
	China	
	Fiji	
	Hong Kong	
	India	
	Japan	
	Malaysia	
	New Zealand	
	Papua New Guinea	
	Taiwan	

Part I

The Americas

Paul Shekelle

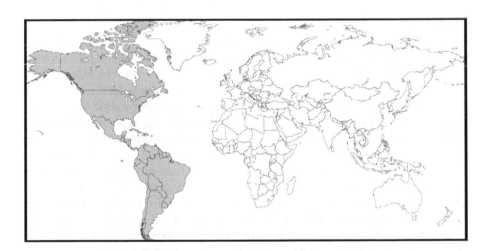

In this first section of the book, we traverse the Americas, a vast landmass ranging from the very northern reaches of Canada, the United States of America, and Greenland, abutting the Arctic, just 700 kilometers from the North Pole, to three desolate islands off the tip of Argentina known as Southern Thule, often considered part of Antarctica. The Americas cover 8% of Earth's total surface area and 28.4% of its land area.

These nine case studies from the Americas are remarkable most for their diversity. The countries we have enrolled reflect this diversity, in size, population, geography, and climate. They span the artic climate in Canada, through the equatorial climate of Guyana and Ecuador, to the Southern Hemisphere climate of Argentina and Chile. They are diverse, too, in how their healthcare systems are organized and financed.

The healthcare success stories being addressed vary greatly: stroke care (Canada), surgical safety (the United States of America), primary care (Venezuela), geriatrics (Guyana), hospital quality and safety (Brazil, Chile, and Ecuador), healthcare access (Mexico), and a number of conditions (Argentina). The funding sources for the initiatives also vary: government-funded initiatives are described in the chapters from Venezuela, Mexico, and Argentina; non-governmental organizations, foundations, and charitable society-funded initiatives are described in the chapters from Guyana, Brazil, Canada, and Argentina; and a professional society-funded initiative is described in the chapter from the United States of America.

The interventions or programs themselves are also extremely diverse. Enrique Ruelas and Octavio Gómez-Dantés describe a Mexican government-funded program to increase access to care; Marcos Iturriaga and Leonel Valdivia in Chile, and Amy Showen and Melinda Maggard-Gibbons in the United States of America, describe performance management systems and their effect on hospital quality and safety; Claudia Travassos, Victor Grabois, and José Noronha describe an Internet-based intervention in Brazil to disseminate safety interventions; Jonathan Mitchell, Qendresa Hasanaj, Hélène Sabourin, Danielle Dorschner, Stephanie Carpenter, Toby Yan, Wendy Nicklin, G. Ross Baker, John Van Aerde, and Sarah Boucaud describe the effect a non-governmental accrediting body had on stroke care in Canada; Jonás Gonseth and Maria Cecilia Acuña describe one hospital's transformation from worst to first in response to a new governmental governing process in Ecuador; William Adu-Krow, Vishwa Mahadeo, Vasha Bachan, and Melissa Ramdeem describe a successful attempt to bring multiple services to geriatric patients in rural Guyana; Pedro Delgado and Luis Azpurua describe an attempt to increase access to primary care for underserved populations; while Hugo Arce, Ezequiel García-Elorrio, and Viviana Rodríguez catalog a number of initiatives in Argentina. A theme in many of the chapters is the vital need for strong leadership and adequate resources in order to be successful. How success is accomplished in different settings is a key learning point.

1

Argentina

Successful Initiatives in Quality and Patient Safety in Argentina

Hugo Arce, Ezequiel García-Elorrio, and Viviana Rodríguez

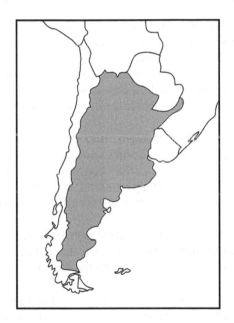

CONTENTS

Background

The Argentine Republic, as defined by its constitution, has a federal structure, whereby the provinces are independent from the federal government regarding health and education. Public health services (hospitals, outpatient centers) and prevention programs are administered by provincial authorities, while the National Health Ministry establishes priorities and general policies, funds strategic programs, and exercises the administration of the health system. Argentina's healthcare system is a mixed system consisting of public, private, and social security subsectors.

A number of healthcare government initiatives and a great many non-government projects are currently being developed and implemented. Among these is the Categorizing Authorization Program (CAP), which aims to unify standards for the licensing of public and private services across the country while developing the operational and technological capacity of healthcare services. The CAP is also tasked with the development of government-sponsored supplementary coverage for at-risk populations, the development of practice guidelines for prevalent diseases, and the assessment of healthcare technologies in order to rationalize investments and determine quality requirements.

There are also a number of non-governmental organizations currently in development: three accreditation bodies and two International Organization for Standardization (ISO) certification boards; two institutes specializing in teaching and research; four specialized scientific societies; two quality awards; and at least seven university training programs in quality and safety.

Despite the wide availability of public services, which represent 55% of installed capacity in inpatient beds, the private sector, as provider of social security and health insurance plans, is the most dynamic sector of the health system.

While quality of care and patient safety has not been the central focus of Argentinian health policy, successive administrations, regardless of political affiliation, have managed to implement a number of government and non-government health system initiatives, with varying degrees of success.

Description of Selected Government Activities that Proved to be Successful in the Field of Quality of Care

One of the Argentinian system's most enduring challenges has been convincing the individual provinces' legislative regimes to authorize the operation of new private assistance services (Arce, 1998). Inconsistencies in the response capacity and technological capability of Argentinian institutions have exacerbated this problem. To resolve this problem, the CAP was developed through the Federal Health Plan (2003–2007) and approved by the Federal Health Council (CoFeSa*) (Arce, 1999). The CAP was developed to unify the different licensing rules, for both public and private services, and to set the response capacity for each institution. This program is currently administered by provincial ministries.

In 1983, the National Health Ministry established the National Program of Epidemiology and Hospital Infection Control to address the problem of healthcare-associated infections (HAIs) in Argentina. Following an initiative of the Argentine Society of Infectious Diseases (SADI) in the late 1990s, the government mandated the registration and classification of HAIs in public and private hospitals through the National Program of Hospital Infections Surveillance in Argentina (VIHDA). The VIHDA program, which received support through external financing, is part of the development of the National Program of Epidemiology and Hospital Infection Control. Its objective is the monitoring of HAIs in healthcare public organizations. The program manages incidence surveillance and conducts an annual prevalence study in which both public and private healthcare organizations participate.

Similarly, in 1993, the National Health Ministry, with the cooperation of several scientific societies, created the National Program of Quality Assurance of Healthcare (PNGCAM). This program developed multiple clinical practice protocols for diagnostic procedures and guidelines aimed at reducing treatment variability.

In 2005, after a severe economic and institutional crisis, the government implemented a program of subsidies for maternal and child care, called the NACER Plan. This plan secured coverage of pregnancy, childbirth, postpartum care, and pediatric care up to 5 years of age. Under the NACER Plan, which involved over 7000 healthcare facilities, more than 4.7 million pregnant women and children received coverage, and 37 million preventive interventions were undertaken. The plan's provisions include access to care during pregnancy and the postnatal period, and for children under 6 years old.

The good results of the NACER Plan led to the development and implementation of the SUMAR Plan, which extended coverage into adolescence up until the age of 18, and until 64 years of age for the female population. One of the objectives of the SUMAR plan is to improve quality of primary care. A pay-for-performance strategy has been used in order to accomplish this objective. The program involves important collaboration between social security and the private and public health sectors. This plan is financed

---

* Denotes acronyms in Spanish.

by the World Bank as well as the national government and the provinces. Outcomes are not available at the time of writing.

External Quality and Patient Safety Evaluation Initiatives

In 1994, the group that drafted the Accreditation Manual for Hospitals in Latin America and the Caribbean established the Technical Institute for the Accreditation of Healthcare Organizations (ITAES), which develops accreditation programs for inpatient healthcare organizations, chronic dialysis centers, and outpatient diagnostic services (laboratory and imaging). In 2014, ITAES received International Society for Quality in Healthcare (ISQua) accreditation for both standards and on-site institutional assessment. In 1995, the Argentine Biochemistry Foundation (FBA) initiated an accreditation program, with its own standards, for clinical laboratories. In 1998, a new accreditation body was created, the Specialized Center for Standardization and Accreditation in Healthcare (CENAS), dedicated to the evaluation of healthcare organizations, with or without inpatient services, as well as the performance of social security organizations. As in most Latin American countries, there were no incentives for accredited organizations in Argentina. Therefore, accreditation programs had no significant results in relation to the 3323 public and private hospitals, except for the FBA program where accreditation was linked to contracts for the provision of services. ITAES and CENAS have different programs from the inpatient organizations (see Tables 1.1 and 1.2).

The Argentine Institute for Standardization (IRAM) is responsible for Argentinian ISO standards certification, with the local health department applying specific rules for the different imaging services. Moreover, with governmental support, the Argentine Organization of Accreditation (OAA)

TABLE 1.1

Number of Hospitals and Accreditation Status in 2016

Accrediting Bodies	Current	Unaccredited	Expired	Accumulated Hospitals Evaluated
ITAES	33	1	14	48
CENAS	38	2	72	112

TABLE 1.2

Number of Clinical Laboratories Accredited by FBA, by Year

Year	95/97	98/99	00/01	02/03	04/05	06/07	08/09	10/11	12/13	14/15
FBA	2.276	2.128	2.303	2.322	2.296	2.171	2.176	2.227	2.250	2.170

Source: Data provided by the accreditation bodies.

works alongside the FBA to ensure that ISO Norm 15.189 is the standard in medical laboratories.

It should be noted that, because the first draft for the accreditation manual promoted by the Pan American Health Organization (PAHO) originated in Argentina, the standards of these three accreditation entities were initially influenced by this model. Something similar happened with the National Accreditation Organization (ONA) in Brazil, although this phenomenon has not been observed in other countries in the region. Moreover, CENAS and ITAES leaders joined the executive board of ISQua during the first decade of the twenty-first century.

Training Initiatives on Quality and Patient Safety

Two organizations dedicated to teaching and clinical research have had a significant impact in the country. Since the 1990s, the Epidemiologic Research Institute of the National Academy of Medicine (IIE-ANM), first established in the 1970s, has been promoting the identification and registration of adverse events, investigations about medical error, and practice guidelines and training in epidemiology.

The Institute for Clinical Effectiveness and Health Policy (IECS), established in 2000, has had a further significant impact on quality and patient safety. Working in collaboration with Harvard University, the IECS promotes training activities in healthcare, along with primary care research programs, clinical practice guidelines, and health technology assessment. An active participant in ISQua, the institute has an international focus, and was instrumental in the creation of the Latin American Consortium for Innovation, Quality and Safety in Healthcare (CLICSS). In 2008, members of IECS organized the Latin American Collaborative Forum on Quality and Safety in Healthcare (CICSP), with the objective of disseminating information, promoting different cultural aspects, training healthcare professionals, and promoting interaction. The annual conference of the CICSP forum helps to connect professionals in quality and patient safety with directors of healthcare organizations from across Latin America.

Since 2008, the University Institute of Health Sciences (IUCS), Barceló Foundation, has delivered an online Diploma in Quality of Health Services, originally devised for Dominican Ministry of Health officers, to Argentine and Latin American professionals. Thus far, eight cohorts have enrolled, with a total of 176 students enrolled and 101 graduated.

A number of specialized scientific societies have also contributed to the promotion of quality and patient safety in Argentina over the last quarter century. These include

- The Argentine Medical Audit Society (SADAM), established in 1972, which was the first to promote quality in healthcare in the country; it currently trains insurance entities in the evaluation of healthcare.
- The Argentine Society for Quality in Healthcare (SACAS), which holds an annual conference on quality and safety and was the host organization for the 18th International Conference of ISQua in Buenos Aires in 2001.
- The Medical Association for Audit and Quality of Córdoba (ASACAM), with a wider scope in other provinces, which holds events and participates in educational activities at local public health schools.
- The Avedis Donabedian Foundation (FAD), which began with a series of conferences organized by Professor Donabedian himself in Buenos Aires in 1993. The foundation sponsors research and events.

Health Technology Assessment

In Argentina, health technology assessments are conducted by both the private and public sector. In the public sector, the Department of Health Technology Assessment works within the structure of the strategic management of the Superintendence of Health Services (SHS) and in the Ministry of Health. Operational since the year 2000, the department has been working on reforms to the Compulsory Medical Program (PMO), the analysis and authorization of services needed by exception, and support in decision-making of SHS. In addition, the National Cancer Institute conducts evaluative research to provide guidelines for medical practice and public sector health policy, and for the regulatory body of the Social Security Sector (SHS).

In the private sector, the Department of Health Technology Assessment of IECS works in collaboration with international organizations, governments, ministries and health departments, academic institutions, and along with health systems in many neighboring countries, including Bolivia, Brazil, Chile, Colombia, México, Panamá, Perú, Uruguay, and Venezuela. The department conducts systematic reviews, burden of disease studies, economic evaluations based on individual patients or using decision models, cost studies, health-related quality-of-life research, clinical guidelines, and other projects related to health systems and health economics. The department has published more than 100 scientific articles in international journals and more than 300 HTA reports, which are indexed in the International Network of Agencies for Health Technology

Assessment (INAHTA) and in the Centre for Reviews and Dissemination of the University of York.

Advances in the field of quality and patient safety are gradual, and Argentina is still working to establish an official framework for the deployment of improvement initiatives. While the impact of these numerous efforts to improve the system has thus far been limited, due to their fragmented and often disconnected nature, the quest to create a safer and more efficient healthcare system continues.

2

Brazil

Knowledge Management for Quality Improvement in Brazil

Claudia Travassos, Victor Grabois, and José Noronha

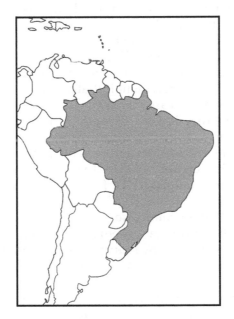

CONTENTS

Background

Since the decision to universalize healthcare coverage was made in 1988, Brazil has struggled to meet the challenge of achieving uniformly distributed quality of care in a middle-income country that is highly populated and geographically vast. A brief account of healthcare reform and quality of care initiatives in Brazil has been provided by Noronha et al. (2015). The Improving Quality and Access to Primary Care Program and the National Humanization Policy exemplify these initiatives.

Like many countries, Brazil is facing changes in demographic and epidemiological patterns, rapidly shifting towards an aging population and predominantly non-communicable diseases. While significant improvements have been made to the access and utilization of services, inequities remain. This new epidemiological profile has created stress on existing facilities and personnel, as services move from an acute care model toward an integrated, patient-centered, and continuous care model (WHO, 2015b). Quality improvement initiatives should be developed and adapted for this new healthcare scenario.

The Brazilian territory is very diverse in terms of population size, density and structure, epidemiological profile, biomes and land use, and social and economic infrastructure. The distribution of health services throughout the territory is also diversified in terms of quantity, size, and the level of complexity of facilities and personnel. Around 13% of the population of Brazil (200 million) lives in the Amazon Region—an area that encompasses over 4 million square kilometers, or roughly 49% of the geographical territory. This population is largely dispersed in an immense rainforest area, where malaria is still endemic and the healthcare infrastructure is precarious. In contrast, the Metropolitan Region of Sao Paulo, the wealthiest region of the country, where the best and more complex health facilities are located, has a similar population (around 21 million), but in an area of less than 8000 square kilometers.

In 2013, there were more than 44,000 health centers, about 41,000 specialty clinics, and 6,600 inpatient facilities in Brazil. Most of the inpatient facilities were small units dispersed throughout 3500 (out of a total 5565) municipalities across the country. Sixty percent of inpatient units had less than 50 beds and only 5.8% had more than 200 beds (Martins et al., 2014). There were more than 350,000 physicians and 287,000 registered nurses. Professional healthcare administrators are very scarce, and there are vast differences in qualifications and expertize. The extent and quality of healthcare resources also vary, and they correlate strongly with wealth distribution.

Collaborative Center for Quality of Care and Patient Safety

Despite extensive scientific literature and a growing awareness of the need to implement evidence-based quality initiatives to achieve better outcomes (Øvretveit, 2015), there has been limited circulation of quality improvement (QI) research among healthcare professionals and managers in Brazil. That knowledge transfer can change behavior has long been recognized; the effective dissemination of information is therefore a strategy for triggering professional awareness of QI theory and practice, and encouraging innovation across organizations (Guptill, 2005). Knowledge transfer depends upon the implementation of a systematic process of identification and selection of evidence-based information, learning objects, success stories, and tools. A critical mass of experts and supporters need to be identified to provide the culture and knowledge base for the selection and editing of material with an eye to the target population. A digital system can provide adequate technical infrastructure to support the collection, management, access, and retrieval of such material. It is also suitable for a country as large as Brazil with a widespread and diverse supply of healthcare facilities and professionals. The continuously changing environment of QI requires an open process, a work-in-progress approach.

Responding to a demand from the Ministry of Health to address long-standing issues of quality of care and patient safety, the Collaborative Center for Quality of Care and Patient Safety (Proqualis) was launched in 2009 by the Oswaldo Cruz Foundation (Fiocruz), a leading scientific and health research institute linked to the ministry. The mission of Proqualis is to contribute to the effective implementation of QI initiatives in healthcare organizations in Brazil by increasing access to health professionals and managers, and by providing patients and their families with relevant, reliable, and up-to-date QI information.

Proqualis was developed in line with the principles of knowledge management (KM), which has been defined as promoting "... an integrated approach to identifying, capturing, evaluating, retrieving, and sharing all of an enterprise's information assets" (Duhon, 1998, cited by Koenig, 2012). Proqualis was initially targeted at hospitals through the development of a web-based portal (www.proqualis.net).

A Successful Pathway

The website is structured with a homepage highlighting the most relevant material related to general topics of QI. The homepage links to a patient safety subportal. This subportal is divided into several sections. The first,

Thematic Pages, addresses cutting-edge issues that matter most directly to management, for example, patient safety culture. The second section, Brazilian Patient Safety Experiences, provides literature on successful QI initiatives related to safety practices in Brazilian hospitals. The objective is to offer health managers and professionals working at the coalface, tools and strategies to support QI in their organizations.

Hospitals with recognized success in safety practices are invited to join the Proqualis network of partner hospitals and to display their QI experience in a particular safety practice on the website. Material is published in designated sections, depending on the theme/safety practice. This information is also registered in a repository that contains all the materials published in the website, organized to make retrieval easier. Specialists and selected hospitals are responsible for the content of specific pages.

The editorial process to select scientific articles to be disseminated uses a unique search strategy developed by Proqualis. The abstracts for material originally written in other languages are first translated into Portuguese. A glossary of terms whose translation is contentious is provided, representing an institutional effort to standardize terminology and support a Portuguese vocabulary in QI. Because the literature in Portuguese is limited, Proqualis has recently assumed the additional role of content producer. Research published by Proqualis Publications will specifically address the needs of the Brazilian healthcare system, such as the development of safety indicators for use in Brazil. In accordance with the open access policies of the respected science and technology health institute, Fiocruz, all material produced by Proqualis is freely available. The communication policy includes replication of materials in other websites.

Social network profiles have also been successfully used to increase interactive communication. The Facebook group, Rede Proqualis, in particular, provides a forum for further support and connection.

Underlying Strategies

Proqualis applies KM strategy directed at healthcare according to Guptill's (2005) framework, which includes five components:

1. Communities of practice
2. Content management
3. Knowledge and capability transfer
4. Performance results tracking
5. Technology and support infrastructure

The organization of communities of practice and the use of social networks allow exchange of experiences and promote user participation. Proqualis publishes a large variety of materials—from scientific articles to guides and reports, protocols, checklists, lectures and videos, journalistic content, brochures, and interviews—to meet the diversity of users' needs. Proqualis is not intended to provide a comprehensive selection of materials and themes in QI. It is designed to publish the most current and relevant QI information, keeping the volume limited and manageable. The editorial policy and architecture is designed to let users find information easily. An efficient search engine facilitates the retrieval of previously published material. Information can be accessed using tablets and mobile phones. The open access policy eliminates any barriers to accessing portal contents.

In the 5 years since its establishment, Proqualis has become highly valued by the medical establishment. It is now one of the most well-known sources of information on QI in the country, particularly regarding patient safety. Proqualis has also become an advisory source for the Ministry of Health, playing a key role in the launching of the National Program for Patient Safety (PNSP). A Proqualis-directed network of specialists and organizations provided the expertise to design the policy and develop its initial tools. Proqualis partners include national and international specialists and organizations, such as the National School of Public Health, Portugal, and the Health Foundation, United Kingdom.

The Proqualis site, which contains nearly 2,000 articles, had 800,000 page views between 2010 and 2014. The average number of hits in 2015 was four times higher than the average between 2010 and 2014. Access to the portal reached 18,000 hits a month in 2015. The Proqualis Facebook page has 5775 members. Online lectures have been viewed by 300,000 users and videos by more than 120,000 users.

Transferability of the Proqualis Model

The dissemination of locally contextualized health system information is desperately needed in low- and middle-income countries. Proqualis provides a model for the dissemination of healthcare information in Brazil and elsewhere. The creation of the Proqualis portal was inspired by international websites such as the Patient Safety Network (PSNet). The open access policy is an important aspect of the model, as is the use of social networks. Countries with resources that are on par with those of Brazil could implement similar initiatives. As with Proqualis, governmental agencies, universities, and health services can collaborate to overcome fragmentation and optimize resources at an acceptable level to apply the KM model.

Prospects for Further Success and Next Steps

Health systems must be able to evolve to meet the challenges of constant change. The Brazilian Unified Health System (SUS) has already moved toward becoming an integrated and patient-centered care organization. In 2011, Presidential Decree 7508 established the guidelines for the organization of regional healthcare networks. Expansion of the scope of the Proqualis portal is planned, with the addition of a section dedicated to information on the streamlining of transitions between points of care. PNSP also increases the requirements for the implementation of safety practices. Challenges for Proqualis include

- Designing contents for more direct use by healthcare providers
- Encouraging greater interactivity among the portal team and users
- Making a greater use of contemporary media and language, consistent with adult learning, such as games, apps and webinars

To improve the quality and safety of care at all organizational levels, it is essential to create an environment where expertise and experience can be shared and utilized. Proqualis has facilitated the development of professional networks that can exchange experiences, compare performance, develop capacities, and continuously improve learning processes. To make healthcare resilient, adjustments to continually changing care requirements will be required, along with a capacity to identify, criticize, and disseminate new conceptual and practical approaches to QI (Hollnagel et al., 2013).

3

Canada

Improving Stroke Outcomes in Canada: The Accreditation Canada Stroke Distinction Program

Jonathan I. Mitchell, Qendresa Hasanaj, Hélène Sabourin, Danielle Dorschner, Stephanie Carpenter, Toby Yan, Wendy Nicklin, G. Ross Baker, John Van Aerde, and Sarah Boucaud

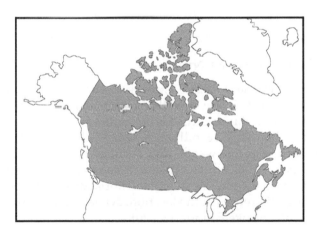

CONTENTS

Background

The social and economic burden of stroke* is a global concern. Stroke is the second leading cause of death in the world (Heart and Stroke Foundation, 2014). Contributing risk factors for the high prevalence of stroke include underuse of strategies for primary prevention, a significant increase in the number of young adults affected by stroke, and an increasing epidemic of risk factors worldwide, including obesity and diabetes mellitus (Feigin et al., 2015). To address this burden, the 2014 World Health Organization (WHO) Global Status Report on Noncommunicable Diseases targeted stroke care with a goal of having at least 50% of eligible people receiving drug therapy and counseling to prevent heart attacks and stroke by the year 2025 (WHO, 2014).

Stroke in Canada: By the Numbers

In Canada, an estimated 50,000 strokes occur each year and 315,000 Canadians are currently living with the impacts of stroke, which frequently involve a degree of disability. Stroke is estimated to cost the Canadian economy CAD$3.6 billion (US$2.8 billion) a year in direct costs for physician services, hospital costs, lost wages, and decreased productivity (Heart and Stroke Foundation, 2014). While stroke is a national concern, there are significant variations in the provincial and territorial death rates resulting from stroke, reflecting differences in the location, availability, and coordination of services (Heart and Stroke Foundation, 2014).

Canadian Context

Canada is a vast country of 10 million square kilometers, with a population of 35 million residing in 10 provinces and three territories. The Canadian healthcare system is universal and decentralized, with both federal and provincial/territorial governments playing key roles. The federal government's role in healthcare includes setting some policy at the national level, administering the Canada Health Act, and funding support to the provinces and territories. It is also responsible for the regulation of drugs and the delivery

---

* A stroke is defined as a sudden loss of brain function, often caused by the interruption of blood flow to parts of the brain (Heart and Stroke Foundation, 2014).

of services to certain groups, including First Nations and Inuit peoples, members of the Canadian Forces, veterans, inmates in federal penitentiaries, and refugees. The main responsibility for organizing and delivering health services belongs to provincial/territorial ministries of health and social services. As a result, each province/territory has its own distinct healthcare system (Marchildon, 2013).

Efforts to enhance health services in Canada are driven by multiple factors. Partnerships between governments, along with national, provincial/territorial, and local healthcare organizations allow for the pooling of resources and expertise. The consolidation of drug procurement power through provincial–territorial purchasing alliances is one such example. Quality improvement (QI) initiatives aimed at improving the timeliness of care as well as the patient experience (Marchildon, 2013) often begin when innovative ideas are adopted within and across organizations with assistance from a number of agencies, including provincial quality councils, and national and provincial associations.

Like many other high-income countries, the Canadian healthcare system is also heavily influenced by demographic changes due to an aging population. Canada is experiencing growth in its senior population, with individuals aged 65 and older expected to reach 25% of the population by 2036 (Canadian Institute for Health Information, 2011). These demographic shifts will require increased stroke prevention and care efforts. Increasingly, attention is being paid to whether and how resources can be better distributed and optimized to deal with the reality of an aging population. Supporting improvements in stroke care requires the development and spread of effective stroke care models across the country.

Accreditation Canada Distinction Program

Accreditation Canada is a not-for-profit, independent organization that provides national and international health organizations with quality-focused, comprehensive accreditation services. The Stroke Distinction program was created to recognize organizations for their outstanding commitment to excellence and leadership in stroke care. The program is one of several highly specialized accreditation programs that serve to improve quality and drive excellence in services. These services have a significant impact on population health and generate high costs in the healthcare system.

The Stroke Distinction program builds on the mainstream Qmentum accreditation program, which is designed to focus on quality and safety throughout all aspects of an organization's services—from governance and leadership to direct care—for the benefit of patients, clients, residents, direct care providers, and staff. Released in 2010, the Stroke Distinction program recognizes excellence in stroke care through a rigorous review process. The Stroke Distinction program identifies healthcare organizations with initiatives supporting risk mitigation, reducing adverse events, and identifying opportunities to standardize care and improve efficiency. Five program components are used to determine stroke distinction:

1. Compliance with the standards
2. Performance indicators
3. Stroke protocols or clinical practice guidelines implementation
4. Excellence and innovation
5. Client and family education

Stroke Distinction Program in Action

In 2012 and 2014, the Kingston General Hospital in Kingston, Ontario, received Accreditation Canada's Stroke Distinction Award. The program contributed to the following improvements:

- The proportion of patients treated on a dedicated stroke unit has improved from 62% in 2010 to 76% annually since 2012.
- The 30-day mortality absolute rate decrease of 5% was sustained from 2010 to 2016.
- The 90-day readmission rate has improved from 8% readmissions in 2010 to less than 4% annually since 2012, in part due to the decreased wait time for transient ischemic attack (TIA) management in the Stroke Prevention Clinic.

There have been several other improvements in care for stroke patients over this period. These include the implementation of the urinary catheter removal protocol, which was associated with a reduction in the number of catheter days for a set number of stroke patients over a 2-week period from 147 in 2013 to 95 days in 2014, along with a decrease in the urinary tract infection rates from 21% in 2013 to 11% in 2014. The use of the standard dysphagia screening process has been associated with a 15% increase in the use of this swallowing screening tool since 2010.

Staff members and direct care providers have noted that the Stroke Distinction program helps "recognize and celebrate the good work we are already doing" as well as "identify opportunities for improvement against objective and evidence-based national standards ... [therefore the program] helps us to improve stroke patient outcomes."

TABLE 3.1

Stroke Distinction Program Outcomes

Indicator	Before[a]	After[b]
Stroke patients in a stroke unit (%)	97	100
Median length of stay (days)	33.2	27
Stroke patients with antithrombotic treatment (%)	95	100
Stroke patients with dysphagia screening on admission (%)	96	100
Median number of days from stroke onset to rehabilitation admission	22	12

[a] April 2010 to September 2010.
[b] April 2015 to September 2015.

As of 2016, the Stroke Distinction program has been implemented by 15 healthcare organizations in Canada. The reported outcome improvements described for the Kingston General Hospital are not limited to a particular health sector or organization type. The Stroke Distinction program applies as well to rehabilitation facilities using customized standards and performance indicators. For example, the Toronto Rehabilitation Institute (part of University Health Network in Toronto) reported similar improvements in outcomes. The results are summarized in Table 3.1.

The improvements in care following participation in the Stroke Distinction program are attributable to many factors. These include increased awareness of best practices shared through the Accreditation Canada Stroke Distinction program and inter-professional team collaboration. While the Stroke Distinction program has been followed by specific healthcare organizations, it focuses on the continuum of stroke care and therefore encourages stroke programs to apply for distinction as a network. These networks cross the continuum of stroke care, with an approach that includes all stakeholders, from first response to rehabilitation. Evaluation occurs at the individual and site level and as an integrated system (Mitchell et al., 2014).

Responses from direct care providers have been positive, with increased confidence in skills, expertise, and care provided. The program brings a focus on continuous learning as well as celebrating team achievements. In the words of direct care providers:

> "I am more confident and knowledgeable to work with geriatric stroke clients. The accreditation process has given me credibility and confidence with my work."
> "Being part of a Stroke Distinction work group allowed me to stay on top of stroke best practice guidelines, evaluate and improve upon our current practice, and highlight the work our team has accomplished."
> "Stroke Distinction has allowed our entire team to evaluate our current practices to celebrate the successful steps we have already taken to enhance patient and family care, and to drive the development of new practices, which may further assist in meeting (or exceeding!) best practice guidelines."

Lessons Learned: How to Spread This Canadian Success Internationally

With 15 healthcare organizations across Canada currently participating in the Stroke Distinction program, this Canadian success in stroke outcomes is also being operationalized internationally. The Stroke Distinction program has been implemented in three client organizations of Accreditation Canada International, two acute care organizations in Brazil, and one health system in Italy. In so doing, Accreditation Canada continues to embed feedback from client organizations and surveyors into future program developments. This includes keeping organizations fully engaged in the program when clients have gone through several cycles of Stroke Distinction, continually updating the program using the latest Stroke Best Practice Guidelines, and moving to a 4-year cycle with mid-cycle touch points to ensure optimal value from each on-site visit.

Several factors have contributed to the success of healthcare organizations participating in the Stroke Distinction program. These include

- A focus on the client/patient at all times as key to improving the care experience. Family members and friends are included in the rehabilitation process. Quality is a team effort.
- Visible leadership commitment across the organization and team. From senior leadership to the unit manager, leadership must communicate the importance of and support recommendations for change. Direct care providers can lead different working groups with broad representation and physician engagement.
- Communication. There is a need to improve the clinical information given to clients and their loved ones. For direct care providers and staff, "tip of the day" e-mails, team huddles for all shifts, debrief on results, targeted education, and posters work well.
- Fostering a culture that sustains quality and positive change. There is a need to encourage the continuous improvement of processes through regular assessments using appropriate indicators.
- Making the process rewarding by focusing on learning and by celebrating successes and achievements. The client, their loved ones, the care team, and leaders must celebrate achievements. Efforts must be acknowledged in order to achieve success.

The importance of collaboration to the positive impact of the Stroke Distinction program on patient and staff experience cannot be overstated. In the words of a direct care provider: "Alone, I cannot accomplish much.

In partnership, we can start to make changes. Within an integrated stroke continuum, all is possible."

Acknowledgments

Special thanks to Chris Niro, at Accreditation Canada, for her helpful review comments.

4

Chile

Constructing Symbolic Capital: A Case Study from Chile

Marcos Vergara Iturriaga and Leonel Valdivia

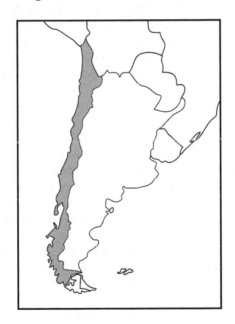

CONTENTS

Background

Chile has a mix of both private and publicly financed healthcare. Prior to 2004, as an inheritance of the Pinochet dictatorship, the public sector, which primarily served only the poorest groups, was underfunded and institutionally weak. With the return of democracy, various pieces of legislation established the financial basis for a more robust system of publicly financed hospitals. Currently, about 75% of Chileans receive care through the public system and 25% receive private care. Law No. 19,966 of 2004 established a system of universal access with explicit guarantees in health (*Acceso Universal con Garantías Explícitas*, or AUGE), covering access, opportunity, quality of services, and financial protection for a number of predefined health conditions (Cunill Grau et al., 2011; Solimano and Valdivia, 2015). Soon after, Law No. 19,937 authorized the implementation of a network of self-managed hospitals (*Establecimientos de Autogestión en Red-EAR*) comprising public hospitals with a higher level of service complexity—that is, hospitals that have the capacity to provide care for patients with serious critical and trauma conditions (Ministerio de Salud [MINSAL], 2005).

Organizationally, these institutions are required to comply with established guidelines relating to cost measurement and containment, quality of care, and user satisfaction, in addition to progressive improvement in staff working conditions and pay. Hospital directors are responsible for directing the execution of programs, designing future plans, and overseeing the institution's internal organization. Each institution must set up a consultative council, made up of five representatives from the local community and two staff representatives, to play an advisory role in the design and evaluation of institutional plans.

Thus, while the AUGE system represents the macro-level reform of the Chilean Health System, the establishment of these self-managed hospitals (57 at present), represents the meso-level reform. All self-managed hospitals belong to the state/public sector. That is, they are institutions managed under the Chilean system of public administration—the administrative statutes that limit their operations to what is explicitly allowed under this administrative framework. This means that the public are both the drivers and the stakeholders in this particular scenario.

Details of the Success Story

Following the methodology of the balanced scorecard (BSC) (Kaplan and Norton, 2000), the Ministry of Health (MOH) and the Ministry of Finance (MOF) established a set of indicators and defined 75% compliance with such indicators as the threshold measure to maintain an institution's status as a self-managed hospital. The 48 indicators relate to four management and healthcare dimensions: clinical management, financial sustainability, operational efficiency, and quality of services. Additionally, the score obtained in the achievement of these indicators determines ranking among the self-managed institutions (Benavente, n.d.). The list of indicators for 2016 is as follows:

Clinical Management

1. Percentage achievement of the Clinical Management Plan as defined in the Strategic Plan
2. Percentage achievement of the medical protocol checklists
3. Percentage of potential organ donor notification
4. Functional index
5. Percentage of discharge after superior prolonged in-hospital stays
6. Percentage of new specialist ambulatory consultations
7. Percentage achievement of the Program of Network Coordination

Financial Sustainability

1. Information system in operation and delivering statistical records
2. Percentage use of diagnosis-related group (DRG) coding for major ambulatory surgeries
3. Use of Management Information System for Windows (WinSIG) for production, efficiency, resources, costs (PERC) as required by MOH
4. Percentage of purchase via public tender Type L1 bidding and via direct purchase
5. Percentage of debt reduction
6. Percentage of service costs properly allocated
7. Percentage of timely accrual of bills
8. Financial equilibrium
9. Timely payment of invoices
10. Percentage of self-generated revenues
11. Percentage achievement of annual programming of specialist medical consultations
12. Percentage achievement of AUGE opportunity guarantees
13. Average wait days for surgeries
14. Percentage of daily dosage implementation

Operational Efficiency

1. Number of days of labor absenteeism due to sick leave
2. Percentage of trained employees in leadership positions
3. Percentage of major ambulatory surgery in patients over the age of 15
4. Emergency room demand categorization
5. Admission opportunity (waiting period) for patients in emergency room
6. Percentage of full and timely prescription filling
7. Percentage implementation of daily dosage drug distribution system
8. Percentage use of pharmaceutical stocks
9. Percentage implementation of Medical Equipment Preventive Maintenance Plan
10. Turnover of inventory of medical devices
11. Percentage of postponed surgical procedures
12. Average number of days of pre-surgery hospitalization
13. Performance per contracted hours
14. Percentage bed day occupancy for patients of risk dependency level D2, D3
15. Bed occupancy rate
16. Percentage availability of critical care beds
17. Percentage use of elective surgery rooms
18. Expenditures in overtime payments
19. Percentages of complaints resolved in a timely fashion
20. Community participation

Quality of Care

1. Percentage achievement of accreditation standards
2. Percentage compliance with audit plan
3. Percentage of audit recommendations fulfilled
4. Percentage of unplanned surgical readmissions
5. Number of patients with pressure ulcers or lesions
6. Percentage of emergency room under 7-day readmission of patients under same major diagnostic category
7. Compliance with standards to qualify as a friendly hospital
8. User satisfaction rates in emergency and ambulatory departments

The ranking results do not provide any awards or special recognition, such as salary increases or bonuses, for those achieving higher scores. However, high rankings, which are publicly reported, create important symbolic capital, and help to further institutional ambitions. For instance, when the upper management team of the Institute of Neurosurgery wanted to reposition the hospital as a recognized national referral entity, achieving a high ranking among self-managed hospitals became a strategic objective of the institute. The current hospital management team assumed its functions in October 2012. At that time, the Institute of Neurosurgery was ranked 45th out of 57 among the country's hospitals, and was below the minimum 75% requirement to maintain its categorization as a self-managed institution.

Once the strategic decision was made, efforts were undertaken to help alleviate the institute's dire situation. These efforts led to the institute increasing its achievement threshold to 82.7% in 2013, easily exceeding the 75% required, and thus improving its national ranking. Most crucially, in terms of the hospital's future direction, the new management team also determined that the hospital's previous evaluations had been substandard, and were able to better coordinate subsequent measurements of internal processes and productivity. The realization that higher rankings, based on internal evaluation, can also be used as a tool for institutional development led to significant changes in the institute's culture. As a result, the hospital began working toward further increasing their ranking, aiming to move into the top 10 in 2013.

In 2013, the Institute of Neurosurgery was ranked second on the national hospital ranking scale and then moved into first place in the years 2014 and 2015 (Figure 4.1). The prevailing message within the institute during these 3 years was that collective effort and shared commitment to institutional improvement would result not only in increased prestige, but also in the provision of better service, along with a vastly improved work environment.

The success story of the Institute of Neurosurgery was based on the application of a two-pronged approach, involving transformations of both a cultural and technical nature. Shifts in the cultural climate of the organization were achieved through the deliberate application of Bourdieu's (1986) principle of symbolic capital accumulation, whereby the importance of institutional recognition and prestige is instilled among all members of the hospital community. On the technical side, an innovative hospital management system, based on the application of the BSC tool, was installed. Some of its main features include

- A focus on quality and safety through patient-focused care management (patient/user participation in the Consultative Council)
- Close coordination between clinical, administrative, and financial management (regular meetings of the directing committee, with representatives from all sections)
- A focus on financial equilibria (e.g., debt reduction and cost-containment measures)

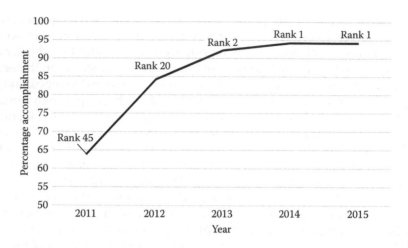

FIGURE 4.1
Evolution of the Institute of Neurosurgery's ranking among self-managed hospitals of the National Health Services System, Chile, 2011–2015. (Prepared by Marcos Vergara, MD. From Ministry of Health, Chile.)

Although the high ranking of the institute did not generate a greater allocation of resources from the government, it did lead to significantly increased financial equilibrium and consolidation, which was partially achieved by reducing institutional debt to zero. The spending reforms demanded by the quest for better rankings generated surpluses that have been used to update technological platforms to further improve institutional management—creating a most satisfying virtuous circle.

Implementation: Transferability of Exemplar

The leadership team of the Institute of Neurosurgery was convinced that striving for high positioning in the ranking of hospitals would be a value-added enterprise for the institute, its employees, and patients, generating significant gains in symbolic capital. The institute's improvement strategies, which basically involved the application of a management evaluation system based on defined indicators, are eminently transferable to all public hospitals in Chile and to neighboring countries. As the system, Sys-Q, has been in use for the past 5 years, there is valuable cumulative experience to support those who wish to adopt it in other contexts.

Efficient hospital administration is not a choice but a necessity, especially for public hospitals that normally operate within the constraints of limited resources and high-service demand. The Institute of Neurosurgery's successful efforts to improve their national ranking provide a useful guide to reforming such institutions effectively and without great expense. This is particularly important when public institutions must compete with privately owned institutions for both patients and financial and human resources (Porter and Teisberg, 2004).

Prospects for Further Success and Next Steps

Striving for service and managerial excellence may produce additional and sometimes unexpected benefits, which should be explored in greater detail. For instance, monthly evaluation sessions with all departmental leaders, as required by the application of the BSC system, encourages questioning, collaboration, and a coordination of efforts that may have otherwise been overlooked.

In both Chile and South America, public hospital management does not figure very prominently in public administration science and practice, at least not in its better-known trends or schools of thought. This may be due to the idea that state provision of public services, such as healthcare, is not considered an essential component of public administration. Rather, the analysis of healthcare is traditionally limited to its significance in terms of the 'public good' and public health (Muñoz et al., 2000). Thus, there is a knowledge gap in relation to public hospital management in the field of public administration, a gap that the experience described in this chapter may help to fill.

Conclusion

Public hospital performance evaluations, which use the BSC method and are based on defined indicators, offer valuable possibilities for future development. The routine application of performance evaluations produces an important by-product, namely teamwork, which constitutes an essential institutional competency—one that must become a central feature in the management of public healthcare institutions (Vergara et al., 2012).

5

Ecuador

Improving Hospital Management as Part of the Health Reform Process in Ecuador: The Case of Abel Gilbert Pontón Hospital

Jonás Gonseth and Maria Cecilia Acuña

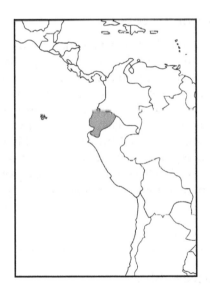

CONTENTS

Background

In 2006, Ecuador set in motion profound state reforms aimed at increasing the role of the public sector in society, strengthening the power of the executive branch and Congress over interest groups, and providing equitable and universal access to good quality social services, in particular healthcare and education. This all-encompassing reform is known as *La Revolución Ciudadana* (The Citizens' Revolution). As part of this process, a new constitution was established in 2008 by means of a national referendum, and the government launched the National Plan for Good Living in 2009.

Health Sector Reform Process

In response to the new conditions established by the constitution and the objectives of the National Plan for Good Living, the Ministry of Health started a reform process in February 2012. The goals of the reform were to strengthen the Ministry of Health's steering role, to consolidate the public health services provision network, to improve quality of care, and to expand health coverage. To achieve these goals, a new organic statute was devised to allow for the reorganization of the Ministry of Health, which resulted in the establishment of a new organizational plan. After these changes, the Health Law also came under revision to provide the Ministry of Health with a wider set of attributes that made for a more robust regulatory capacity.

Beginning of a Success Story

Abel Gilbert Pontón (AGP) Hospital was founded in 1973. Located in a low-income area of Guayaquil, the most populous city in Ecuador, it was the first public hospital in the city built by the Ministry of Health. AGP Hospital receives patients whose medical expenses aren't covered by social security and who don't have the economic resources to pay for private medical care. Over time, AGP Hospital deteriorated due to successive governments' neglect of the public health system. This was further aggravated by the Ecuadorian economic crisis of the late 1990s. Scarce economic resources were frequently misused and quality of care was lacking. The hospital fell into a chronic state of disarray.

In 2012, the Regulation for Hospital Process Management was passed by the Ministry of Public Health (Ministry of Public Health [Ecuador], 2012). This was to have a significant impact on the future of AGP Hospital. Hospitals with over 70 beds were classified as either a general or a specialty hospital. Specialty hospitals could focus on a specific group of diseases (e.g., infectious, respiratory) or a particular specialization (e.g., pediatrics). The term *specialty hospital* also refers to a hospital portfolio that covers a wide range of specialties with a high level of complexity. AGP Hospital, with 260 beds, was categorized as a specialty hospital in 2012.

Under the new regulation, all Ecuadorian hospital activities were classified under one of the following processes:

- Governing processes: the new position of hospital manager was created for hospitals with more than 70 beds.
- Added value processes: this includes all healthcare divisions, the medical director, and coordinators of clinical, surgical, nursing, and diagnostic services.
- Support processes: this covers all the administrative areas of the hospital, including human resources, financial department, procurement, information technology, and maintenance. All these departments are under the supervision of the administrative director. In addition, two departments were strengthened: admissions and patient service (including social workers).
- Advisory processes: this includes the Quality Management Unit (QM), the Planning Follow-up and Evaluation Unit (PFE), the legal department, and the communications department. Legal and communications departments already existed, but the QM and PFE are new. Significantly, QM includes a hospital-acquired infectious control subunit.

An international selection process for all hospital manager positions was conducted in parallel with the implementation of the new regulations, and managers/directors were appointed to 42 Ministry of Health–dependent hospitals. These positions were tendered internationally, in the expectation that outside expertise would assist in the implementation of the new vision and enrich the process. Despite the international scope of the selection process, 40 of the 42 managers hired were Ecuadorians resident in Ecuador. One international manager (Colombian) undertook the task of managing Eugenio Espejo (EE) Hospital in Quito, the capital of Ecuador, and the other international manager (Spanish) was appointed to AGP Hospital in Guayaquil. These hospitals are the largest specialty hospitals in Ecuador: EE Hospital covers the highlands region, while AGP Hospital covers the coastal region. Because of Ecuador's historical centralism, the highlands region, with its center in the capital, Quito, has a more structured health system than that of the coastal region, which is chronically underfinanced and underdeveloped. Thus, in 2012, the situation of EE Hospital was significantly better than that of AGP Hospital.

Prior to the application of the new regulatory framework, AGP Hospital was considered the most notorious hospital in the country because of the poor quality of patient care and widespread internal corruption. For example, the most notorious cases involved corrupt procurement processes, with frequent instances of health technologies, drugs, and medical devices being bought unnecessarily at inflated prices through illicit arrangements. Resource theft involving fake patients and even fake healthcare professionals was also discovered.

While there were many attempts to improve the situation, with local directors appointed and corrupt doctors removed, the critical state of affairs continued. Even budget increases, along with an official declaration of a state of emergency to facilitate procurement, failed to improve matters. Over this period, failure and confrontation had become deeply rooted in the culture of the hospital.

With support from the Pan American Health Organization/World Health Organization Ecuador (PAHO/WHO Ecuador), which was involved in developing the conceptual framework and logistics of the process, all newly appointed hospital managers took part in an induction week in Quito in order to apply the new regulatory framework. Because AGP Hospital and EE Hospital are both specialty hospitals and are expected to serve as role models for the country, they worked to establish a common approach. Again, their efforts involved specific support from PAHO/WHO.

Although the international manager appointed to EE Hospital resigned by the end of 2012 and a new international manager was appointed, the hospital has still exhibited a degree of improvement to date. However, management proved more stable at AGP Hospital, and improvements over the last 3 years have been outstanding in both hospitals. The outsider standing of the manager has helped to highlight negative aspects of the prevalent culture, and has probably played a significant role in facilitating change.

Pathway

A plan with precise milestones to be accomplished has become the rational pathway to the overhaul of the hospital. The three major milestones comprise:

Milestone 1

Guarantee of the provision of drugs and working equipment. This includes process management of hospital procurement, warehouse, and information technologies so that recorded data are consistent with the actual quantities of drugs and equipment. Fighting corruption and working toward transparency were fundamental in this phase. In addition to the provision of physical tools, the guarantee also includes improving points of care and providing dignity in care. This includes refurbishments that facilitate respect for patient privacy. This process was carried out over a period of 6 months to 1 year.

Milestone 2

Redefining the hospital portfolio. This entails discussion of the mission of the hospital as a higher complexity node of care in the local and national health system. The needs and culture of the community were considered, along with expectations. Patient empowerment and engagement was fundamental during this phase. This process was carried out over a period of 1–2 years.

Milestone 3

Pathway to excellence. One of the fundamental aspects of the pathway to excellence is the sharing of responsibility between professionals and patients. A culture of broad empowerment and clinical leadership has been established. The role of the hospital manager has become more supervisory as members of staff take greater responsibility and demonstrate leadership skills. Improvements are sustainably enhanced through staff involvement in defining priorities and decision-making. These efforts are complemented by a broad hospital patient literacy strategy encompassing all specialties, focusing on disease management and the appropriate use of the health system.

Depending on each particular phase, the whole process of improvement has focused on the different milestones. Every milestone must be reviewed so that it is sustained and evolves coherently along with the hospital.

The Impact

Strong evidence of AGP Hospital's improvement is supported by the hospital portfolio. In 2012, only 12 specialties were offered, whereas today 14 clinical specialties and 14 surgical specialties are offered. In 2012, the hospital emergency room was overcrowded with primary care patients, accepting a mean of 1200 patients per day. Today, patients in the emergency room are triaged and a mean of 300 patients per day is accepted, while all primary care patients are transferred to the emergency departments of the healthcare centers. Improved patient literacy, a result of intensive communications initiatives, has also significantly contributed to this improvement.

In June 2012, only 58 doctors had the necessary qualifications to be considered specialists, while 180 doctors had those qualifications in 2015. Additionally, only 23 nurses were registered in 2012, while in 2015 the number of registered nurses had increased to 160. The new departments (QM, PFE) were staffed, and many others were reinforced. Ecuador suffers from a profound lack of specialist doctors, partly because formal training programs were suspended during the 2009–2012 period. The only way for new doctors to specialize was to study abroad. However, from 2012 to 2015, a new government initiative, *Ecuador Saludable Vuelvo Por Ti*, offered Ecuadorian and foreign specialized doctors economic and administrative incentives to join the national health system.

All this investment accounts for an increase of only 15% in the salary budget. The salary budget for 2012 was US$23,808,476 versus a salary budget for 2015 of US$27,160,727.

Patient satisfaction increased from less than 50% of those surveyed who regarded it as "fair" in 2012, to more than 70% who regarded it as "fair" in 2015. The media's perception of the hospital has also changed significantly for the better (Hospital de Especialidades Abel Gibert Pontón, 2016).

In 2015, AGP Hospital was accredited by Canada Accreditation International (Accreditation Canada, 2015).

Transferability

The same initiative has been transferred to Guayaquil's social security specialty hospital, Teodoro Maldonado Carbo Hospital (Hospital de Especialidades Teodoro Maldonado Carbo, 2016). In February 2015, the reform process was prompted by a surprise visit of the president of Ecuador to this hospital, which was found to be significantly below required standards. Milestone 1 was initiated almost immediately, and since April 2016, efforts have been focused on successfully implementing Milestone 2.

Components that worked as strong facilitators of change and are potentially transferable to any other critical hospital in low- and middle-income countries looking for a pathway to improvement include

- Conceptual framework of process management
- Outsider professional in an executive position in charge of the transformation
- Fighting corruption and enhancing transparency
- Patient engagement
- Clinical/staff leadership participation
- Outsider technical support as from the World Health Organization (WHO) representation in the country, external experts, consultants, or collaborating centers

- Enhancing the vision of healthcare networks, where the hospital plays a distinctive role, in the context of integration and continuum of care: empowering primary care levels
- Implementation of sound initiatives that work as triggers for general improvement (e.g., patient safety initiatives, such as the alcohol rub hand hygiene model and the surgical safety checklist)
- Strong political support

All these very concrete initiatives have been implemented, overcoming the most relevant barrier: licit and illicit conflicts of interest, along with many other human factors that result from change. Strong political support is critical to success. Sharing and celebrating achievements smooths the transition. The turning point for change may be the arrival of a manager who is an outsider with no previous links to the hospital and with no interest beyond the institution's improvement. The managers need strong support from those in power to do whatever is needed to bring about change.

Conclusion

The intervention has led to significant improvements to the patient experience with the hospital. Before changes can be made, corruption must be tackled and strong internal and external collaboration must be established. Transferability has proved possible in Ecuador, and many of the components analyzed here may be transferable to other low- and middle-income countries.

6

Guyana

Holistic Geriatric Mega-Clinics for Care of the Elderly in Guyana

William Adu-Krow, Vishwa Mahadeo, Vasha Elizabeth Bachan, and Melissa Ramdeen

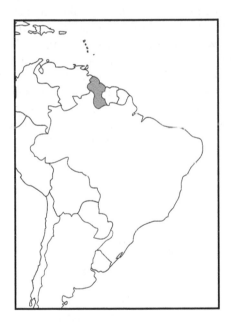

CONTENTS

Background

Guyana, like most countries, is experiencing an increase in its aged population due to improved medical care and increased lifespan (American Geriatrics Society, 2005). Current estimates suggest that about 55,000 Guyanese (7%) are aged over 60. The physiological and pathophysiological changes that are inherent to the aging process mean that there are unique social needs and healthcare challenges within the geriatric population, many of which are currently not being met (Eng et al., 1997). This can be attributed, in part, to the increased mobility of the younger population, which has led to an erosion of the extended family that once provided significant support and care for older people within the community (Bhatia, 1983; Goel et al., 2003). Furthermore, although Guyana's primary healthcare system aims to provide care for the entire population, the relative isolation and lack of mobility that comes with age means that the provision of care to the elderly can be challenging, and is not always satisfactory (Natarajan, 1987).

To fill some of the more evident gaps, the Care for the Elderly program was established in Guyana's Region 6 (East Berbice-Corentyne) in November 2013 to provide low-cost holistic geriatric mega-clinics in the community (see Figure 6.1). The program was specifically geared at improving the quality of life for the elderly within their own community, ultimately enabling them to live longer (Bigelow et al., 1991; Felce and Perry, 1995).

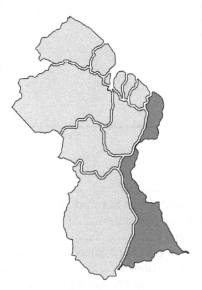

FIGURE 6.1
Map of Guyana showing Region 6.

Development: Initial Training and Support Partnerships

To ensure the success of the program, support was provided by the Pan American Health Organization/World Health Organization (PAHO/WHO) in the training of healthcare workers (HCWs) and social workers in entitlement care and other programs to promote "activities of daily living" (ADL) (American Psychological Association, 1996). HCWs were recruited from relevant specialties and divisions, including internal medicine, geriatric care, nutrition, mental health services, and social services. The aim of the training sessions was to build capacity to complement each other's work. Partnerships were also established with faith-based organizations (FBOs), women's groups (Women's Progressive Organization), and other non-governmental organizations (NGOs), both international and domestic, such as Food for the Poor (FFP) and Guyana Medical Relief (GMR), in order to develop well-functioning and properly coordinated local entities (Chaubey and Vij, 1999).

Geriatric Mega-Clinic Implementation

Initially, the community to be served was identified by the Berbice Regional Health Authority (BRHA), which was charged with developing the program. Catchment areas near already existing health centers were chosen to facilitate subsequent follow-up. Meetings were then held with local medical and administrative staff who could help set up such mega-clinics. Wheelchair-accessible facilities able to cater to a minimum of 50 persons were identified as potential mega-clinic sites.

Involvement with community groups was essential for the success of the program. All mega-clinics were hosted by FBO entities, either individually or in groups, and they provided significant financial and in-kind support, such as physical spaces and volunteers to serve as orderlies. Meetings were held with local community leaders who could help promote the program. The mega-clinics were promoted through public announcements, which were made using vehicle-mounted loudspeakers, and local media were also engaged.

The availability of necessary supplies was then ascertained. Most over-the-counter drugs and medical supplies were provided by NGOs, and the remainder were government supplied. Equipment and supplies, such as tents, wheelchairs, tables, chairs, and so forth, were provided by the health centers, NGOs, and FBOs. Healthy meals and snacks for clients and volunteers were generally provided by the FBOs. Volunteers prepared the site 1 day prior to the clinic.

The transportation of patients was provided by FBOs and NGOs, supplemented by health authority vehicles. The elderly attendees were transported from their homes or from pick-up points to the clinic sites and back. Guaranteed transportation meant that the clients were also able to socialize with one another after their clinic visits.

During the clinics, trained medical teams provided basic physical checks and offered treatments where required. The mental health team screened the elderly and provided counseling and care. Social workers, nurses, and support staff then provided special care and noted when any specific material requirements such as walkers, bedpans, or urinals were required, and offered educational advice on diet and nutrition.

Formal clinical support included rehabilitative services, exercises, and on-site physiotherapy. The informal support sessions included massages and "pamper sessions" carried out by voluntary groups such as beauticians. A spirit of volunteerism was encouraged among the staff so that the whole program was executed at a minimal additional cost to the healthcare system. Usually, there were around 10 trained volunteers for the 50–70 elderly clients who attended the clinics (see Figures 6.2 and 6.3). Relevant data collected during the program was shared with health officials in the patients' neighborhood.

Impact of the Success Story

According to a self-assessed questionnaire, the mega-clinic visits generally had a positive impact, with 40% of the elderly clients feeling that they had greater knowledge of issues pertaining to their health following the visit. Such knowledge is known to have a number of flow-on benefits, including improved self-esteem, greater sense of control over health, and positive behavior change (Woodall et al., 2010). The organizations involved, which were also evaluated, were likewise empowered, with 35% stating that they had experienced an increased sense of community involvement, broadened social networking, and social support.

Again, according to subsequent evaluations, clients' subjective assessment of their quality of life (QoL) (WHO, 2006) also improved following their clinic visits, with the "good" and "very good" categories moving from 48% to 82% (Goel et al., 2003; Donald and Berman, 2015). The QoL scale was made up of a five-dimension scale that measured physical, material, and social and emotional well-being, as well as development and activity. It is pertinent to note that some of these assessments were done during the second round of the mega-clinics, while others were the result of follow-up by community nurses and other health workers attached to the health centers in the catchment area of the patients.

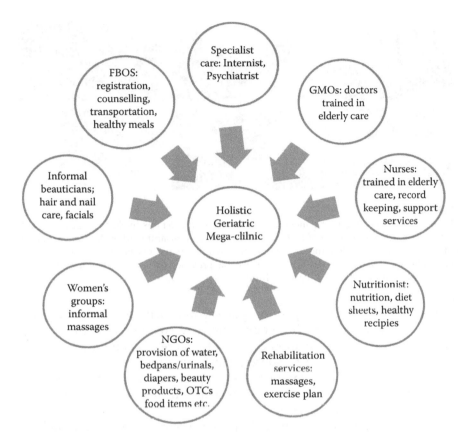

FIGURE 6.2
Schematic diagram showing the holistic, multidisciplinary approach to providing care for the elderly in the community through provision of geriatric mega-clinics.

The mega-clinics led to increased networking on an individual level as well as collaborative partnerships between previously isolated community organizations, thus improving communication and general efficiency.

In all, 2148 elderly clients were managed within 8 months of the start of the program. The clinics made care more accessible to the elderly in the community, many of whom tend to stay in their homes until their health deteriorates. The program brought a comprehensive service to them in their own communities, making it accessible and cost-effective (Rao, 1984).

A number of previously undiagnosed conditions, including diabetes mellitus and high blood pressure (3%) and respiratory tract infections (6%), were detected in individuals. Many patients were therefore able to benefit from early detection and treatment, avoiding long-term organ damage and disability.

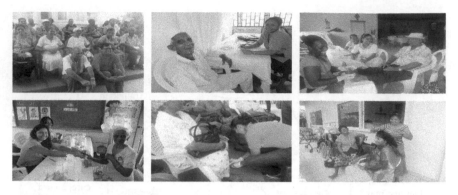

FIGURE 6.3
Photographs taken at geriatric mega-clinics at different locations in Berbice, Guyana. (a) Dr. Vishwa Mahadeo (then CEO of BRHA) and Dr. Leslie Ramsammy (then Minister of Health) with elderly patients attending a geriatric mega-clinic. (b and c) Consultation with medical and professional staff. (d–f) Additional treatments provided by volunteers to members of the geriatric population attending a mega-clinic.

There was a positive impact on participants' self-esteem. Many elderly persons living alone have little opportunity to communicate and socialize with their peers. Such isolation can lead to depression and associated loss of self-esteem. According to subsequent focus group evaluation sessions, the medical services and pamper sessions provided at the mega-clinics led many participants to experience an increase in their sense of self-esteem (Ramamurti and Jamuna, 1993).

The mega-clinics also facilitated efficient information sharing and data management with the local health services. Many individuals were able to get information regarding their official entitlements and received advice on various medico-legal matters.

Why Has the Selected Program Been Successful?

The BRHA approach to holistic and integrated care for the elderly in the community has been successful because it adds little in terms of cost to an already over-burdened healthcare system. The program not only provides much-needed care for a vulnerable and increasingly isolated group within our society, but it also builds self-esteem and provides a forum or meeting place where the elderly population can meet others in their own community to share views, ideas, and even advice, thereby fostering a sense of belonging.

Implementation and Replication

This is the first time that a mobile holistic approach to health and social services delivery has been successfully used to provide care to a specific population whose needs were, until now, largely unmet. This program involved collaboration between the public health system, volunteers, and community groups, including diverse organizations such as women's groups, NGOs, and FBOs. As this approach has been tested over an 8-month implementation period, and has proved, through qualitative assessment, to be highly successful in providing much-needed care in the local community, it should be considered as a template for effective care of the elderly.

Prospects for Further Success and Next Steps

Every government needs to take a systematic approach to addressing the needs of these unique, vulnerable, and ofter overlooked members of our community. Successful implementation of such programs requires a team effort, so governments should identify team players who can use the previously identified core strategies, such as partnerships with all the various entities, community involvement, empowerment, social inclusion, and capacity and confidence building. Potentially, various other marginalized populations could also be supported by the adoption of the aforementioned strategies.

Conclusion

The Care for the Elderly program initiated by the BRHA in Region 6, Guyana, has been a unique and successful program that has improved access to care, led to early detections of some ailments, and improved the quality of care and life of the elderly population served (Eng et al., 1997).

7

Mexico

Monitoring and Evaluation Strategy of Mexican Health Reform: Content, Conditions for Implementation, and Sustainability

Enrique Ruelas and Octavio Gómez-Dantés

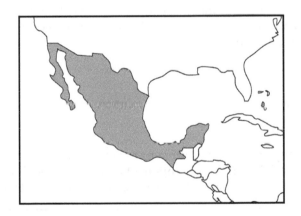

CONTENTS

Background

In 2003, the Mexican Congress approved a reform whose purpose was to expand social protection in health to half of the total population: those working in the informal sector of the economy, the self-employed, and the unemployed (Frenk et al., 2006). Between 2004 and 2013, more than 50 million people were enrolled in a new public insurance scheme called Popular Health Insurance or *Seguro Popular* (SP) (Knaul et al., 2012). This insurance scheme guarantees access to a package of 250 essential interventions delivered in public ambulatory facilities and general hospitals, and around 60 costly interventions, including treatment for cancer in children, cervical and breast cancer, HIV/AIDS, and heart attack in adults under 60. These interventions were selected making use of cost-effectiveness analysis, in addition to social acceptability criteria, which was introduced to conform to the norms of behavior of health professions and to broader social preferences ascertained through consultative processes (Frenk and Gómez-Dantés, 2009). The reform comprised several components including a monitoring and evaluation (M&E) strategy.*

The purpose of this chapter is to discuss this strategy by answering three basic questions: what was done (in terms of M&E)? What were the implementation requirements? And what remains of what we did? We conclude our chapter with a brief discussion of the main lessons of this M&E experience for developing countries.

What Was Done?

The M&E strategy of Mexican health reform was based on a very simple framework (see Figure 7.1) with three components for each of the three levels of the health system: the organizational level, the program level, and the policy level.

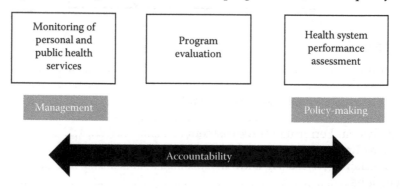

FIGURE 7.1
Monitoring and evaluation framework of Mexican health reform.

---

* This strategy was designed and implemented by a group headed by the authors of this chapter, who worked for the Ministry of Health, one as a vice minister and the other as director general for performance evaluation, which at the time was a newly created position within the ministry.

Our first objective was to monitor, at the organizational level, the way in which personal and public health services were being provided. Next, we planned to evaluate the most important programs of the administration. Finally, we wanted to assess the performance of the national health system and 32 state health systems. We assumed that M&E activities would be useful largely at the management level, and that program evaluation and assessment of health system performance would be useful for policy-making at the highest levels of the system. We also assumed that the information produced by M&E activities would be valuable for accountability purposes.

Monitoring of Personal and Public Health Services

In terms of the monitoring of health services, we had originally planned to design three observatories to monitor ambulatory services, hospital services, and public health services; however, there was only time and resources to monitor the performance of public hospitals. Three annual reports on the performance of public hospitals in Mexico, *Observatory of Hospital Services*, were published between 2003 and 2005 (Secretaría de Salud, 2004a, 2005a, 2006a). These reports offered information on resources and services provided by all public hospitals, which took into account the following:

- Patient and staff safety: including data on accreditation, mechanisms for the disposal of toxic waste, and hospital-acquired infections
- Quality: including information on the average length of stay, in addition to details of complications following a set of hospital interventions (births, C-sections, appendectomies, cholecystectomies, hernias, and pneumonia)
- Patient satisfaction

The sources of information for this report were the hospital discharge information system, which is one of the modules of the national health information system, along with ad hoc satisfaction and responsiveness surveys.

Program Evaluation

In terms of program evaluation, we conducted external evaluations of at least three important programs: Fair Start in Life, which was a program dealing with child and maternal health; National Crusade for Quality in Healthcare; and *Seguro Popular*, a new public health insurance scheme intended to provide social protection in health to the non-salaried population. The evaluations of the first two programs were designed and implemented by researchers from the National Institute of Public Health of Mexico. To evaluate SP, we hired a group of researchers from Harvard University to develop an observational evaluation and a randomized evaluation. The design and implementation of the controlled evaluation were monitored by an external advisory committee that included experts in evaluation of social programs from academic institutions, international organizations, and private foundations.

For the observational evaluation of SP, we followed the evolution of a set of indicators relating to health services utilization, responsiveness, effective coverage, and financial protection (Gakidou et al., 2006), simply by measuring the changes in the values of these indicators before and after the intervention. The problem with this type of evaluation is that it wasn't possible to attribute the changes in the values of these indicators to the intervention under study. For this reason, we also decided to do an external evaluation of SP using a randomized design, taking advantage of the fact that full enrollment in SP would take at least 7 years.

The original plan for the quasi-experimental evaluation involved taking a baseline measurement of selected variables related to the utilization of services and expenditure in healthcare in 2005 and follow-up measurements in 2006, 2008, and 2010. The advantage of this controlled design was that it allowed a longitudinal comparison between households receiving the intervention in an initial phase and those households receiving the interventions in future phases. We first identified 1000 paired health clusters (the population assigned to an ambulatory health unit) in seven states (see Figure 7.2). These clusters were matched on the basis of socioeconomic and demographic characteristics. We then randomly selected 100 paired clusters in areas where affiliation to SP was active. Fifty clusters were randomly selected to receive the intervention, which involved the promotion of affiliation to SP, in a first stage (treatment group) and the other 50 clusters, in a second stage (control group). In each cluster, we randomly selected 380 households, which were surveyed at baseline to collect information on several expected outcomes but focused initially on financial protection. The baseline measurement was done in 2005 and the first follow-up measurement in 2006. From this second measurement, we were able to determine that program resources were reaching the poor, that there was an increased utilization of health services by those enrolled in SP, and that there was a statistically significant reduction in catastrophic health expenditures in the treatment group (King et al., 2009).

Health System Performance Assessment

Finally, in terms of health system evaluation, the central idea was to use the World Health Organization (WHO) framework for the assessment of health

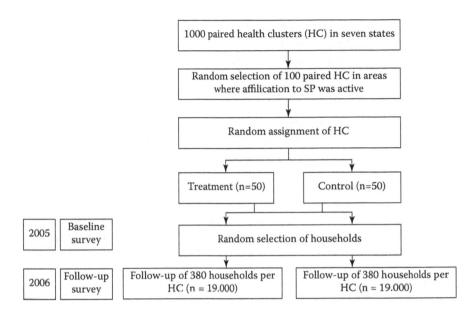

FIGURE 7.2
Controlled evaluation of *Seguro Popular*.

system performance to make periodical comparative assessments of the performance of national and state health systems, making use of health conditions, responsiveness, and fair financing indicators (Murray and Frenk, 2000). Our sources of information were the national information system, various national satisfaction and responsiveness surveys, and the national income and expenditure surveys, which provide information on household expenditure every 2 years. We published this information in five annual reports called *Mexico: Salud*, which were presented in a very well publicized event in Mexico City by the minister of health and, on three occasions, by the president of Mexico (Secretaría de Salud, 2002, 2003, 2004b, 2005b, 2006b).

What Was Required?

A number of factors helped us execute such an ambitious M&E strategy. The legal framework was accommodating: two laws were passed by Congress during that particular administration: the Access to Public Information and Transparency Law (2002) and the Social Development Law (2004). The latter created the National Evaluation Council, which was established to coordinate and monitor the evaluation of all social development programs in Mexico, which were mandatory from that date.

There was also a strong high-level commitment to transparency, accountability, and evaluation. Both the president of Mexico and the minister of health were convinced that transparency, accountability, and evaluation were crucial for democracy and essential for the success of public policies.

This commitment was translated into institutional, financial, and political support. The minister of health turned a small evaluation department nested in the General Directorate for Health Information into a General Directorate for Performance Evaluation, which was given institutional independence and a proper budget. We also received direct support from the minister of health to face and overcome resistance by those who were evaluated and, eventually, to promote the adoption of recommendations.

Strong design and hard evidence are essential components in the effective evaluation of services, programs, and policies, and we were able to overcome resistance through strong technical expertise. Our evaluation support team comprised two PhDs in epidemiology, three health economists, two experts in health systems, and one actuary. We also maintained strong links with academic institutions that provided technical advice and support, such as the Mexican Health Foundation, the National Institute of Public Health, and the Harvard School of Public Health.

What Remains of What We Did?

Ten years after its initial implementation, the M&E strategy remains in place; however, the strength of its various components is uneven. The evaluation of the personal and public health services component was improved during the subsequent political administration (2007–2012) with the addition of an observatory of ambulatory services. While still active, both components lost impetus after a new administration took over in 2013.

The program evaluation component remains in good shape. This is largely because the evaluation of social development programs is now mandatory. Nonetheless, because of budgetary constraints, the 2008 and 2010 follow-up rounds of the SP controlled evaluation were not implemented.

The comparative health system performance assessment was abandoned in 2007. In addition to the new administration's lack of interest in this type of evaluation, a significant number of civil servants familiar with the methodologies required to develop this kind of report abandoned the ministry of health following the change of government.

Although annual comprehensive reports, essential to the dissemination of evaluation results, were published during the 2006–2012 political administration, they were not well publicized, and were discontinued after the change of government in 2013. Somewhat surprisingly, however, a similar report was published at the end of 2015.

Conclusions

A number of conclusions can be drawn from the M&E experience of the recent Mexican health reform:

- M&E activities should be implemented early in the reform process; this gives the research the necessary longitudinal depth, so that results can be used to support and/or stimulate change.
- M&E initiatives demand high-level support to finance them, overcome resistance, and eventually promote the adoption of recommendations.
- The design and implementation of M&E strategies require broad technical expertise to generate reliable results.
- Meaningful change should be the final goal of M&E. However, it is usually difficult to achieve, especially in the context of a decentralized health system.
- Long-term sustainability of M&E efforts is an elusive goal and requires strong institutions and high social visibility.

While these lessons illustrate the successful establishment of an M&E system, a thorough impact analysis of the Mexican evaluation system is still needed.

Conclusions

8

The United States of America

The Use of Report Cards and Outcome Measurements to Improve the Safety of Surgical Care: The American College of Surgeons National Surgical Quality Improvement Program

Amy Showen and Melinda Maggard-Gibbons

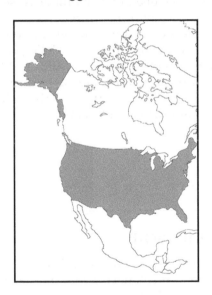

CONTENTS

Background

Over 30 million operative procedures are performed in the United States annually (United States Department of Health and Human Services, Centers for Disease Control and Prevention, National Center for Health Statistics, 2010). Unfortunately, postoperative adverse events occur frequently. Even in common, non-complex cases such as a colectomy, surgical site infections occur more than 10% of the time (Englesbe, 2010). These adverse events increase hospitalization length and cost. The cost of a surgical site infection is over US$27,000, while a ventilator-associated pneumonia can cost US$50,000 (American College of Surgeons [ACS], 2011; Dimick et al., 2004). Length of stay increases when complications occur, ranging from 3 to 11 days for respiratory events, for example (Damrauer et al., 2015; Silber et al., 2005). Nationally, there is great interest in providing optimal patient care. Since the Affordable Care Act was signed into law in 2010, payments have been reduced for adverse events such as central line infections and 30-day readmissions.

The largest and best-known intervention for reporting surgical outcomes in the United States is the American College of Surgeons National Surgical Quality Improvement Project (ACS NSQIP). This program provides risk-adjusted postoperative outcomes as benchmarks intended to spur local quality improvement efforts. This review summarizes the program's history, components, and evidence of its impact on surgical care.

Development of ACS NSQIP

ACS NSQIP grew, in part, out of efforts initiated by Veterans Affairs (VA) health system researchers and clinicians. In response to concerns about high complication rates, VA NSQIP was launched in 1994 to collect and report clinical variables and outcomes across all VA hospitals (Khuri et al., 1995).

With growing attention paid to surgical outcomes reporting, non-VA hospitals became interested in applying the VA experience more widely in the late 1990s. A pilot study in three civilian hospitals showed feasibility in the private sector (Fink et al., 2002). The ACS expanded efforts to a broader group of hospitals (14 sites), and in 2004, ACS NSQIP began (Khuri et al., 2008). Now more than 700 sites, or 15% of the almost 4500 hospitals in the United States, are participating. Because sites tend to be high volume, they account for a third of procedures performed nationally.

Components of the Program

ACS NSQIP consists of four main components:

1. A surgeon champion, at the participating site, helps establish and oversee the program locally.
2. A trained surgical clinical reviewer, generally a nurse, collects data on preoperative clinical variables and on 30-day outcomes.
3. Risk-adjusted models of expected mortality and morbidity are generated by procedure type.
4. Data are reported to the individual sites alongside masked data for the other sites.

The data are presented so that sites are displayed as being high outliers (worse than expected) or low outliers (better than expected) for each procedure and outcome. Lastly, the sites are encouraged to address and correct problem areas of clinical care.

While the responsibility for making changes remains with the sites, the administrative ACS NSQIP staff provide support via case reports, best practices, national meetings, and monthly conference calls with the surgeon champions and clinical reviewers. Staff connect sites with others who have made improvements in an area of interest. The annual national meeting serves as a critical forum for sites to discuss quality improvement efforts and successes. The majority of the participating hospitals send a representative each year, and most send more than one (the past meeting had 1400 attendees for approximately 700 participating sites).

Impact

Morbidity and Mortality

The rationale for how ACS NSQIP improves care is multifaceted. To improve care and reduce complications, surgeons must know the outcomes of their procedures. The data must be high quality and reliable, and the risk adjustment must be adequate to allay concerns about comparing "apples to oranges." This allows surgeons and hospitals to see how they compare in terms of outcomes, which promotes accountability and stimulates work on corrective measures. Of the sites surveyed, 59% were unaware of their hospital's adverse event rates, let alone how they compared with other hospitals, until after they had enrolled in ACS NSQIP (ACS, 2011).

Although no randomized trials have assessed the impact of ACS NSQIP participation, there is general evidence that the use of outcome reporting is associated with improvements in operative mortality and morbidity. This evidence includes the strong theoretical rationale for why it should work, the evidence that outcome reporting has improved surgical outcomes in other settings (e.g., the New York State CSRS), peer-reviewed studies, and numerous reports from ACS NSQIP sites of quality initiatives following the identification of high outlier status with ensuing, sometimes dramatic, improvements in those outcomes.

A 2015 study examining outcome trends among hospitals participating in ACS NSQIP for at least 3 years found that 69%, 79%, and 71% had improved their mortality, morbidity, and surgical site infection rates, respectively. The authors estimated annual reductions of 0.8% in mortality, 3.1% in morbidity, and 2.6% in surgical site infections. As these are annual reductions, the magnitude of quality improvement increases with time in the program (Cohen et al., 2016).

A longitudinal study of 118 hospitals participating in ACS NSQIP in 2005–2007 found similar results, with 66% and 82% of hospitals improving mortality and morbidity, respectively (Hall et al., 2009). The adjusted absolute difference in the observed-to-expected (O/E) ratio was –0.174 for mortality and –0.114 for morbidity (negative numbers mean less morbidity and mortality). Comparable results were seen across hospital type (academic vs. community, urban vs. rural, large vs. small, etc.). The number of high outliers (poorer performers) decreased over time and low outliers (better performers) increased. High outliers were more likely to improve and had larger mean changes in outcomes. A limitation of these longitudinal studies is the lack of a non-ACS NSQIP-participating control group, and the potential influence of "secular trends" cannot be ruled out.

Two studies came to less favorable conclusions about the utility of ACS NSQIP. The first study looked at national Medicare administrative data to evaluate whether participation was associated with improved outcomes compared with otherwise similar non-participating hospitals. After controlling for patient risk and preexisting temporal trends, the study did not find significant improvements in outcomes following enrollment in ACS NSQIP (Osborne et al., 2015). Likewise, the second study compared University Health System Consortium (UHC) hospitals with ACS NSQIP hospitals, and found no significant differences in outcomes over time between the two groups (Etzioni et al., 2015). A limitation of both studies is that this kind of analysis misses the one-on-one targeting of morbidities by specific hospitals. An individual hospital's improvement may be statistically and clinically significant, but undetectable when their data are aggregated with dozens of other hospitals, some of which may not elect to target the same outcomes. Furthermore, both studies are limited by their use of administrative data, which may inadequately capture the very complications that ACS NSQIP aims to help reduce (i.e., recent research found that ACS NSQIP identified

97% more surgical site infections and 100% more urinary tract infections than UHC) (Steinberg et al., 2008).

Cost Saving

The cost to participating hospitals includes an annual administrative fee to support the statistical methods and the generation of reports, a salary for the surgical clinical reviewer, and sometimes bonus payments to support the surgeon champion or quality improvement teams. Since the overarching goal of ACS NSQIP is to reduce complications, which are expensive, the business case for participating is that the program generates savings for the hospital. Reductions in one complication alone, surgical pneumonia, are estimated to have saved the VA US$9.3 million annually (Arozullah et al., 2003; Khuri et al., 1995). Furthermore, the longer an institution participates in ACS NSQIP, the more cost-effective the program becomes (Hollenbeak et al., 2011). Pre-post study design limits inference of causal relationships.

Harm

Few studies assessed the potential and actual harm of this program. A primary concern is that surgeons will avoid high-risk cases for fear of adversely affecting their outcome assessments (Omoigui et al., 1996). However, analyses found, on the contrary, that the severity of illness and comorbidities has increased (Hannan and Chassin, 2005). The longitudinal ACS NSQIP study found that the risk profile and illness severity for surgical patients in NSQIP-participating hospitals has increased over time (Hall et al., 2009). Thus, surgeons in NSQIP-participating hospitals do not appear to be declining to operate on higher-risk cases.

Transferability

It became apparent that a variety of program models were needed to accommodate different clinical settings, and ACS NSQIP has been flexible in terms of fitting these needs. Program options vary in terms of the number of variables collected, surgical specialty, targeted procedures, and case sampling. The specifics can be adapted for variable hospital sizes, large versus small collaboratives, vastly different modules for specific procedures, and even a new program for a specific surgical population—ACS NSQIP Pediatric for pediatric surgery reporting (Raval et al., 2011). Thus, a great deal of experiential evidence exists on how to implement ACS NSQIP in heterogeneous settings.

ACS NSQIP was developed for surgery. Like other surgical reporting systems, the conceptual model behind ACS NSQIP works best in situations where outcomes are measureable within a short time frame from the care that is meant to influence them, and there are reasonably good means to adjust for case-mix differences. This may not be generalizable to all of healthcare, such as primary care, chronic care, and so on. However, it may translate well to certain aspects of healthcare that share these properties, such as treatment provided in intensive care units.

9

Venezuela

Misión Barrio Adentro: Universal Health Coverage Efforts in Venezuela

Pedro Delgado and Luis Azpurua

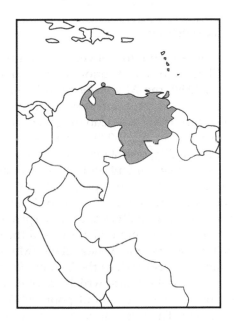

CONTENTS

Background

Since 1998, when the late Hugo Chavez was sworn in as president of Venezuela, more than a dozen ministers of health have come and gone. Chavez's successor, Nicolas Maduro, has already rotated ministers four times in less than 3 years (Wilson, 2015). The populist approach of Maduro's ruling United Socialist Party promised universal coverage as a constitutional right, but at present it is failing to provide even the most basic levels of care (Constitution of the Bolivarian Republic of Venezuela, 1999).

Details of the Success Story

Designed to improve access and to deliver on the promise of universal health coverage described in the constitution (Constitution of the Bolivarian Republic of Venezuela, 1999), the *Misión Barrio Adentro* (Inside the Ghetto Mission) national primary care program was launched by the Venezuelan government, with support from the Cuban government in 2003, under their cooperation agreement. In April 2003, a Chavez ally, the mayor of the Caracas Libertador Municipality, one of poorest and most densely populated areas of the city, reached an agreement with the Cuban government for the implementation of a primary care pilot project. In 2004, the program was expanded nationwide, with the public support of Chavez. Its overarching aims were to bring free, in situ healthcare to underprivileged populations, and to provide a primary care system that addressed the immediate healthcare needs of the many low-income Venezuelans (Muntaner et al., 2006). Additionally, the initiative would reduce the burden on the hospital system by reducing the need for hospital visits, which are often challenging due to the precarious transport infrastructure and poor public hospital management of access to treatment. The population welcomed the program, which challenged the prevailing "health as a commodity" paradigm, redefining it as a social right (Organización Panamericana de la Salud Oficina, Regional de la Organización Mundial de la Salud, 2006).

Misión Barrio Adentro sought to improve access and revolutionize the concept of health in communities across Venezuela, encompassing not only health, but also education, culture, sports, food security, and other areas of community need. It built on the Cuban experience where a similar program was put in place in 1984 when they launched the primary healthcare model plan, *del Médico y Enfermera de Familia* (Family Doctor's and Nurse's plan) (Delgado-García, 1996; Santos-Briones et al., 2004). The original model entailed healthcare workers living and working in the same place, as well as engaging with the community. While a combination of high levels of criminality in the *Misión Barrio Adentro* locations meant that shifts could only be scheduled during selected days and times, the fact that doctors were living in the community meant that they were considered *doctores del pueblo* (doctors of the people), and the community took care of them. This symbiosis meant that, early on, the program was embedded in and therefore valued by the community.

The development of physical infrastructure included both primary care centers, which provided care and sometimes living quarters for doctors, and diagnostic centers called *Centros Diagnósticos Integrales* (Figure 9.1). *Misión Barrio Adentro* facilities were categorized as Level I and Level II (launched in 2004) or Level III and Level IV (launched in 2006), depending on the number and degree of specialization of services provided in each. To provide a sense of scale, by May 2007, approximately 2700 Level I centers (out of 8500 planned) had been built, with a further 3300 under construction, along with 417 Level II comprehensive diagnostic centers (of 600 planned), 576 comprehensive rehabilitation centers (of 600 planned), and 22 advanced technology centers (of 35 planned) (Jones, 2008). These facilities were staffed by 31,439 healthcare professionals, including 1,234 Venezuelan and 15,356 Cuban doctors who had been brought in to expedite the implementation of the program. Many of the disproportionately large number of Cuban doctors were *médicos integrales comunitarios*, a type of primary-level physician without a counterpart in Venezuela. While these doctors initially practiced without Venezuelan medical licenses, medical practice laws were subsequently changed to accommodate them (Pan American Health Organization, 2006).

Despite the sometimes fraught nature of the working and living conditions in the barrios, enlisting local doctors to work in the program was reasonably

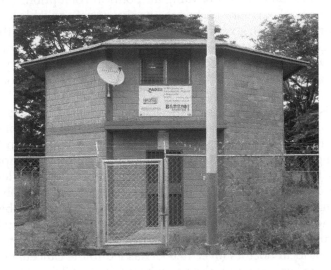

FIGURE 9.1
Misión Barrio Adentro primary care facility.

unproblematic. Because medical training is free in Venezuela, *Misión Barrio Adentro* was able to leverage the fact that residents are legally required to spend a year doing community service in primary care in order to have their medical degree conferred (República Bolivariana de Venezuela, 2011).

Details of the Impact of the Success Story

While it is estimated that around US$29.7 billion has been invested over the last 12 years, due to the lack of available data it is impossible to provide an accurate evaluation of the program's health impact (Transparencia Venezuela, 2015). The program reports 705 million visits during the 12 years of activity (2003–2015), but no epidemiological data are available to investigate either morbidity trends or quality measures for safety, efficiency, or effectiveness (Telesur, 2015). In 2014, the government claimed that over 10,000 clinics had been created; however, they provided no further statistics on effective access or health impact (Venezolana de Televisión, 2014). As of December 2014, it was estimated that 80% of *Misión Barrio Adentro* establishments had been abandoned, with a large number of Venezuelan doctors not participating due to insecurity, and most Cuban doctors having left the country given the existing financial crisis and challenging living conditions (La Patilla, 2014; Sonneland, 2016). Complaints are now ever-present (El Universal, 2014).

Sadly, the *Misión Barrio Adentro* program has failed just when it is most needed. A fatal combination of rampant political corruption, unsuccessful attempts to control currency exchange, the absence of a reliable legal system, long-standing populist government policies that disempower the population while generating dependency on the government, short-term planning, combined with the recent sharp decrease in oil prices (the country's finances depend almost exclusively on oil income), have all led to the worst crisis in Venezuela's history.

This crisis has seen complete financial collapse, food scarcity, shortages of medicines and medical supplies (including condoms), scarcity of water and electricity, and deepening social inequity, which has resulted in Venezuela experiencing the highest levels of criminality (including kidnappings and intentional homicides) in the world (The Economist, 2015; Gillespie, 2016; Sonneland, 2016). This crisis has had a dire effect on the Republic's healthcare system. Since Chavez took office, a number of communicable diseases such as dengue fever, malaria (the worst rates in the last 50 years), measles, and tuberculosis have reappeared; AIDS figures have skyrocketed; and the emigration of local doctors (over 13,000) has led to the cancellation of some residency programs due to lack of numbers (Boston Globe, 2015; Fox News Latino, 2014; Lohman, 2015; Pardo, 2014). In early 2015, it was estimated that only 35% of hospital beds were available and 50% of surgical theaters could not be used due to a lack of resources (Boston Globe, 2015).

Implementation: Transferability of the Exemplar

With recent global demographic and epidemiological trends placing huge pressures on health systems, upstream solutions that include prevention and easily accessible primary care have been factored into many countries' health policies. Hence, *Misión Barrio Adentro*'s innovative approach to comprehensive health and healthcare close to people's homes is (in theory) highly relevant and aligned with emerging global priorities around universal health coverage. However, without the ability to measure its impact, we cannot advocate for its transferability.

Conclusion

If the health of our population is to be improved and health systems are to be strengthened, adequate planning, implementation, and transparent and effective governance, along with effective measurement mechanisms, are required. As the failed *Misión Barrio Adentro* program has shown, without these we run the risk of wasting valuable limited resources that result in derelict physical infrastructures and disgruntled low-income populations who remain without access to much-needed health and care.

Part II

Africa

Stuart Whittaker

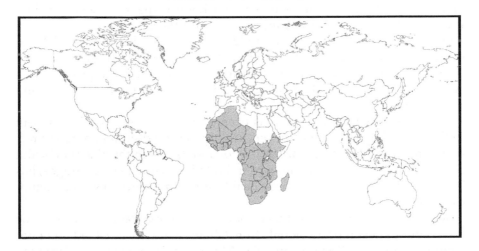

Africa is the world's second largest continent, with 54 independent countries and an estimated total population of 700 million. Although it is among the fastest growing regions, Africa's growth rate slowed to 3% in 2015, accompanied by a low per capita income growth, high population growth, and high rates of extreme poverty, estimated at 43% in 2012.

Africa is a low carbon-emitter, but suffers the most from the effects of climate change, through droughts, coastal erosion, and flooding. Rising violence and conflicts are causing increasing forced displacement, along with trafficking, piracy, and religious extremism. The risk of pandemics is high, and the lessons of the Ebola crisis highlight the importance of developing strong health systems and supporting regional disease surveillance and coordination. South Africa, with its well-developed infrastructure and deep-water ports, is the economic powerhouse of Africa south of the Sahara Desert.

Lizo Mazwai, Grace Labadarios, Bafana Msibi, and Stuart Whittaker describe the legislative reforms that have been implemented to provide equity in healthcare and have resulted in the establishment of the Office of Health Standards Compliance (OHSC). This organization is required to inspect South Africa's 4010 health establishments every 4 years to determine their compliance with a minimum set of quality standards, promulgated as regulations, to ensure the provision of quality healthcare services.

From Namibia, a neighboring country of South Africa, Apollo Basenero, Christine S. Gordon, Ndapewa Hamunime, Joshua Bardfield, and Bruce Agins tell the story of how the Ministry of Health and Social Services has built a national quality program, using their HIV quality-management program, as the platform for spreading quality management throughout the public health system.

The Economic Community of West African States is a solid geographical bloc of 15 states from Nigeria in the east to Mauritania in the west. As a result of their respective colonial histories, these countries are divided into French-speaking states, like Guinea, and English-speaking states, including Nigeria, Ghana, Liberia, Sierra Leone, and the Gambia. In this region, an outbreak of Ebola virus began in December 2013, where a total of 28,616 confirmed, probable, and suspected Ebola cases were reported with 11,310 deaths. Shamsuzzoha Syed and Edward Kelley describe the process from recovery to resilience in the Ebola-affected countries of Guinea, Liberia, and Sierra Leone.

In oil-rich Nigeria, the focus has been on various systems improvement initiatives to improve its health services, the most important being the recognition of the value of the private sector and its role in the Nigerian health sector as a whole. A key initiative, as indicated by Emmanuel Aiyenigba, has been the revitalization of primary healthcare with a move toward demand-driven health delivery.

Sodzi Sodzi-Tettey, Richard Selormey, and Cynthia Bannerman describe the exodus of health professionals from Ghana, a heavily indebted and poor country, to mainly Western countries. This brain drain took place from the 1990s to mid-2000s. The authors describe the efforts by the government of Ghana to arrest it and the impact that this had on improving the health of citizens and the health system in general.

The small landlocked central African countries of Rwanda and Burundi form part of an economic union of countries in the central African region. Roger Bayingana and Edward Chappy describe how in Rwanda, after the 1994 genocide against the Tutsi, different health system initiatives have been put in place to improve health service provision. These included community-based health insurance, performance-based financing, a community health worker program, e-health technologies, and quality improvement methodologies. They also describe the associated role of the Economic Development and Poverty Reduction Strategy 2013–2018 in bringing about the accelerated attainment of the Millennium Development Goals, increased access to healthcare services, and the reduction in financial catastrophes due to out-of-pocket expenditure for healthcare.

10

Ghana

Arresting the Brain Drain in Ghana

Sodzi Sodzi-Tettey, Richard Selormey, and Cynthia Bannerman

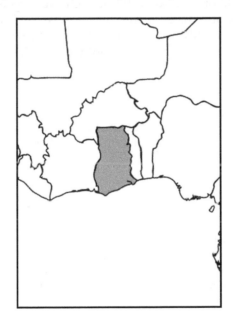

CONTENTS

Introduction

By 2001, Ghana was declared a heavily indebted and poor country (HIPC) (International Monetary Fund, 2001). Like other countries, Ghana had signed up to the United Nation (UN) Millennium Project Development Goals, a set of development goals to be achieved between 1990 and 2015. Among other challenges, the planning and management of human resources were identified as the weakest link in the quest by these HIPC countries to achieve equity and cost-effective funding mechanisms (Martinez and Martineau, 2002).

Ghana, a country of some 26 million people, is now a low-to-middle-income country. Although Ghana did not achieve targets in maternal and child health, the country made significant progress. By 2014, Ghana's under-five and maternal mortality rates had both been reduced to half of their 1990 baselines (see Table 10.1). Among pregnant women, 74% now deliver under

TABLE 10.1

Ghana Country Profile

Population and Health	1990s	2014
Total population	17 million	25.9 million
GDP per capita in USD	403	1858
Poor as percentage of total population	51.7%	24.2%
Life expectancy at birth	56.8 years	61 (2012)
Under-five mortality rate per 1000	119	60
Infant mortality rate per 1000	66	41
Maternal mortality rate (per 100,000 live births)	760	380
Immunization coverage: measles	64%	89%
Births attended by skilled staff	44%	74%
Health System and Expenditure		
Total expenditure on health per capita (public and private) in USD	19	100
Total expenditure on health (public and private) as % of GDP	3.1	5.4
Ghana Government total expenditure on health in USD	100 million	1500 million (2013)
Health budget as percentage of total government spending	7%	11%
Of this: donors' share	30%	10%
Number of doctors	1115	3016
Number of nurses	16,000	28,000

Source: From World Bank, Ghana Statistical Service, demographic and health surveys extracted from DANIDA. (2016). Ghana-Denmark 1994–2016: A healthy partnership: An account of 22 years of life-saving cooperation in the health sector. Retrieved from http://um.dk/en/~/media/Ghana/Documents/Ghana%20E-Paper%20UK%20health.pdf

the care of skilled attendants. HIV prevalence is low at 1.85%, down from 3.6% in 2003. Overall life expectancy has consistently increased for both men and women, from 56.8 to 61 years. By 2013, government spending in the health sector had increased by 1400% from US$100 million in the mid-1990s to US$1500 million.

Human resources are critical for the delivery of quality health services, and the shortage of human resources was identified as the most critical public health constraint in achieving the UN Millennium Development Goals. A good human resource base is also the foundation for universal health coverage. Improvements in the planning and management of human resources in the health sector were critical to the improvements recorded by Ghana. In this chapter, we explore the exodus of health professionals from Ghana to mainly Western countries (brain drain) that took place from the 1990s to the mid-2000s, and the efforts by the government of Ghana and stakeholders to arrest this phenomenon.

Brain Drain: Patterns Observed in the Early 1990s

Brain drain, according to Mutume (2003), is said to occur when a country becomes short of skills because people with such expertise emigrate. Lowell and Findlay (2001) also define brain drain as the "emigration abroad of tertiary educated persons at such levels and for such durations that their losses are not offset by their remittances home, by transfer of technology, or by investment or trade from the recipient country." According to the International Organization for Migration, at perhaps the height of the brain drain in the early to mid-1990s, Africa lost one-third of its human capital, including over 20,000 doctors, university lecturers, engineers, and other professionals. At the same time, Africa spent US$4 billion per year (representing 35% of total official development aid to the continent) to employ some 100,000 Western experts performing functions generically described as technical assistance (African Renaissance Ambassador Corporation, n.d.).

During the 1980s, Ghana lost 60% of its medical doctors, with around 600–700 Ghanaian physicians reportedly practicing in the United States alone—a figure that at the time represented roughly 50% of the total population of doctors in Ghana. A 2005 survey established that 60% of doctors trained in Ghana left the country (DANIDA, 2016).

In 2006, Ghana's doctor to population ratio was 1:14,733, while the health sector workforce density per 1000 population in Africa was recorded by the World Health Organization at 2.3 compared with 24.8 in the Americas (Alhassan et al., 2013).

Reasons for Brain Drain: Pull and Push Factors

According to Dovlo (2003), "push" factors are those factors that occur within the country of origin, motivating professionals to leave. "Pull" factors, on the other hand, are the deliberate and/or unintended actions of the recipient country (i.e., policies) that attract health professionals from other countries.

These pull factors were found to be influenced by demographic changes including aging populations in some of these recipient countries. Other pull factors were the generally increased demand for health professionals, the use of a common language, and similarities in professional systems in originating and recipient countries. The push factors included low remuneration and poor economic conditions, poor working conditions, and low job satisfaction, inability to acquire social amenities, and poor governance or perceived poor governance (Clarke, 2003; Dovlo, 2003).

Effects of Brain Drain

In Ghana, the brain drain resulted in a severe shortage of health professionals and maldistribution of the remaining staff, and it contributed to the poor health indicators at that time.

In addition to the high doctor–population ratios, increased workload, burnout, and reduced quality of care, there was also weak or poor supervision from more experienced colleagues and great financial loss to the host countries. Between 1986 and 1995, Ghana lost an estimated US$5,960,000 in tuition costs alone from the 61% of medical graduates who emigrated from just one medical school (Dovlo and Nyonator, 1999). These losses from the school aggregated costs from training from primary to tertiary, lost contributions to gross domestic product (GDP) and taxes, the costs of illness/morbidity caused or aggravated by staff shortages, and costs arising from substituting less-qualified staff or importing expatriates to fill the vacant posts (Dovlo, 2003).

Ghanaian expatriates, on the other hand, remitted almost US$400 million annually to Ghana. These remittances represented the fourth highest foreign exchange earning to the nation (Amuakwa-Mensah and Nelson, 2014).

Interventions

Nyonator et al. (2004) published a number of recommendations for remedying the situation. These included increasing training opportunities; improving salaries; providing cheap mortgages, car loans, and educational subsidies; and increasing the age of retirement (WHO, 2005b). At the national level, various conversations were held among professional associations, within the political leadership, and among development partners on how to reverse the brain drain. Two interventions proved critical. These were the establishment of a postgraduate medical college in 2004 and significant increases in the salaries of health professionals in Ghana in 1998, 2006, and 2010.

Allowances and Wages

In 1998, the government introduced the additional duty hours allowance (ADHA) to compensate health professionals for long hours of work. As these were not sustainable, the Ministry of Health commissioned further health sector salary reforms in 2005.

In 2006, government rolled out a new health sector salary structure, followed in 2010 by the single spine salary structure, targeting the wider public sector. Both structures had embedded within them a premium component, which paid health professionals an extra allowance above the base pay in acknowledgment of their scarce skills (Sodzi-Tettey, 2015). Overall, studies conducted by the World Bank in Ghana showed that higher wages reduced attrition from the public sector payroll. It estimated that "a ten percent increase in wages decreases annual attrition from the public payroll by 0.9–1.6 percentage points (from a mean of eight percentage points) among 20–35 year-olds" (Antwi and Phillips, 2012) (Figure 10.1).

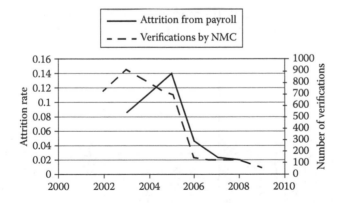

FIGURE 10.1
Migration and attrition of nurses from Ghana. (From Antwi, J. and Phillips, D. (2012). *Wages and Health Worker Retention in Ghana*. World Bank. Retrieved from https://openknowledge. worldbank.org/bitstream/handle/10986/13581/691070WP00PUBL0GhanaMigrationSalary. pdf?sequence=1)

Establishment of a Postgraduate Medical College

In 2004, the Ghana College of Physicians and Surgeons (GCPS) was established to provide an avenue for doctors seeking to specialize and hone their professional and academic skills. Figure 10.2 shows the increasing enrollments in the college between 2004 and 2012.

In 2014, Amuakwa-Mensah and Nelson assessed the perception among the residents of the college of the quality of training. The results showed that most of the interviewed residents were highly satisfied with the quality of the clinical curriculum and instruction and the duration of the program. However, fewer were satisfied with the availability of study resources to enhance studies (Amuakwa-Mensah and Nelson, 2014).

These findings have possible implications for the future direction of the brain drain, given that satisfaction with specialist training programs significantly impacts the decision to leave or stay (Amuakwa-Mensah and Nelson, 2014) (Table 10.2).

Other Interventions

A review of the 2007–2011 human resource strategy of the Ministry of Health shows other interventions that have been implemented. These include

- Establishment of a ministerial committee on human resources to allocate quotas of health graduates to the various service agencies
- Establishment of health training institutions in each of the regions, with emphasis on nursing and midwifery training programs

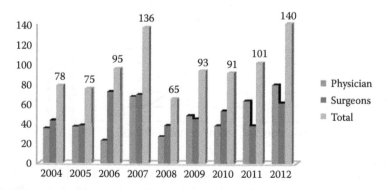

FIGURE 10.2
Residents (membership) enrollment, September 2012.

TABLE 10.2

Physician Opinion of Program Quality and Duration

	Rating	Frequency	Percent
Quality of clinical curriculum	Below expectation	6	11.5
	Normal	34	65.4
	Well prepared	12	23.1
	Total	52	100
Quality of clinical instruction	Below expectation	6	14.3
	Normal	30	71.4
	Well supervised	6	14.3
	Total	42	100
Satisfied with the duration of	No	6	11.5
program	Yes	46	88.5
	Total	52	100

Source: Amuakwa-Mensah, F. and Nelson, A. A. (2014). *Journal of Education and Practice,* 5, 5. Retrieved from http://pub.epsilon.slu.se/11597/11/amukava_mensah_f_ayesua_ama_n_150116.pdf

- Increased intake into the community health training schools and production and recruitment of community health nurses from 2009
- Formulation of the policy of posting 70% of regionally trained new graduates within their originating region
- Revitalization of the health workforce observatory as the principal stakeholder forum for policy dialogue and coordination
- Piloting of the human resource information system in the northern region to enable national scale-up
- Development of staffing norms
- Establishment of advisory boards for health training institutions
- Establishment of an allied health task force to begin the regulation of allied health professionals

Current Situation

After more than 2 decades of extensive brain drain by Ghanaian health professionals, the migration of health workers has finally slowed. Between 1999 and 2014, the population to doctor ratio has improved from 15,246:1 to 8587:1, while the population to nurse ratio has also improved from 1062:1 to 925:1. These numbers are derived from Table 10.1, which was created by DANIDA (Denmark's International Development Agency) in 2016 as a composite from three data sources: the World Bank, the Ghana Statistical Service, and the demographic and health surveys. This is based on an account of 22 years of partnership in the health sector by DANIDA.

While the interventions outlined previously appear to have stemmed the brain drain, inequity in the distribution of health workers continues to be a major challenge. According to Snow et al. (2011), career development opportunities are the strongest factors influencing doctors to stay in urban centers. To address this, they propose that physicians perform short-term service in rural areas linked to special mentoring and/or training, and leading to career advancement (Snow et al., 2011).

Continually increasing wages are also a problem for the government, with salaries reportedly making up almost 90% of the health budget. One challenge, it would appear, has been replaced with another.

To counter these difficulties, the current human resource strategy and implementation plan has outlined the following policy thrusts: increase the production and quality of middle-level health professionals, ensure equity in the distribution of health workers, and improve health worker productivity (Ministry of Health [Ghana], 2013).

Conclusion

Arresting the brain drain has been achieved by creating postgraduate training opportunities and enhancing the compensation packages of health professionals. There is more to be done, however, particularly when it comes to redressing inequitable distribution and dealing with increasing salary costs.

11

Namibia

A Public Health Approach to Quality Management:
How a Disease-Specific Improvement Program Propelled
a National Health-Systems-Wide Quality Program
in Namibia

Apollo Basenero, Christine S. Gordon, Ndapewa Hamunime, Joshua
Bardfield, and Bruce Agins

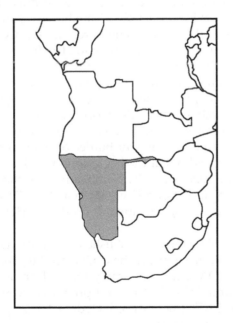

CONTENTS

Background

With a population of approximately 2.4 million, Namibia is an expansive country located in southwestern Africa bordering the Atlantic coast. Independence from South Africa was achieved in 1990, preceded by a formal constitution adopted in that same year. Namibia's HIV epidemic is generalized: transmission primarily occurs through heterosexual and mother-to-child transmission. The HIV prevalence rate in adults aged 15–49 is 13.3% (12.2–14.5%) and the number of people living with HIV in Namibia is 210,000 (200,000–230,000) (Joint United Nations Programme on HIV/AIDS [UNAIDS], 2015).

Distinguished by a decentralized model of healthcare delivery, the Ministry of Health and Social Services (MoHSS) in Namibia is organized into four levels. In 1999, the National AIDS Coordination Program (NACOP) was established to oversee the different sectors responding to HIV. In 2002, the Directorate of Special Programs (DSP) was established within NACOP. Access to antiretroviral therapy (ART) and mainstreaming of HIV programs have occurred in all sectors with the coordination of government offices, ministries/agencies, regions, nongovernmental organizations, and faith-based organizations through MoHSS. The private sector and various development partners also play a distinct role in addressing the causes and reducing the burden of HIV/AIDS.

ART was rapidly rolled out at the beginning of 2003 and was available in all state hospitals by 2006. By 2006, Namibia had reached its World Health Organization "3 by 5" targets, and by 2009, more than 70,000 adults and children were treated, with 135,000 patients enrolled in HIV care in the public sector.

In 2003, the Namibia MoHSS established a quality assurance (QA) unit (see Figure 11.1) as a subunit under the Undersecretary for Health and Social Welfare Policy. The QA unit was mainly focused on audit, accountability, and setting standards. Initially, this unit primarily oversaw infection, prevention, and control (IPC) activities, including the implementation of the medical injection safety project.

Introduction of Quality Improvement in Namibia

The principles of quality improvement (QI) and quality management (QM) in Namibia were not formally introduced until 2007, within the context of a

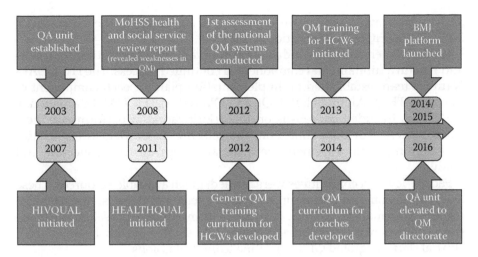

FIGURE 11.1
Timeline of national QM structures and programs in Namibia.

disease-specific program focusing on HIV, when the MoHSS, with support from the U.S. President's Emergency Plan for AIDS Relief (PEPFAR), piloted a HIV-specific QM program, HIVQUAL-Namibia. Independent of the QA unit and overseen by the HIV unit in the DSP, HIVQUAL-Namibia was designed to build capacity and systems for HIV care and treatment to scale-up ART and accelerate quality of care for people living with HIV (PLHIV) using modern improvement methods.

Development and Implementation of a Disease-Specific QI Program

HIVQUAL-Namibia was initiated in 16 clinics, with performance measurement (PM) data collection and QI project implementation expanding to 38 HIV care and treatment facilities in all 34 districts. Ten consecutive rounds of performance data collection were submitted between July 2007 and March 2013, representing more than 37,000 individual patient charts sampled across review periods. During this period, aggregate mean improvement was achieved in 10 of 11 performance measures between the first reported review period and the most recent. Core areas of HIV care and treatment demonstrating improvement included ART to eligible patients ($p < .00008$), ART adherence assessment ($p < .01$), CD4 monitoring ($p < .03$), and cotrimoxazole preventive therapy ($p < .01$), among others (Bardfield, 2015; HEALTHQUAL International, 2015).

Leadership engagement and support for planning were critical first steps and remain a fundamental component of continued success. The HIVQUAL-Namibia team established an implementation plan for each component of the HEALTHQUAL model: PM, QI, and QM (HEALTHQUAL International, 2016). This included consensus on the prioritization of performance measures, systems for data collection, the selection of participating facilities and training in improvement methods, and steps for data collection and analysis.

Facility-level QI committees were formed, given available resources. These teams were composed of multidisciplinary teams of doctors, nurses, pharmacists, pharmacy assistants, data clerks, community counselors, and consumer representatives in some facilities. At smaller health facilities, HIV clinical staff integrated QI into routine team discussions.

A process for PM was instituted. Measures based on national guidelines and globally accepted standards of care were adapted to the existing health information technology (IT) platform and electronic patient-monitoring systems (ePMS). Data collection and reporting occur biannually, with results used to drive future improvement activities at both facility and national levels. The MoHSS uses aggregated data to produce national benchmarking reports. Performance scores are reported as mean clinic rates and trended longitudinally to determine national priorities for HIV care and treatment.

To build and sustain the national program, coaching and mentoring visits are routinely conducted by national and regional program managers. Facility teams apply skills and knowledge gained from a cadre of national improvement coaches to adapt methods and strategies to address local and national priorities for HIV care, including skills building for data collection, reporting, and analysis.

The MoHSS has committed leadership and resources in support of peer learning strategies to spread improvement knowledge and skills to achieve scale-up. The national program convenes regional QM groups and improvement workshops at the end of each performance review period as an approach to share both data and improvement strategies, while building capacity at facility level for improvement skills. These peer exchange sessions bolster local improvement knowledge and the dissemination of successful implementation strategies. Improvement workshops include expert plenaries, peer learning through group work, presentation of performance data, writing and updating of improvement work plans, and dedicated time for formal QM planning. The MoHSS leadership is present at these meetings as a demonstration of support for the national quality program, where they also have an opportunity to respond to emergent policy issues.

Evolution from a Disease-Specific Model to a National, Health-Sector-Wide Quality Program

Realization of Namibia's national quality program evolved from a commitment to establish systems for routine improvement in the national HIV care and treatment program. In 2011, this, in turn, catalyzed a focus on expanding the (HIV-specific) HIVQUAL model to a generalized public health approach to quality (HEALTHQUAL) across the public health system through the creation of key formal administrative structures. Principles from this disease-specific model were successfully integrated into the larger system. This transition was further driven by a 2012 assessment of national QM systems undertaken by the MoHSS (MoHSS [Namibia], 2014). Components not present in the national QM system that were identified as important included

- A national quality management policy and strategic plan to guide QM activities
- A systematic approach to quality improvement activities
- QM focal people at all levels of healthcare to support QI initiatives
- A unified understanding of what quality means in most of the healthcare facilities
- A culture of quality care embraced by all healthcare workers
- Systems for appraisal and reward of healthcare workers who excel in their daily activities
- Meaningful consumer engagement in QI activities
- Quality indicators for most of the services in the MoHSS

These findings led directly to the following developments:

- A QA technical working group (TWG) composed of a multidisciplinary team, including the MoHSS and stakeholders, was established to provide expert guidance to the QA unit.
- The MoHSS drafted a national QM policy and strategic plan, which, when approved, will be administered through the QM directorate.
- To support scale-up and spread, a QM training curriculum for health workers was developed targeting core components of QM, including QI methods, principles of PM, QI project implementation, improvement tools and resources, and consumer involvement, among others.
- The curriculum has been used since 2013 to train healthcare managers. A total of 180 healthcare managers have been trained in all 14 regions. In addition, 250 healthcare workers at the implementation level have been trained. The curriculum is accredited by the Health

Professionals Councils of Namibia (HPCNA) with 28 continuous education units, which is an incentive for healthcare workers to participate.

- A QM coaches' curriculum has been developed and will be deployed to train health workers as regional QM coaches to support the peer learning model described previously.

The MoHSS established the Medical Doctors and Dentists Annual Forum, an annual meeting of clinical providers, to exchange knowledge about clinical care in the health system with important opportunities to integrate quality as a thematic area of focus. One example of the aforementioned public health approach is the initiation of an ongoing national maternal and child health (MCH) QI project designed to develop concise, written standard operating procedures (SOPs) and audit tools to ensure consistent management of obstetrics and gynecology conditions. In addition, the project will establish an improvement process to measure performance and ensure that QI efforts focus on reducing maternal mortality, targeting its most common causes. To date, nine MCH SOPs have been developed, each with audit tools and training materials to address the common causes of maternal mortality and morbidity. The MoHSS has also developed key guidelines to ensure the provision of quality healthcare services. Four essential guidelines were identified in 2012 (MoHSS [Namibia], 2015). All four guidelines were launched by the Minister of Health in August 2015 and disseminated to all healthcare facilities.

Achievement of a National Quality Program in Namibia

Applying the HIV QM program as the model, the Namibia MoHSS has successfully built a national QM program using HIV as the platform to spread quality throughout the public health system. Notably, this includes the development of a national QM policy and strategic plan through the establishment of a formal QM directorate (see Figure 11.2).

The QM directorate will be responsible for developing a national QM framework that covers each level of healthcare services in the MoHSS to ensure that the highest quality of care levels are achieved and maintained. The QM directorate structure was carefully designed to ensure major components required for a successful QM program are incorporated, including PM, QI, and QM. The overall goal of the program is to strengthen QM systems at all health administration levels in which the QM directorate will oversee quality of care at multiple levels.

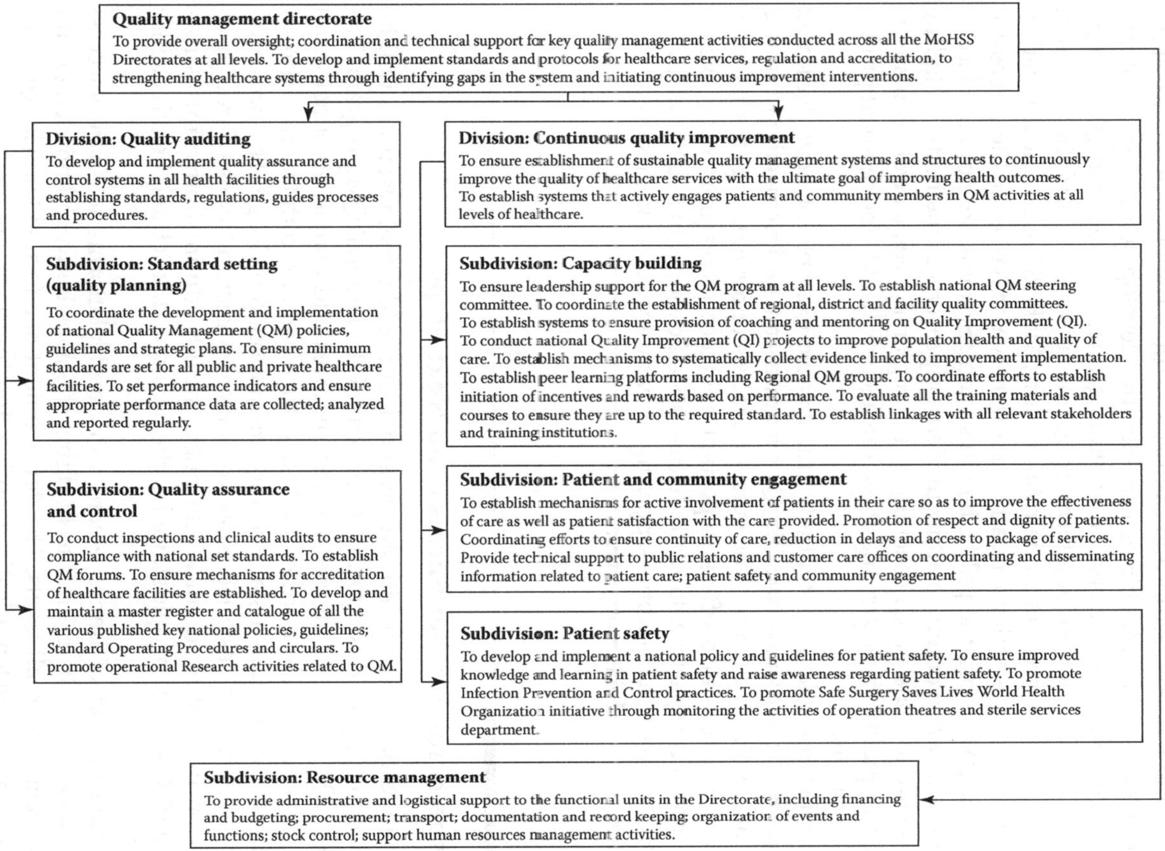

Quality management directorate

To provide overall oversight; coordination and technical support for key quality management activities conducted across all the MoHSS Directorates at all levels. To develop and implement standards and protocols for healthcare services, regulation and accreditation, to strengthening healthcare systems through identifying gaps in the system and initiating continuous improvement interventions.

Division: Quality auditing

To develop and implement quality assurance and control systems in all health facilities through establishing standards, regulations, guides processes and procedures.

Subdivision: Standard setting (quality planning)

To coordinate the development and implementation of national Quality Management (QM) policies, guidelines and strategic plans. To ensure minimum standards are set for all public and private healthcare facilities. To set performance indicators and ensure appropriate performance data are collected, analyzed and reported regularly.

Subdivision: Quality assurance and control

To conduct inspections and clinical audits to ensure compliance with national set standards. To establish QM forums. To ensure mechanisms for accreditation of healthcare facilities are established. To develop and maintain a master register and catalogue of all the various published key national policies, guidelines; Standard Operating Procedures and circulars. To promote operational Research activities related to QM.

Division: Continuous quality improvement

To ensure establishment of sustainable quality management systems and structures to continuously improve the quality of healthcare services with the ultimate goal of improving health outcomes. To establish systems that actively engages patients and community members in QM activities at all levels of healthcare.

Subdivision: Capacity building

To ensure leadership support for the QM program at all levels. To establish national QM steering committee. To coordinate the establishment of regional, district and facility quality committees. To establish systems to ensure provision of coaching and mentoring on Quality Improvement (QI). To conduct national Quality Improvement (QI) Projects to improve population health and quality of care. To establish mechanisms to systematically collect evidence linked to improvement implementation. To establish peer learning platforms including Regional QM groups. To coordinate efforts to establish initiation of incentives and rewards based on performance. To evaluate all the training materials and courses to ensure they are up to the required standard. To establish linkages with all relevant stakeholders and training institutions.

Subdivision: Patient and community engagement

To establish mechanisms for active involvement of patients in their care so as to improve the effectiveness of care as well as patient satisfaction with the care provided. Promotion of respect and dignity of patients. Coordinating efforts to ensure continuity of care, reduction in delays and access to package of services. Provide technical support to public relations and customer care offices on coordinating and disseminating information related to patient care; patient safety and community engagement

Subdivision: Patient safety

To develop and implement a national policy and guidelines for patient safety. To ensure improved knowledge and learning in patient safety and raise awareness regarding patient safety. To promote Infection Prevention and Control practices. To promote Safe Surgery Saves Lives World Health Organization initiative through monitoring the activities of operation theatres and sterile services department.

Subdivision: Resource management

To provide administrative and logistical support to the functional units in the Directorate, including financing and budgeting; procurement; transport; documentation and record keeping; organization of events and functions; stock control; support human resources management activities.

FIGURE 11.2

Directorate: QM organogram with functions.

Leadership continues to be a core contributing element to Namibia's success in building a truly national QM program in the public health arena. Specifically, this has included resource support to implement the work and visible participation in key quality events, such as healthcare worker training and the annual Doctors and Dentists Forum. Promotion of quality at the highest levels of the MoHSS has enabled the development/adaption of systems for measurement, technical working groups, and regional QM groups, all of which are vital to long-term programmatic success and the spread of knowledge for improvement. Fundamentally, MoHSS has promoted institutionalization of the national quality program, which has led to the successful spread of QM across the public health system. Systems are now in place to train healthcare workers to apply modern improvement methods, including a structure to scale-up QI coaching at the regional level, as well as plans to integrate quality into curricula at Namibia's new health and medical professional schools.

Namibia provides a potentially translatable example of how dedicated resources for a disease-specific QI program can be leveraged to build a national quality program. The current process of formalizing this national quality structure also offers important evidence of programmatic expansion from a compartmentalized, disease-specific model to a national public health approach to quality—applying already tested strategies to achieve acceleration of MoHSS objectives.

Prospects for Further Success and Next Steps

Human resources for health are essential, and additional resources will be needed to support this critical component of the national QM program. The current QA unit is understaffed and requires additional personnel at all administrative levels. Further, high staff turnover at health facilities threatens local success and sustained implementation knowledge. The proposed QM directorate is designed to address these structural issues through its focus on integrating quality into public health administrative infrastructure with QM focal people staffed at the regional, district, and health facility levels.

Documentation of improvement work and platforms to share successful strategies will be critical to bridging the gaps between knowledge and implementation at all levels. The development of a formal knowledge management plan—systematically documenting improvement work, synthesizing findings, and disseminating lessons learned locally and throughout the global improvement community—would facilitate this process.

Conclusion

The case of Namibia offers valuable insight into how a disease-specific QI program can evolve into a national quality program supported by key systems, administrative structures, and functions. The imminent launch of the QM directorate should allow the MoHSS to accelerate quality of care across the public health system by ensuring the systematic and coordinated implementation of national efforts across diseases and health conditions under one national agency, driven by a "vision of shared values, attitudes, and beliefs, comprising a 'culture' of QI throughout the MoHSS" (MoHSS, [Namibia], n.d.).

12

Nigeria

Removing the Imaginary Walls That Divide and Limit

Emmanuel Aiyenigba

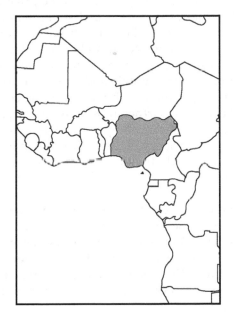

CONTENTS

Background

Nigeria, a country comprising about 177 million people from 371 different ethnic groups, has come a long way in efforts to build resilient healthcare. While health system architecture makes health planning and delivery a herculean task at every level of governance—even more at the points of delivery—the last decade has seen various systems improvement initiatives despite ongoing political upheaval and economic instability (Nigeria Local, 2014; World Bank, 2016c; WHO, 2010b).

Important initiatives include the development of the National Health Bill, passed into law in 2014, which recognized that the private health sector is a crucial component in the restructuring and strengthening of the Nigerian health sector. The private sector had previously not been regarded as a strong player in the push to improve the Nigerian health system. However, despite the relatively excellent results achieved in the private-driven health sector, a lack of collaboration between public and private sectors has contributed to the further worsening of the health indices in the country. Opening up the platform for collaborative partnerships between the government and the private health sector at various levels appears to have had a positive impact on the effectiveness and efficiency of the health system in a number of ways, including the provision of additional capital, alternative management, and implementation skills, along with better identification of needs and optimal use of resources.

The traditional modes of health delivery in Nigeria, comprising a tiered system with very weak structures of communication, have also contributed to the dearth of services. Poor road networks and a skewed distribution of healthcare professionals have left the needy rural population exposed and inadequately catered for. With the creation of a conducive policy environment, health initiatives between state governments and private sector players have proven effective in combating some of the challenges within the Nigerian health space.

Current Efforts to Enhance Care

The Nigerian Federal Ministry of Health (FMoH) has the mandate to formulate, disseminate, promote, implement, monitor, and evaluate the health policies of the federal government of Nigeria (National Health Act, 2014 [Federal Republic of Nigeria]). Current efforts at the FMoH in Nigeria include reforms of the National Primary Healthcare Development Agency (NPHCDA), giving autonomy to each state primary healthcare development agency, and ensuring funds are appropriated directly from federal level to each state

Primary Healthcare Development Agency (PHCDA) (National Health Act, 2014; Federal Ministry of Health [Nigeria], 2014; National Primary Healthcare Development Agency [Nigeria], 2015).

The development of a national health quality strategy is an indication of the government's commitment to building a responsive health system. These efforts aim to ensure that the populace can access care at primary health centers, thus reducing pressure on the secondary and tertiary centers and establishing an efficient continuum of care. Individual states have begun to adopt community-based health insurance programs in a bid to align with the federal government initiative of revitalizing the primary health centers and ensuring that quality and affordable healthcare is directed toward those who really need it.

Economic, Political, Social/Cultural, and Technological Forces Influencing Improvement Efforts

The introduction of a level of autonomy to the state governments in the design and coordination of primary healthcare has had a positive impact on the delivery of quality care.

The health financing structures of most states in the federation were designed with heavy reliance on the federal government. However, through the National Health Act 2014, the creation of the basic healthcare provision fund, financed by a federal government annual grant of not less than 1% of its consolidated revenue fund and by grants from international donor partners, has ensured a more sustainable health financing plan for the country. The funds, to be managed by the NPHCDA, the National Health Insurance Scheme, and the FMoH, have been allocated to the following areas:

- The National Healthcare Development Agency: 45% of the fund is disbursed through each state and the Federal Capital Territory (FCT) Primary Healthcare Development Board for the provision of essential drugs, vaccines, and other consumables.
- The National Health Insurance Scheme receives 50% of the fund for the provision of the basic minimum package of health facilities.
- The FMoH manages 5% of the fund for the provision of the basic minimum package of health facilities.

The National Health Act further creates a structure for the provision of training for human resources for health as well as insurance for underserved populations (National Health Act, 2014).

More than 28 states have begun to put in structures for the implementation of the National Health Act. A few examples include Kwara, Lagos, and Ogun states where programs have been designed in alignment with this National Health Act and results have been seen to support the feasibility of successful implementation.

Somewhat paradoxically, the current downturn in oil prices has provided a much-needed push, forcing the government to consider innovative models of care provision. This, in turn, has led to the development of several models of community-based health insurance schemes with varying degrees of public–private collaboration. The Kwara State Health Insurance Scheme (a partnership between the Health Insurance Fund, the Netherlands, and the Kwara state government) and the ARAYA Program (a partnership between the Shell Petroleum Development Company and the Ogun state government) are examples.

Details of the Success Story

The traditional model of health design and delivery focuses on the provider and not the healthcare user. This format is usually physician-centric, facility-based, and strongly designed with little or no input from the end user. However, one of the innovative models of health design and delivery in Nigeria involves modified "last mile" health delivery initiatives, which provide quality primary healthcare services to those living in remote areas. These models rely on strong community involvement and participation in the design. For instance,

- Community committees are involved in decision-making determining the health package and the selection of health service points.
- Private and public sectors collaborate more effectively.
- Service providers are empowered to deliver quality healthcare services.
- The obstacle of poor access is addressed through various means, namely, community health outreach, mobile clinics, digital health options.

The model connects both the demand and supply sides of the health system and supports patient and family-centered care.

In Kwara and Ogun states, the conceptual phase of the programs included medical due diligence, which involved community disease needs and trends, provider mapping, and gaps analysis against international standards. Concurrently, stakeholders were identified and engaged in the design of insurance schemes that were accessible, affordable, and relevant to the communities. Community involvement and empowerment have been heightened as a result.

The gaps identified in the system were jointly addressed with each stakeholder contributing their expertise and resources. For instance, the initiatives have ensured that providers are able to meet the demands of the community in terms of their capability to provide quality and safe care. With the aid of quality improvement methodologies and regularly supportive supervisory visits, providers are able to cater to the demands of the now-empowered communities as they collaborate to design and deliver health to the people.

Having to attend to what communities need and how healthcare consumers conceptualize quality, means that the government must now map resources before allocation is made. While resource mapping should be a given in the face of resource constraints, this important concept is often ignored. In contrast to the situation 10 years ago, paying attention to the use of available resources now supersedes an unbalanced focus on scarcity of resources. In Kwara state, the State Health Bill, which evolved from successful reform efforts, and the Community Health Insurance Scheme set the platform for government collaboration with local and international development agencies to act in alignment with the needs of the communities.

The mechanism that drives these initiatives is strongly rooted in innovative public–private partnerships. These partnerships were not strong before the government made a bold move toward supporting such collaborative efforts by creating a policy environment conducive to them (such as the National Health Act, 2014) and backed up by resource allocation.

For a country of Nigeria's physical size and population, access to care has been a major challenge. An additional and closely related concern is the quality of care accessed when the services are present. Challenging circumstances, such as poor access and the skewed distribution of qualified health professionals, call for radical and innovative solutions, beginning with the redefinition of the roles of the players in the system. Whatever the proposed intervention, it must be seen to provide the solution to issues of access and quality.

Improvements in access to quality health are already evident in some states in the federation that began to reform their systems prior to the national move toward state-level sustainable health systems. Kwara state and Ogun state both run initiatives that merge access to care with assured quality of care. Delta, Lagos, and Nasarawa states are working toward similar projects (JSI Research and Training, Inc., n.d.; Medical Credit Fund Africa, 2015).

Details of the Impact of the Success Story

The success of these initiatives can be attributed to the following features:

- Patient-centeredness: The shift in focus from provider to consumer has made the method of care delivery more patient focused. The providers are rewarded for providing patient- and family-focused care.

- Community involvement: mechanisms that enhanced community involvement and empowerment were established and continuously monitored.
- Continuous quality improvement, both on technical parameters as well as programmatic indices: the attention on continuous improvement is a rather new concept in the Nigerian health space, but one that is now gaining ground. These initiatives have served as research on the effectiveness of the methodology.
- Government buy-in and effective public–private partnerships play a central role.
- Health delivery reengineering: the limits of possibility have been expanded by innovatively creating opportunities for access to the people (e.g., mobile clinics and mobile health).

The success of these health initiatives can be evaluated from multiple perspectives. Using the systems approach has produced the following:

- Greater population coverage: the remote care project has improved the number of enrollees on the scheme yearly over a period of 5 years.
- The cost of travel, which was frequently greater than the insurance premium, has been significantly reduced or eliminated.
- Utilization rates have been increased and quality improvement ensured with the introduction of a model of healthcare that comes at a cheaper—insurance driven—rate.
- The rate of immunization and healthcare awareness in communities that have a remote care facility has been significantly improved.
- Patient referral for more appropriate care in the nearest bigger facility has been improved.
- Maternal, newborn, and child health (MNCH) emergencies and other conditions that would otherwise have resulted in mortalities are now promptly referred for appropriate care (AIID, 2015).

Implementation: Transferability of the Exemplar

The uniqueness of the initiative is the integration of access to healthcare in a "last mile" community at an affordable price with regular monitoring of quality improvement and patient safety practices by the provider of healthcare. The alignment of community support and government buy-in means that sustainability is guaranteed.

Similar systems are likely replicable in other nations if the model outlined here can be followed and appropriately contextualized. Other health systems could work on process improvement in supply chain logistics that will improve the delivery of services to the "last mile" communities, including the supply of drugs, fuel or power-generating systems, reagents, kits, oxygen, lab wares, machinery, and even manpower. This must be closely monitored and can vary between countries.

Prospects for Further Success and Next Steps

A stronger federal and state government buy-in, along with the active involvement of the government at the local level to guarantee accountability, will ensure sustainability of the transformed "last mile" health delivery model. Local government involvement will enhance community acceptance, participation, collaboration, and even financial support. The support of community-based health insurance schemes, managed by efficient administrators who can balance quality, affordability, and accessibility, will further strengthen the scheme (PharmAccess Nigeria, 2015).

Conclusion

Every successful health model has core ingredients, integrating multistakeholder initiatives with the alignment of political will, resources, and talents. The blend of a demand-driven healthcare system with appropriate resource allocation and continuous provider empowerment in quality and business training will go a long way to making any healthcare model sustainable. Government buy-in and community support must be achieved in all models of healthcare to ensure success. The role of community health workers and the concept of facility-based care must continuously evolve to encourage the dynamism that the health system needs to be effective and efficient.

13

Rwanda

Community-Based Health Insurance in Rwanda: How It Fostered Achievement of the Millennium Development Goals

Roger Bayingana and Edward Chappy

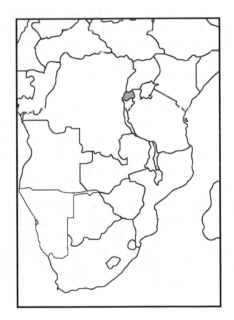

CONTENTS

Background

After the 1994 genocide against the Tutsi, Rwanda embarked on a reconstruction of the country. Rwandan leaders realized that health equity was central to the country's Vision 2020, which invokes the principles of inclusive, people-centered development, and social cohesion (Ministry of Finance and Economic Planning [Rwanda 2000]). Since 1994, different health system initiatives have been put in place. These initiatives include community-based health insurance, performance-based financing, adding community health workers to the healthcare workforce, e-health technologies such as telemedicine, and quality assurance and accreditation initiatives.

Since 1994, the government of Rwanda has significantly reduced poverty by implementing the Economic Development and Poverty Reduction Strategy 2013–2018 (Ministry of Finance and Economic Planning [Rwanda], 2013). A key strategy to reducing poverty was the realization of universal health coverage. Data show that because of health insurance schemes like the community-based health insurance, which covered 90% of the population in 2011, there has been significant improvement in healthcare utilization and significant reduction in financial catastrophe and impoverishment caused by out-of-pocket spending (Lu, 2012).

Other efforts that have been key to improving the healthcare system in Rwanda include performance-based initiatives, and the use of e-health technologies to track childhood and maternal morbidities, monitor epidemic outbreaks, and map vaccination coverage. In addition, there have been improvements in capturing and analyzing health-related data and using it to inform policymakers for better decision-making. Most importantly, the leadership of the country has shown the political will to strengthen the health sector through improved coordination of donors and external aid, and then monitoring the effectiveness of this aid. As a result of these efforts, Rwanda has come close to meeting all the health targets under the United Nations Millennium Development Goals (MDGs) (see Table 13.1) (United Nations Development Programme, 2014b).

Details of the Success Story

Rwanda has used several strategies to improve its health system and each has contributed to the achievement of the MDGs. However, one strategy, *Mutuelles de Santé*/community-based health insurance (CBHI) appears to have impacted significantly on the general improvement of health indicators in Rwanda (Schneider and Diop, 2004). In 1996, utilization of healthcare services was 0.28 contacts per capita, a quarter of what is recommended by

TABLE 13.1

Progress of Achievement of the Millennium Development Goals in Rwanda

	MDGs 4 and 5: Maternal and child mortality				
Indicator	2000	2005/2006	2010/2011	Target 2015	Status
Infant mortality rate (per 1000 births)	107	86	50	28	On track
Under-5 mortality	196	152	72 (2012)	47	On track
Percentage of 1-year-olds immunized against measles	87	75.2	95	100	On track
Percentage of children aged 12–23 months fully vaccinated	76	75.2	95	100	On track
Percentage of births attended by skilled health personnel	31	39	69	—	—
Percentage of women aged 15–49 using a modern contraceptive method	4.3	10.3	49	—	—
Antenatal care coverage (at least one visit)	92.5	94.4	98	100	On track
Unmet need for family planning	17.7	37.9	18.9	—	—
Contraceptive prevalence rate	4.3	16.3	45.1	—	—

Source: United Nations Development Programme. (2014b). Rwanda Millennium Development Goals—Final Progress Report: 2013. Retrieved from http://www.undp.org/content/dam/undp/library/MDG/english/MDG%20Country%20Reports/Rwanda/Rwanda_MDGR_2015.pdf

the World Health Organization (WHO) (Ataguba and Kalisa, 2014). By 2013, utilization had risen to 1.23 contacts per capita partly due to the implementation of CBHI.

In addition to the increased utilization rate, the results from a household survey in 2013, conducted among CBHI beneficiaries, showed that CBHI improves access to health services for the population (Ataguba and Kalisa, 2014). In addition, 78% of the households indicated that CBHI covers most of their healthcare needs, including access to medicines. Also, most members reported that they do not have to delay seeking care when needed.

According to a study carried out by the University of Rwanda, together with the Ministry of Health (MoH), financial catastrophe due to out-of-pocket expenditure was significantly reduced from 10% in 2000 to 2% in 2010. As a result, impoverishment due to out-of-pocket expenses was reduced from 2.4% in 2000 to 0.6% in 2010, due to the expansion of health insurance coverage nationally (National Institute of Statistics of Rwanda, 2012), Today, Rwanda's CBHI covers 90% of the population (Odeyemi, 2014).

From 2005 to 2011, due to CBHI and other initiatives such as performance-based financing, deaths from malaria dropped by 87% (Binagwaho et al., 2012). Between 2000 and 2010, Rwanda's maternal mortality ratio fell by 59.5%. From 2000 to 2011, the under 5 years' deaths decreased by 70.4%, falling below half of the regional average and approaching the global mean (Farmer et al., 2013). During the same period, the absolute number of child deaths fell by 62.8% annually, even though the population increased by 35.1%. Rwanda's regional ranking for child mortality went from 42nd in 2000 to 7th in 2011 and the average annual rate of reduction of 11.1% for this period was the world's highest.

After 1994, the government, with the help of donors, covered all healthcare costs so that patients did not need to pay when they sought healthcare services. However, in 1996, due to a reduction in donor support, the MoH reintroduced user fees for health services. The consequence was a reduction in health service utilization and a lack of financial protection for users. In 1999, the MoH piloted a community health insurance scheme with successful results. For example, in the first pilot year, 88,303, 7.9% of the total population of the three districts, enrolled in the program (Ministry of Health [Rwanda], 2012). Due to the success of the pilot scheme in three districts, CBHI was scaled up nationally in 2005. Today, the Rwandan CBHI is widely recognized by WHO and the World Bank as one of the most successful national insurance schemes in Africa, with coverage increasing from 7% of the population in 2003 to 90% in 2010 (National Institute of Statistics of Rwanda, 2011; Nyinawankunsi et al., 2015; World Bank, 2009).

Rwanda's macroeconomic stability has been strengthened through the implementation of various initiatives like the *Ubudehe* (the deep-rooted Rwandan practice and culture of collective action and mutual support to solve problems within a community), which is aimed at fighting poverty, as well as programs such as CBHI, which are aimed at ensuring that Rwandan citizens can access affordable healthcare programs (Niringiye and Ayebale, 2012). These important initiatives, along with many others, have established the base for sustained growth and further poverty reduction as well as accelerating overall progress toward most of the MDGs. This progress has been achieved due to a strong and sustained political commitment at the highest level in government along with significant international support in developing well-designed and efficiently managed national programs.

Why Has CBHI Been a Success?

CBHI has been a success story because of the strong political commitment from both central and decentralized governments. CBHI coverage has become one of the most important indicators for districts when looking at signing performance contracts. Because the health system in Rwanda is decentralized, with a network of health facilities in all districts, national coverage, along with the tackling of other health issues, is achievable. In addition, one of the objectives of the national health policy is to improve financial accessibility to health services (Nyinawankunsi et al., 2015). CBHI constitutes an important pillar of this objective and allows for the promotion of community financing mechanisms and risk sharing. CBHI has greatly improved access to healthcare, as members do not have to delay seeking care when it is needed and it covers the majority of the healthcare needs of its members.

Transferability of CBHI

Since its inception, Rwanda's success in implementing CBHI has relied on consensus from the population that access to healthcare must be equitable and affordable. CBHIs success has also been due to it being a national program, given financial and legislative support from the government—with laws requiring the provision of basic healthcare to the uninsured. A decentralized health system has helped to ensure that there are *Mutuelle* sections in nearly all health facilities in the country and members are entitled to a comprehensive list of curative and preventive services.

Originally, contributions of households to *Mutuelles* were not based on their ability to pay. They were based on a flat rate premium and were therefore strongly regressive. The system was considered by WHO to be unfair, and to some degree excluded those, often poor, who work in the informal sector (MoH [Rwanda], 2014). In April 2010, a change in *Mutuelle* policy introduced a new CBHI premium schedule using a system of stratification. The new stratification system was based on individual assets rather than on the local leaders' assessment. This new system of contribution ensured that those who are extremely poor had access to care.

The Rwandan CBHI experience offers valuable lessons to other low-income countries. The rapid expansion of the *Mutuelles* program and high rates of enrollment suggest a strong societal consensus regarding equal opportunity for all citizens to access healthcare with financial protection. Although studies elsewhere show similar results, the commitment at the highest level of government makes the *Mutuelles* program in Rwanda unique. It is important to note that the government has played a crucial role through increased financial investment in the health sector, successful legislation of the entitlement of basic care for the uninsured population, and an intensive nationwide campaign. The positive results of the *Mutuelles* program in promoting medical care utilization and financial risk protection suggests that the community-based health insurance scheme, together with other policy instruments, can be an effective tool for achieving universal health coverage (Basinga et al., 2011). The success of the program is also due to the government's close collaboration with development partners—a factor that can be easily replicated in other countries.

Prospects for Further Success of CBHI

Although the extension of the CBHI system to the national level in Rwanda occurred at a very fast pace, it still faces some challenges. There is a need to

- Improve the current pooling mechanisms
- Empower *Mutuelle* staff with management capabilities
- Increase public awareness about *Mutuelles* so as to reach the large number of people in the informal sector with capacity to contribute
- Continue to improve the ability of the healthcare system to meet the demand for services

The CBHI experience has shown that once there is investment in healthcare services and the people of the country are part of the decision-making process regarding the healthcare services, health system improvement can be achieved. The Rwandan experience, where MDGs and other health targets were incorporated into the national vision and strategy, provides an example of what other countries can do to improve their systems.

Conclusion

Rwanda has demonstrated how agreed goals and government determination can lead to real improvements in healthcare for its citizens. Although several healthcare initiatives have been introduced in Rwanda, the introduction of CBHI has had the most demonstrably positive impact. Translating the UN's MDGs into the Economic Development and Poverty Reduction Strategies (EDPRS I and II), and introducing CBHI as a means of reducing poverty, appears to have both accelerated the attainment of the MDGs and helped to reduce poverty. CBHI has increased access to healthcare services and allowed people to seek early treatment, thereby reducing chronic illness, and has significantly reduced financial catastrophe due to out-of-pocket expenditure on healthcare.

14

South Africa

The Development of an Equitable National Juristic Body to Regulate Public and Private Healthcare Establishments in South Africa: A Progress Report

Lizo Mazwai, Grace Labadarios, Bafana Msibi, and Stuart Whittaker

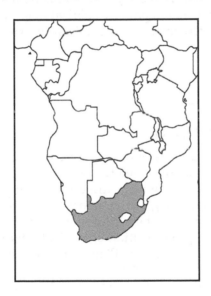

CONTENTS

Historical Background

In 1994, the newly established Democratic Government of South Africa was faced with the challenge of modernizing a fragmented and hugely inequitable healthcare system. The inequitable South African health system was a legacy of early twentieth-century colonial and missionary ideologies, with their ostensibly "philanthropic" attitudes toward providing healthcare to indigenous people. These attitudes created a dual system of healthcare in which both mission hospitals and public hospitals were established, each with different sets of values and standards.

These systems were entrenched by subsequent political regimes and finally legislated into the Apartheid system after 1948. The Homeland policy of separate development perpetuated inequities between rural and urban facilities (Khunou, 2009). While the inequitable dual system of healthcare continued along racial, geographic, or political lines, it is now perpetuated by socioeconomic differences, which manifest in private and public sector inequities.

Movement toward Equity

Since 1994, South Africa has worked to transform its highly inequitable health system into a national health system that incorporates both the public and private sectors, with a drive toward universal coverage. To achieve this, a number of legislative reforms have been made, culminating in the establishment of the Office of Health Standards Compliance (OHSC) following the promulgation of the National Health Amendment Act in September 2013 (National Planning Commission [South Africa], n.d.; Republic of South Africa, 2004, 2013). The OHSC is required to inspect South Africa's 4010 health establishments (HEs) every 4 years to determine their compliance with a minimum set of quality standards, which will be promulgated as regulations, to ensure the provision of quality healthcare services.

OHSC Composition, Mandate, Vision, Mission, Values, and Principles

Figure 14.1 summarizes the structure of the OHSC. The OHSC mandate is to "protect and promote the health and safety of users of health services" by

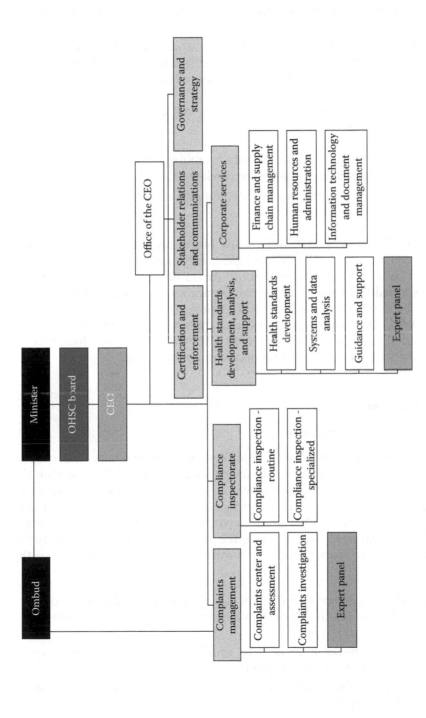

FIGURE 14.1
Organogram showing the staffing structure of the Office of Health Standards Compliance.

- Monitoring and enforcing compliance by HEs with norms and standards prescribed by the minister in relation to the national health system.
- Ensuring consideration, investigation, and disposal of complaints relating to non-compliance with prescribed norms and standards in a procedurally fair, economical, and expeditious manner.

This mandate contributes to two distinct but interdependent regulatory outcomes. These are

- Reductions in avoidable mortality, morbidity, and harm within HEs through reliable and safe health services
- Improvements in the availability, responsiveness, and acceptability of health services for users

The OHSC vision is safe and quality healthcare for all South Africans, and the OHSC mission is to act independently, impartially, fairly, and fearlessly on behalf of the people of South Africa in guiding, monitoring, and enforcing healthcare safety and quality standards in HEs (Office of Health Standards Compliance [OHSC] [South Africa], 2015b).

The OHSC (2014) values and principles are informed by the South African Constitution and Batho Pele Principles: "Human dignity; freedom, and the achievement of equality; and that people must come first."

National Core Standards

The National Core Standards (NCS) were developed by the precursor to the OHSC, the Office of Standards Compliance (OSC), within the National Department of Health over a period of 3 years. Initially, these were generic standards, which were publicized nationally for all HEs to adopt and implement (National Department of Health [South Africa], 2011a). After national consultation, the standards were approved by the National Health Council and the minister in 2011. The purpose of the NCS is to

- Develop a common definition of quality care, which should be found in all HEs in South Africa, as a guide to the public and to managers and staff at all levels
- Establish a benchmark against which HEs can be assessed, gaps identified, and strengths appraised
- Provide for the national certification of compliance of HEs with mandatory standards

A subset of these standards, focusing on six critical areas of most concern to patients, has been prioritized throughout the public health system. These areas are

1. Values and attitudes
2. Waiting times
3. Cleanliness
4. Patient and staff safety and security
5. Infection prevention and control
6. Availability of medicine and supplies

Inspectorate Unit of the OHSC

The aim of the Inspectorate Unit of the OHSC is to inspect HEs in order to assess and encourage compliance with regulated standards. Its objectives are to monitor the compliance of regulated standards and to raise healthcare provider awareness of the need to meet regulated standards. The inspections of HEs are conducted using the following data collection methods:

- Document review and analysis
- Observation
- Patient interview
- Patient record assessment
- Staff interview

During the development phase of the norms and standards, regulations, and their promulgation, which are likely to take place during 2017, mock inspections, using the NCS, are carried out. The ongoing inspections provide experience for inspectors in preparation for the implementation of regulated norms and standards, which will lead to the certification of HEs. Inspection teams, composed of a team leader, four to five inspectors, and a data-capturer, are each required to complete one of the following three combinations of health establishment inspections in a five day working week:

1. Eight clinics
2. Six clinics and one Community Health Centre
3. One hospital and two clinics

All facilities inspected are in the same geographical location for logistical efficiency.

An annual performance plan has been developed requiring that the OHSC carries out a number of annual inspections (OHSC, 2015a). These include

- A random 10% sample of the 3816 public HEs at selected sites across the nine provinces by six teams of inspectors.
- A 30% sample of HEs found to be non-compliant at inspections within the previous 6 months for re-inspection within the provinces.

Facilities are identified by means of early warning indicators as potentially presenting an unacceptably high risk to patient safety and/or routinely reported outcome data such as mortality rates, average length of stay, utilization rates, readmission rates, and media reporting, and by means of whistleblowing by personnel or the public.

Using this approach, in the 2015/2016 financial year, a total of 627 inspections were carried out across the country. This included four central hospitals, 11 provincial tertiary hospitals, nine regional hospitals, 27 district hospitals, nine CHC, and 567 clinics. Of these, 132 were re-inspections.

Inspection Results

The baseline inspections of the healthcare establishments inspected revealed that all healthcare establishments required improvements, especially the clinics, which were found to have the lowest level of standard compliance.

The re-inspections carried out in the 2015/2016 financial year revealed that the four central hospitals and 12 of the provincial and tertiary hospitals had improved their performance. However, while the 27 re-inspected district hospitals were found to have improved in some areas, many weaknesses remained.

In contrast to the improvements shown in the hospitals, the 567 re-inspected clinics showed little improvement. Problem areas included poor infrastructure, lack of medication, and severe staff shortages. In addition, policies and procedures relating to adverse event and disaster management (including risk management) were either missing or poorly implemented, with little support in relation to training or guidance on how to carry out necessary processes.

In general, both new inspections and repeat inspections revealed that clinics supported by feeder hospitals did better than those with district office oversight. The re-inspections indicated that there was lack of guidance and support by the provincial governments. In particular, HE personnel have not been encouraged to perform self-assessments to monitor and sustain compliance with the NCS. In addition, the provision of resources required to enable compliance with the NCS is beyond the delegation of HEs.

The OHSC will continue to carry out mock and repeat inspections at HEs using the current NCS while the draft regulated norms and standards and associated procedural regulations are processed for promulgation.

Following formal promulgation of the regulations, the law requires that procedures must be carried out in cases of continued non-compliance with regulated standards. In such cases of continued non-compliance, OHSC inspectors may issue a notice of non-compliance to the person in charge of the establishment, which must reflect

- Any prescribed norm and standard that has not been rated as compliant
- Details of the nature and extent of non-compliance
- Steps that are required to remedy identified shortfalls and the period over which such steps must be taken
- The penalties that may be imposed in the event of continued non-compliance

The notice of non-compliance will take into account the nature, extent, and gravity of the contravention and consequently the OHSC may take any of the following actions:

- Issue a written warning with a prescribed time frame to achieve compliance
- Require a written response from the HE, providing evidence as to why it is not possible for them to comply, that is, factors beyond their control
- Recommend to the relevant authority any appropriate and suitable action, including disciplinary proceedings
- Recommend to the minister the temporary or permanent closure of an establishment or part thereof if it constitutes a serious risk to public health or to health service users
- Impose upon accountable persons or HEs a fine
- Refer the matter to the national prosecuting authority for prosecution, for example, where criminal activities are found (such as fraudulent activity, criminal negligence of patients, etc.)

OHSC Regulatory Principles

Five principles guide the daily operations and regulatory decisions of the OHSC in line with good regulatory practice, and enable evaluation of its performance as a regulator. The five principles are as follows:

1. All regulations must foster greater accountability
2. All regulations must be clear and transparent
3. All regulations should be targeted
4. Regulatory interventions should be proportionate
5. All regulations should be applied consistently and yield reliable decisions

OHSC and National Health Insurance

In *A National Health Plan for South Africa*, published in May 1994, the ANC government committed to the creation of a single comprehensive, equitable, and integrated national health system (African National Congress [ANC], 1994). In August 2011, the green paper on national health insurance was published, outlining the government's intended policy for the delivery of universal health coverage (National Department of Health [South Africa], 2011b). A green paper is a discussion document published by government to invite public comment on their intended policy. In this green paper, it was announced that HEs wishing to provide services under the envisaged national health insurance (NHI) scheme will be required to achieve certification against the regulated standards. HEs that do not achieve certification will not be able to receive payment from the NHI fund.

In December 2015, the white paper on NHI was published (National Department of Health [South Africa], 2015). With the implementation of NHI, the government seeks to achieve the following key objectives for the entire population of South Africa:

- Ensuring universal health coverage for all South Africans
- Improving the quality of healthcare services irrespective of socio-economic status
- Promoting equity and social solidarity through the pooling of risks and funds
- Creating one public health fund with adequate resources and funds to plan for and to effectively meet the health needs of the entire population
- Creating a single, strategic health purchaser that will ensure that health services and health products are purchased and procured at reasonable costs

The implementation of NHI will be phased in over a 14-year period, during which time there will be a progressive realization of the right to health by extending coverage of health benefits to the entire population. NHI seeks to benefit from efficiency gains in service delivery to offset resource constraints in an environment of resource constraint.

Summary of Achievements of the OHSC to Date

The OHSC has now been established within a legislated framework, and basic systems and processes are nearing completion. The repeat mock surveys show an emerging pattern of improving compliance within HEs in the program. The following improvements are currently underway:

- The process for the promulgation of the draft regulatory standards is reaching an advanced stage.
- An advanced IT system that will be used for the capture, collation, and analysis of inspection data, the calculation of certification status by means of a predetermined algorithm, and the generation of inspection reports, has been procured and is nearing completion.
- Systems for setting up the certification of HEs for the determination of compliance thresholds are at an advanced stage.
- The development of a comprehensive, accredited inspector-training program is nearing completion.

Challenges

In an over-burdened and under-resourced health system, it is challenging for healthcare workers of all cadres to engage with quality improvement initiatives. Despite these constraints, many HEs within South Africa have demonstrated that compliance with the NCS is possible and that improvements made can be sustained.

To facilitate compliance with regulated standards and the achievement of certification, adequate training and support must be provided to assist healthcare workers to understand the requirements of the regulated standards as well as to understand and successfully implement quality and risk management processes.

Governing bodies must recognize their fundamental role in assisting HEs to achieve certification by providing efficient and effective accountability structures, effective management systems—particularly in relation to the supply of goods and services—effective leadership, equitable distribution of human resources for health, in addition to the creation, distribution, and implementation of policies and guidelines.

15

West Africa (Guinea, Liberia, and Sierra Leone)

Quality Improvement in Ebola-Affected Countries: From Recovery to Resilience

Shamsuzzoha B. Syed and Edward T. Kelley

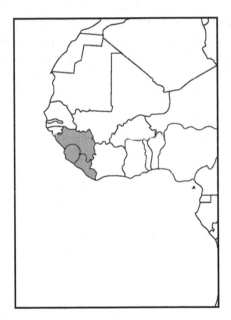

CONTENTS

Background

The outbreak of Ebola virus disease (EVD) in West Africa has been unprecedented in scale and impact. As of May 2016, a total of 28,616 confirmed, probable, and suspected Ebola cases were reported in Guinea, Liberia, and Sierra Leone, with 11,310 deaths (WHO, 2016b). At the height of the outbreak (between 1 January 2014 and 31 March 2015), 815 confirmed and probable health worker EVD cases were recorded; among the health workers for whom the final outcome is known, two-thirds of those infected died (WHO, 2016c).

In addition to the human suffering and deaths caused by Ebola, morbidity and mortality from other priority diseases were significantly affected. Indeed, health service utilization was severely compromised. For example, in Liberia, between August and December 2014, compared with the same period in 2013, the number of outpatient visits decreased by 61%, antenatal consultations decreased by 40%, institutional deliveries decreased by 37%, and measles vaccinations decreased by 45% (United Nations Development Programme, 2015). All this occurred in health systems that faced severe quality challenges pre-Ebola in terms of structures, processes, and outcomes.

The concept of resilience has been brought to prominence in an age where global health security faces enormous threats posed by infectious diseases, outbreaks, and other shocks. Resilience has been defined as "the ability of a system exposed to a shock to resist, absorb, accommodate, and recover from the effects of the shock in a timely and efficient manner, including through the preservation and restoration of its essential basic structures and functions" (WHO, 2011). The stronger the health system, the better it will be able to absorb shocks and implement risk-reduction measures alongside a strong health emergency and epidemic risk-management program. The same strong health system can address increased health needs and restore access to quality services promptly. Resilience requires that long-term investments are undertaken during the recovery phase, if not planned previously, for addressing underlying weaknesses in the system. Indeed, the Ebola epidemic has shown the fundamental structures that should exist for health systems, progressively moving toward universal health coverage with resilience as a key outcome. The need for a more applied definition of resilience thus becomes apparent.

It is within this context that recovery and resilience plans were developed in each of the three Ebola-affected countries. Front-line experiences were considered central; the heightened awareness of the critical importance of quality improvement was strikingly evident in this process. The convergence of the discourse on quality, universal health coverage, and resilience was particularly poignant in understanding the relationship between the macro, meso, and micro levels in enhancing the delivery of care. The harsh realities of recovery in the post-Ebola context may not be the natural place to look for a success story on improvement; however, that is exactly what we are examining here.

Success Story

Reflecting back on the Ebola experience in West Africa, recovering from the outbreak required national authorities to drive the safe reactivation of essential health services—such as maternity services and routine immunizations—within the context of ongoing response activities. This balancing act was no easy task, with recovery-focused efforts often viewed with some skepticism in the heat of a local, national, and global crisis. Yet, recovery served as a link between immediate outbreak response and the path to rebuilding the health system for the long-term. Recovery efforts were designed to address the most important health system constraints that existed prior to the epidemic and that contributed to the late detection and delayed declaration of the Ebola epidemic. Indeed, recovery sought to address limitations in capacity to respond to future epidemics, moving the health system toward resilience. What were the key ingredients of the recovery planning in the Ebola-affected countries and what lessons can be extracted for the future, particularly within the context of health improvement efforts in post-shock settings? Six stand out:

1. First, and most crucially, there must be an emphasis on the importance of recovery processes in the midst of the response effort through senior national leadership endorsement. For example, in Sierra Leone, a national team conducted recovery analyses in the field as early as October 2014, at the height of the crisis, and this laid the ground for future recovery and resilience planning.

2. Second, systematic post-disaster needs assessments, which focus on quality parameters, with a particular emphasis on the delivery of essential health services, must be conducted. For instance, the multi-country Ebola recovery assessment provided an entry point for this micro-level approach and allowed linkage between local and global efforts.

3. Third, infection prevention and control (IPC) was a key linkage between the emergency response teams and health worker safety. For example, in Liberia, IPC facility assessments during the response provided the foundation for a more sustained approach to patient safety for the longer term. Health worker protection became a key area of focus as summarized within the first-of-a-kind synthesis on health worker infections in the Ebola-affected countries (WHO, 2015d).

4. Fourth, community perspectives must be incorporated within recovery planning. Perceptions of the quality of health services captured directly from communities during the crisis in all three Ebola-affected countries were critical to "ground-truthing" the recovery plans that would otherwise have been made in distant board rooms.

5. Next, a clear focus on the links between quality improvement and district health management must be ensured. All three Ebola-affected countries recognized this early on and have focused on building management capacity at the sub-national level, an incredibly difficult but necessary task for quality improvement.

6. Finally, structures for quality must be focused on if discourse on improvement is not to sound empty. For example, Liberia adopted water, sanitation, and hygiene (WASH) standards for healthcare facilities in late 2015, which were supplemented with the development of a national training package using a risk-based continuous improvement approach to enable district health management teams and health facility staff to understand and begin incremental WASH improvements (WHO, 2015e).

As shown above, developments in quality improvement during the recovery phase need to be considered within a wider context of national health policy and planning. The role and importance of universal health coverage (UHC) becomes critical here. Each of the Ebola-affected countries has a clearly articulated vision for UHC. This promise of UHC, however, needs to be grounded by the quality of care being delivered. Quality care is what helps to build and maintain the trust of people. When people are placed at the center and engaged as active participants—an approach greatly appreciated in the Ebola response—care is better delivered and utilized. In order to maintain essential health services while dealing with the shifting priorities that may be required during times of crisis, health systems must develop strong health emergency and epidemic risk-management programs during times of relative stability. This requires strong leadership and guidance, with well-developed, implementation-informed national policies, along with open communication channels and support at the sub-national and local levels. Indeed, the move toward UHC can be a driver toward resilience.

Where does public health fit within this equation? Essential public health functions (EPHF) is a concept used to describe the core set of activities that a government should have in place to create a comprehensive public health system that protects and promotes the health of their population. The relations between essential public health functions, UHC, quality, and resilience are crucial, multiple, and complex (WHO, 2016d). Quality of health services is essential to several EPHFs and in particular for achieving effective preparedness, detection, and response capacities. The strong emphasis on the development of national public health institutions in the Ebola-affected countries, for example by the Liberian national authorities, is noteworthy. Needless to say—but important to reiterate—is the necessity for these public health institutions to be strongly interconnected with the organization of health service delivery; there is little capacity to have parallel public health and health service organization.

Quality of service delivery can be considered the final common destination in efforts to strengthen health systems. It is here that efforts are now being concentrated in order for the foundational efforts in each of the Ebola-affected countries to be translated into operational realities. Now that attention has shifted away from West Africa, creating support systems for healthcare delivery teams is more important than ever. One innovative approach supported by the World Health Organization (WHO) and other partners has been twinning partnerships between hospitals in the Ebola-affected countries and other countries, such as France, Japan, the United Kingdom, and the United States (WHO, n.d.c.).

Impact of the Success Story

The true impact of the success described previously is yet to be seen. The nature of the success, however, is focused on foundational efforts within Ebola-affected countries on quality improvement; such experiences from post-shock scenarios are rarely described.

Yet the potential impact of systematic national planning on quality improvement that moves the system from recovery to resilience cannot be overstated. In particular, this provides an excellent opportunity for the global pool of knowledge and expertise to support nationally driven efforts that focus on the front-line of health services. For example, the recovery toolkit developed by WHO has been designed to support national plans, an example of local driving global, as opposed to the usual supply-driven approach to global, technical assistance on quality improvement (WHO, 2016e).

Implementation: Transferability of the Exemplar

In terms of transferability, each of the Ebola-affected countries has been sharing valuable lessons between their health systems. For example, a technical meeting hosted in Kobe, Japan, earlier in 2016 explored the inter-connections between quality, recovery, resilience, and UHC from the perspectives of country teams (WHO, n.d.d.). With dozens of countries across the world facing acute and protracted emergencies, there is clear scope for the transferability of the foundational efforts described.

Kruk et al. (2015: 1910) state that "health systems that earn the trust and support of the population and local political leaders by reliably providing high-quality services before crisis have a powerful resilience advantage." The experience from the Ebola-affected countries described previously provides an opportunity to inform the global knowledge pool on this subject.

Prospects for Further Success and Next Steps

Quality improvement endeavors within Ebola-affected countries are just now starting to take shape. For example, in Liberia there is a simultaneous focus on facility-level quality improvement and the step-wise development of a national quality strategy to drive action for the coming years. There is a clear need to prospectively track the progress in these countries to ascertain whether and how the foundational efforts taken on quality during the recovery phase impact the long-term resilience of the health system. With this in mind, there is a continued need to track key parameters of health service delivery.

Further, efforts to strengthen country capacity under the International Health Regulations (WHO, 2005a) to prevent, detect, and rapidly respond to public health threats—for example through the joint external evaluation (JEE) and subsequent action planning—needs to place quality of service delivery centrally. Indeed, just as there can be no global health security without local health security, there can be no local health security without quality.

Conclusion

The human suffering caused by the Ebola crisis left a dent in the global health arena and has been acknowledged as a collective failure to prevent mortality and morbidity that could have been averted. Yet, even within the depths of sorrow, national efforts toward quality improvement to build for the future provide a window for local and global exploration with a view to improvement. These experiences and explorations need to feed into a global learning laboratory for quality UHC for maximal impact on population health (WHO, n.d.e.).

Part III

Europe

Russell Mannion

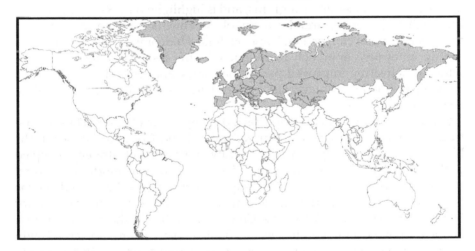

In our extended tour of the world's health systems, we now arrive in the World Health Organization (WHO) European region. The 23 countries covered in Section III vary widely in terms of their land mass, size of population, per capita income, sociopolitical systems, and in the organization, structure, and financing of their respective health and social care systems. The success stories discussed in this section are wide ranging, spanning interventions to improve patient care at the macro, meso, and micro levels. Nevertheless, some common themes can be discerned in the success stories contributed by different countries.

First, a key feature of the narratives of success of many of the countries is a clear focus on achieving better integration and collaboration among the different sectors, organizations, and agencies responsible for delivering care. Serbia, through work reported by Mirjana Živković Šulović, Ivan Ivanovic, and Milena Vasic, has implemented a raft of integrated national policies that have been shown to improve the protection of vulnerable children from abuse and neglect. Denmark, according to Janne Lehmann Knudsen, Carsten Engel, and Jesper Eriksen, has streamlined care pathways for cancer patients, resulting in reduced delays in diagnosis and treatment. In the chapter by Andrew Thompson and David Steel, from Scotland, partnership and collaboration have become the watchwords of recent health policy with new supporting initiatives introduced, including the development of Managed Clinical Networks and enhanced support for staff governance and public involvement. The discussion led by Kaja Põlluste, Ruth Kalda, and Margus Lember shows how Estonia has made great strides in strengthening its primary healthcare system with a range of positive outcomes for staff and patients. Spain is the only country in the world that has experienced a continuous improvement in deceased organ donation over many years. This has been achieved through better integration and collaboration among national and regional agencies and programs, and is highlighted by Rafael Matesanz, Elisabeth Coll Torres, and Rosa Suñol. Meanwhile, Germany, according to Oliver Groene, Holger Pfaff, and Helmut Hildebrandt, has pioneered a highly innovative approach to integrated care systems at regional level, which is delivering improved patient outcomes, and Ireland has developed a successful model of integrated care for patients with hemophilia (author: Feargal McGroarty)

Second, a number of countries have developed novel approaches to continuous quality improvement. For Roland Bal and Cordula Wagner in the Netherlands, for example, a new quality improvement strategy, coupled with external incentives, has reduced rates of hospital mortality. Several countries have developed quality improvement approaches based on the Breakthrough Collaborative model initially developed by the Institute for Health Improvement (IHI) in the United States. In Northern Ireland (in a chapter from Levette Lamb, Denise Boulter, Ann Hamilton, and Gavin Lavery), a new strategy for maternity care based on an Improvement Collaborative model has helped to lever positive cultural and behavioral change among health professionals. Portugal has pioneered a Breakthrough Collaborative approach to quality improvement, which has helped to reduce rates of hospital-acquired infections (authors: Paulo Sousa and José-Artur Paiva). Similarly, in Switzerland, Anthony Staines, Patricia Albisetti, and Paula Bezzola describe the Breakthrough Collaborative model, which has been used to facilitate multidisciplinary teams working to improve patient safety. In Austria, Maria Hofmarcher, Judit Simon, and Gerald Haidinger analyze the creation of specialized stroke units, which have been associated with a dramatic decline in stroke mortality.

Third, a number of success stories involve the use of new information technology alongside improved healthcare data collection, analysis, and sharing. Persephone Doupi, Jorma Komulainen, Minna Kaila, and Ilkka Kunnamo highlight that Finland has invested significantly in the development of new technological platforms, including the use of electronic patient records and electronic prescribing. These have had a positive impact on nurturing new ways of working and have improved quality of care. Norway, as presented by Ellen Tveter Deilkås, Geir Bukholm, and Ånen Ringard, has improved patient safety through the development and use of more sophisticated methods for measuring and monitoring the incidence of adverse events in accident and emergency departments (A&E). John Øvretveit and Mats Brommels show how Sweden has built over 100 new databases (national registers) for collating, storing, and informing the use of clinical data. And Israel, according to Eyal Zimlichman, has promoted the sharing of data between organizations through a novel health information exchange program, which has improved patient outcomes

Fourth, several countries have introduced national procedural initiatives related to guideline development, external regulation, and accreditation. In England, Martin Powell and Russell Mannion report how the setting up of the National Institute for Clinical Excellence (NICE) has proved effective in promoting cost-effective treatments. Meanwhile, Sandra Buttigieg, Kenneth Grech, and Natasha Azzopardi-Muscat illuminate how, in Malta, reforms in medical practitioner training and regulation have helped to reverse the "brain drain" with fewer doctors now leaving Malta to work in other countries. Russia has introduced a set of evidence-based guidelines, which have helped to reduce unnecessary treatments and improved quality of care (authors: Vasily Vlassov and Alexander Lindenbraten). Turkey has introduced a national accreditation system for healthcare services with the aim of improving standards in hospitals, as shown by Mustafa Berktaş and İbrahim H. Kayral. Italy, as outlined by Americo Cicchetti, Silvia Coretti, Valentina Iacopino, Simona Montilla, Entela Xoxi, and Luca Pani, has developed a new pricing and reimbursement system that has proved successful in stimulating pharmaceutical innovation.

Finally, the promotion of the patient perspective has been used as a key driver of reform. According to René Amalberti and Thomas le Ludec, in France the introduction of new patient rights and increased support for patient voice have been used as successful levers for improving quality and patient safety. Wales (author: Adrian Edwards) has implemented an innovative shared decision-making process by which clinicians and patients work together to select treatments and care pathways based on clinical evidence and patients' informed preferences. This has been shown to improve patient satisfaction, and in some cases, drive more cost-effective care.

16

Austria

Stroke Units in Austria: Incubators for Improved Health Outcomes

Maria M. Hofmarcher, Judit Simon, and Gerald Haidinger

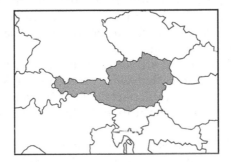

CONTENTS

Background

In 1990, Austria ranked 14th among selected high-income countries in terms of disease burden due to stroke; by 2010, this ranking had improved significantly, with Austria moving to 7th place. This was an unprecedented improvement when looking at the 25 leading causes of disease burden internationally (Institute for Health Metrics and Evaluation, 2010). This progress was achieved despite increasing incidence of stroke in Austria over the same time period and therefore can be linked to improved therapeutic and care options in the country (Austrian Ministry of Health, 2015a). The establishment of stroke units, specialist multidisciplinary units that are increasingly regarded as necessary to enable timely diagnosis and therapy, has been instrumental to these improved outcomes (OECD, 2014a).

In Austria, healthcare responsibilities are shared between the federal administration and the nine federal states with their municipalities. There is also a high degree of delegation of responsibility to health insurance funds, which has led to a mixed model of financing combined with a tradition of supply planning. In recent years, plans have been drawn up to build capacity. Planners looked at hospital service volumes and began planning for stroke units (Hofmarcher, 2010). Since 1997, inpatient stroke care has been remunerated by case rates financed through nine regional health funds. These funds are sourced jointly by the social health insurance companies responsible mainly for outpatient care and by federal tax money (Hofmarcher, 2013). This financing structure facilitates the capital-intense healthcare sector that is characteristic of Austria and that supports the establishment of stroke units.

A hospital-based survey of stroke care in Austria, performed in 1990, showed that in 146 hospitals that were caring for stroke patients, 69% of patients had been admitted to departments of internal medicine and 31% to neurological departments (Brainin and Klinger, 1992; Brainin and Lang, 2008).

Currently, about 25,000 cases of stroke occur each year in Austria (population in 2014 was 8.5 million) (Gesundheit Österreich GmbH, 2016; Statistics Austria, 2016). Ischemic stroke represents around 85% of all cerebrovascular disease cases. Ischemic strokes occur when blood supply to a section of the brain is interrupted, leading to necrosis of the affected part. Treatment for ischemic stroke has advanced dramatically over the last decade. Clinical trials have demonstrated clear benefits of thrombolytic interventions (OECD, 2014a). While the recommended time window for thrombolytic therapy is 3 hours from symptom onset, recent data suggest that there are still treatment benefits even up to 4.5 hours after onset (Robinson et al., 2011). Beyond immediate healthcare issues, stroke impacts all dimensions of quality of life, including physical, psychological, and social functioning (Austrian Ministry of Health, 2015a).

Details of the Success Story

In 1997, Austria established a national network of acute care stroke units. Throughout the country, centrally organized stroke units with a uniformly high structural quality, and connected to an online stroke registry, were established. Stroke units comprise four to eight beds within an area of the hospital that is exclusively used for stroke patients and is usually affiliated with the hospital's neurology department. Essential personnel include a board-certified neurologist as the responsible physician. In addition, one neurologist in training has to be present for 24 hours. An internist must be available or at least on call for 24 hours. A minimum of one nurse per bed is required. In addition, at least one physiotherapist, one occupational therapist, and one speech therapist must be assigned to the stroke unit, with each position responsible for six beds (Steiner and Brainin, 2003). These criteria must be fulfilled, and structural and process quality must be assessed for accreditation by regional health authorities.

Currently, 35 stroke units, located in 33 hospitals, guarantee a nationwide optimal acute treatment of those affected. As a result, most patients can now be admitted to a stroke unit within 45 minutes of the incident (Brainin, 2006). In less than 4% of the Austrian municipalities, accessibility is currently over 90 minutes (Austrian Ministry of Health, 2016).

By 2006, 57% of all ischemic stroke patients hospitalized in Austria were admitted to stroke units, and only 32% to departments of internal medicine (Brainin and Lang, 2008). In 2013, 88.5% of patients who had suffered a stroke were admitted to a hospital with a stroke unit, and about 80% of all cases were transported to the hospital by ambulance. About 63% of all patients received thrombolytic treatment, depending on age and time span between incident and lysis (Gesundheit Österreich GmbH, n.d.).

Details of the Impact of the Success Story

Since the establishment of the stroke units, data show improvements in a number of areas. Between 1980 and 2008, age-adjusted mortality for both hemorrhagic and ischemic strokes declined strongly for both sexes (77.3% for males and 76.7% for females) and in all age groups (Bajaj, 2010). While both the magnitude and trend of mortality reduction were pronounced for ischemic stroke, for hemorrhagic stroke these were much less defined. In terms of disease-specific years of life lost (YLLs), this corresponds to an overall 53% reduction between 1990 and 2010 (Institute for Health Metrics and Evaluation, 2010).

The rate of stroke mortality decline in Austria between 2000 and 2012 exceeded the pace of decline in other EU-28 countries, and was greater than in the frontrunner country, France (OECD, 2014a). Between 2000 and 2010, when stroke units were gradually established, the decline in stroke mortality was almost five times greater than between 1970 and 1980 and twice as high as between 1990 and 2000 (Statistics Austria, 2016).

In addition, 30-day mortality after admission, which was at 6.4 per 100 admissions in 2011, dropped almost 40% after 2003, while the corresponding drop in 31 OECD countries was about 18% (OECD, 2015a). Austria performed well against Germany and Switzerland when national data on case fatality were compared (Austrian Ministry of Health, 2015b).

There is evidence that stroke mortality declines with rising health expenditure (see Figure 16.1) (Sposato and Saposnik, 2012). A recent disease-specific comparative analysis found that stroke survival rates improve with increased spending even though the relationship between cost and outcome is not always consistent (Häkkinen et al., 2015).

The well-equipped and accessible Austrian hospital sector, working in tandem with effective emergency services, has been instrumental in Austria's stroke care success. The establishment of stroke units reflects enhanced efforts to concentrate care for high-burden diseases in specialized units. Additional investments in the strategic expansion of stroke care seem to have the potential to enhance survival (see Figures 16.1 and 16.2).

Between 2006 and 2009, direct stroke care cost per capita increased by about 50% in Austria, exceeding national health expenditure growth rates substantially (Nichols et al., 2012). At the same time, stroke mortality began to decline strongly. Extrapolating this difference beyond 2009 shows that with no initial additional investments in stroke care, the absolute direct stroke care cost growth would have been visibly lower (see Figure 16.2). For example, with no investments in stroke care, costs growth would be visibly lower, yielding a difference of €13 (US$14.70) per capita in 2009. Overall, strokes in Austria cost an estimated €780 million (US$880.9 million) in 2009. Of this total amount, direct medical costs comprised about 57%, while the

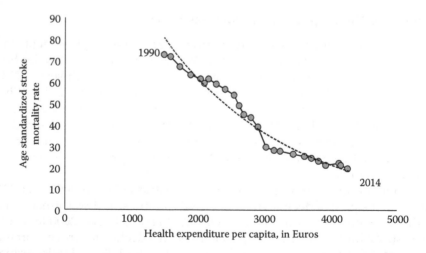

FIGURE 16.1

Per capita health spending and stroke mortality (ICD-10: I60–I69) in Austria 1990–2014. (From Statistics Austria. (2016). *Jahrbuch der Gesundheitsstatistik 2014* [Yearbook of Health Statistics]. Verlag Ö sterreich, Vienna, Austria; SHA. (2016). [System of Health Accounts] Data.

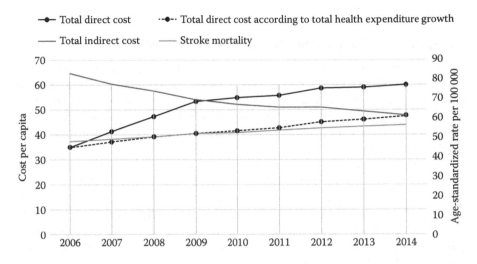

FIGURE 16.2

Care costs and mortality of stroke. National age-standardized stroke mortality data (left axis) and the development of per capita direct and indirect cost (right axis). (From Nichols et al. (2012). *European Cardiovascular Disease Statistics.* European Heart Network, Brussels; Statistics Austria. (2016). *Jahrbuch der Gesundheitsstatistik 2014* [Yearbook of Health Statistics], Verlag Österreich, Vienna, Austria.)

cost of informal care was 29%. The remaining costs were indirect costs due to productivity losses caused by mortality (10%) and morbidity (4%).

Implementation: Transferability of the Exemplar

Stroke units improve care through the balanced provision of highly specialized services. This model may well be transferable to other high-burden diseases, such as acute myocardial infarction and cancer, or mental healthcare, particularly as supply-side planning in Austria will continue to be the government's main instrument for streamlining care provision.

While the planning of healthcare capacity in Austria has unique features, methods may well be transferable to other countries. These methods combine volume data coming from activity-based financing (DRGs) and measures of the regional distribution of hospital capacity to ensure equitable access to care. While structural quality has always been factored into planning, indicators of process quality have rarely been used. Currently, a set of outcome indicators is produced to monitor hospital quality including stroke care (Austrian Ministry of Health, 2015b). Since many countries have now implemented activity-based hospital financing, capacity planning based on volumes in stroke care should be increasingly feasible and enable decision makers to better monitor outcomes (Busse et al., 2011).

Prospects for Further Success and Next Steps

A stronger focus is needed on social and long-term care, including post-acute care and rehabilitation. For example, the care of patients discharged from acute hospital care but who still require medical and social care, is often poorly coordinated. Linking of stroke care services at all levels to multidisciplinary primary care teams may also lead to further service improvements (Hofmarcher, 2014).

More effort is needed to expand effective planning of care provision for specific high-disease burden, high-cost patients to improve health outcomes, and ensure cost-effective care across care sectors. While current (hospital) capacity planning in Austria does consider care volumes defined in other sectors of the health system, it has no influence on other areas such as outpatient ambulatory care, as this responsibility, including financing, is delegated to social health insurance.

Activity-based financing, in combination with supply planning, appears to be an important prerequisite for the successful (market) concentration of services for diseases that require immediate secure access to hospitals, up-to-date technical equipment, and skills. This involves a policy environment and administration that is capable of building up reliable data infrastructures and quality checks of data used for reimbursement and planning. More importantly, preventive services, including the treatment of chronic diseases such as diabetes, are largely inadequate (Hofmarcher, 2013). While policymakers and social planners usually focus on access, quality, and efficiency as core objectives in efforts to improve the performance of their health systems, basic investment in these other areas seems crucial.

Conclusion

The introduction of specialized stroke units in Austria has led to significant observable health improvements within a short time frame, and a clear, likely causal relationship between service reforms and health outcome improvements can be established. Strategic planning of and investment in stroke units, in concert with an effective emergency transport system, have been instrumental in enhancing the likelihood of surviving a stroke. Progress in treatment is clearly evident as currently 50% of all stroke cases recover to some extent, while 20 years ago, the figure was only 30%. However, underlying risk factors such as diabetes, high blood pressure, and cholesterol levels leading to stroke have not yet been adequately addressed by primary prevention, and further efforts are required if outcomes are to be further improved.

17

Denmark

Cancer Patient Pathways

Janne Lehmann Knudsen, Carsten Engel, and Jesper Eriksen

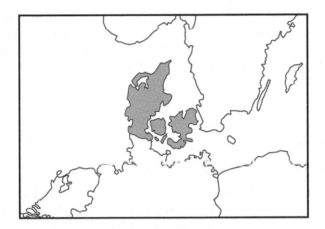

CONTENTS

Introduction

Our story is about a specific regulatory initiative streamlining the care pathway for cancer patients in order to reduce delay and ensure a uniformly high quality of care across the country. The national cancer plan in 2005 had addressed the need in general terms, but to effectively initiate improvement, a political agreement between national and regional politicians was pushed forward by cancer experts and the Danish Cancer Society in 2007.

The agreement caused a paradigm shift in handling cancer patients, and moved cancer toward being regarded as an acute life-threatening disease. The development of cancer-specific patient pathways (CPPs) and national monitoring of treatment wait times against time frames agreed upon by professionals, were both instrumental to this shift. Governmental funding was allocated.

Since the pathways were introduced, delays to diagnosis and treatment have been reduced and negative patient stories are less common. It is generally believed that the cancer pathways have moved Danish cancer care to a higher level of quality in terms of clinical- and patient-reported outcomes, but solid evidence is still needed.

The story demonstrates that a national health plan is not enough to ensure leadership, and that data alone doesn't ensure quality improvement in clinical settings. However, taken together, individual patient stories, clinical cases, and data can create the sense of urgency required to motivate political action.

Background and Development of Commitment

Throughout the world, cancer is a major challenge in terms of potential life years lost, reduction in quality of life for the population, and as a financial burden for society (Organization for Economic Cooperation and Development, 2013). Across the developed world, the incidence and prevalence of cancer will increase over the coming years, mainly due to increased longevity. Denmark aims to provide world-class healthcare, so it was an issue of concern 15 years ago, when it became clear that Danish outcomes in cancer care did not compare favorably internationally. While the incidence of cancer was the highest of all Nordic countries, the 5-year survival rates were the lowest. EUROCARE studies revealed that Denmark also had poorer survival rates across a range of cancer types than other Western European countries (Engholm et al., 2016; Sant et al., 2001).

A National Cancer Steering Group was established in 1998, followed by national cancer plans in 2000, 2005, and 2011. A national network organization, DMCG.dk, was established to coordinate all specialties in cancer care, with a focus on professional collaboration, research, and data-driven quality.

Long waiting times for diagnosis and treatment have been a recurring issue of concern. In 2001, cancer patients were granted a statutory right to treatment within 2 weeks of diagnosis. However, there was no guarantee concerning the time required to reach a diagnosis. In the following years, it became increasingly apparent that organizational obstacles in cancer patients' diagnostic journeys, along with lack of leadership and clear responsibility, were partially responsible for long waiting times. Cancer care is managed by public hospitals in regional settings; however, each patient has to be referred by a general practitioner (GP) in order to be diagnosed and treated for cancer by specialists. Missing or delayed action by the GP, in addition to complex pathways and lack of professional follow-up, caused safety issues, long waiting times, and patient dissatisfaction.

The problems were addressed in 2005 in the second cancer plan. A regional hospital, Vejle Hospital, developed and implemented a diagnostic fast track for their patients. Taking their cue from Vejle's positive experience, the national cancer plan recommended similar cancer care packages—national cancer pathways covering the diagnostic process as well as treatment within specific time frames—be implemented.

Studies that followed verified that Danish patients tend to be at a more advanced stage at diagnosis than those in other Scandinavian countries, and that diagnostic delays were a contributing factor to the low survival rate (Olesen et al., 2009). However, no concrete action was taken. An alliance was formed between DMCG.dk and the Cancer Society, who strongly pushed for improvement. A national conference was held in March 2007, to which high-ranking politicians were invited. A clinical case that was presented to the audience, showing details from scanned pictures that clearly showed a cancer in the jaw progressing in just 2 weeks from a small, localized tumor to an invasive and destructive cancer, led to a widespread sense of urgency. Research data based on 2000 incidents of documented diagnostic delay reinforced the need for action (Hansen, 2008). The key message from the conference was that if even a short delay can reduce treatment availability and the possibility of cure, cancer should be treated as an acute condition.

On August 10, 2007, the Danish Prime Minister publicly committed to taking care of the problem. By August 17, Danish Regions (the umbrella organization of the five regions) had presented a plan embracing seven initiatives, and on August 28, both the central government and Danish Regions issued a press release stating their joint commitment to action: they had agreed that in order to treat cancer as soon as possible, only medically necessary waiting periods should be accepted in the clinical pathway from symptom to treatment. A political agreement was a reality by October 12, and a national taskforce was established to ensure implementation of the following:

- Patient pathways, based on national clinical guidelines and time frames agreed on by experts, were to be developed for every cancer. They were to be implemented within 3 months from release.
- Every pathway was to be continuously monitored, as far as possible, using existing data.
- An identified hospital-based healthcare professional should be available for each patient.

Development and Monitoring of Cancer Patient Pathways

The first set of CPPs were published in 2008. These were revised in 2012 after recommendations in the cancer plan of 2011. In total, 29 specific pathways and one diagnostic pathway—for cases with atypical symptoms—have been launched. CPPs were designed to reshape the pathway from a series of localized actions into an integrated team effort, in order to prevent delays and to ensure a more uniform standard of quality across the country. The key elements were

- A formalized set of alarm-symptoms that should prompt the GP to refer a patient for further investigation
- An algorithm that describes the diagnostic flow that these symptoms should elicit, as well as the flow of treatment, once a cancer is diagnosed

The National Board of Health, in close collaboration with specialists across the country, was in charge of the development of CPPs. A working group of multidisciplinary cancer specialists and clinical leaders was tasked with defining and agreeing upon the clinical treatment for the specific cancer types, within an explicitly defined pathway structure (Probst et al., 2012).

Following this process, a national monitoring system, focusing on the pathway from referral received at hospital to the initiation of treatment, was developed. Since then, three different models have been launched. Only the third was found to be practically feasible. Since 2012, this system has provided information continuously, with data on key indicators published every 3 months. It is a generic model, but the time frames differ between the specific cancers and adapt according to the treatment(s) required, that is, chemotherapy, surgery, and radiation.

In 2008, the government provided a total of 51 million Dkr (US$7,611,656) over 3 fiscal years, to support the implementation of CPPs in the regions, reduce waiting times, and improve the financing system. No system was put in place to ensure money was allocated to the clinical units, an oversight that has led to some criticism by caregivers.

Impact of Cancer Patient Pathways

National monitoring measures the proportion of patients who begin initial treatment within the recommended time frame. There is no official national target, but there is broad political consensus that 90% of the patients should begin treatment within the time frame.

In 2013, the proportion was 72%; by 2014 it had risen to 77%, and it is expected to increase to 78% by 2015. The figures disguise substantial differences between the specific cancers. For example, in 2014, 97% of patients with melanoma received surgical treatment within the time frame, compared with only 27% of patients requiring surgical treatment of bladder cancer. Significant discrepancies between the healthcare regions have also been revealed by the data, provoking serious political debate. It is an objective of the forthcoming cancer plan (IV) to reduce these regional disparities.

Data across the Nordic countries indicates that the CPPs have had an impact on cancer survival rates. Between 1999 and 2003, survival rates for men were 9–13% lower than in Finland, Iceland, Norway, and Sweden. For women, the survival rates were 5–8% lower. These differences have since been reduced: between 2009 and 2013 the gap for men was reduced to 3–7%, and for women to 4–5% (Engholm et al., 2016).

It also appears that the number of negative patient stories about obstacles in the diagnostic and treatment pathways has declined. In 2016, the Danish Cancer Society will carry out the second comprehensive survey, which will illuminate the perspective of the cancer patients.

Reflections on Reasons for Success

CPPs were the response to a clear and well-documented problem. The feasibility of the recommended technical solution was demonstrated by the success of a specific hospital program. But this evidence was not enough to initiate a change. As demonstrated in other settings, a more comprehensive approach was needed to ensure improvement in practice (Dixon-Woods et al., 2011).

In this case, the alliance between prominent cancer experts and the patient organization was critical to ensuring concrete action was taken at the national level. The presentation of individual patients' medical narratives, supported by visual images as well as data, also played a part.

That CPPs have been so widely accepted is primarily due to professional involvement and "ownership" during development. The decision was top-down, but the actual pathways were developed in a bottom-up process, giving clinicians considerable freedom to develop the clinical content. In order to ensure implementation, regional politicians and administrative leaders are held accountable by ongoing monitoring of waiting times, national public reporting on data, and critical feedback provided by the Cancer Society, the press, and the public.

Transferability of the Exemplar

The story illustrates the power of building commitment through a combination of soft and hard intelligence, and through systematic follow-up. But the specific program can be transferred as well.

Integrated pathways are now used in the treatment of acute cardiac disease and mental disorders throughout Denmark. However, some psychiatrists have raised concerns that integrated pathways may be less suitable in their domain, where it is harder to fit treatment options and decisions into a formalized algorithm.

Inspired by the success of the Danish model, Norway and Sweden have established their own cancer patient pathways (Cancer Centrum, 2015; Helsedirektoratet, 2016).

Prospects for Further Success and Next Steps

A more cancer-aware population, greater efforts in local implementation, and improved monitoring are required if objectives are to be met. A public campaign outlining the symptoms of cancer is ongoing and initiatives to improve the skills of Danish GPs have been launched. The monitoring system has to be tuned to assess delays more specifically.

The CPPs will be continually developed to address cancer patients' needs. The biggest challenge is that only 50% of patients initially present cancer-specific symptoms and fit into the pathway referral criteria. It is expected that the upcoming cancer plan will focus on how to deal with patients who do not present specific alarm-symptoms when they contact their GP. It is also expected that the plan will facilitate rapid and early diagnosis by expanding GP access to diagnostic facilities and expertise.

18

England

A NICE Success Story from the English National Health Service

Martin Powell and Russell Mannion

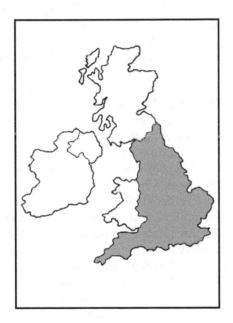

CONTENTS

Introduction and National Policy Context

The British National Health Service (NHS), which was established in 1948, was the "first health system in any Western society to offer free medical care to the entire population through a state-provided, comprehensive service funded largely from national taxation" (Klein, 2013: 1). However, like other systems, it has attempted to square the circle between supply and demand by some form of economic rationing of healthcare interventions.

In 1997, the New Labour government of Tony Blair was elected. One of the major problems facing the NHS at this time was the so-called postcode rationing in which access to treatment was partly determined by area of residence, with some local purchasers of health services denied funding for interventions that were provided to patients living elsewhere in the country, with some cases contested and resulting in litigation (Syrett, 2003).

The Labour government's response was to increase the "National" in the NHS. Within some 6 months of taking office, Health Secretary Frank Dobson issued a white paper, The New NHS (Department of Health [DH] [UK], 1997). This stressed two major themes. The first involved greater equity, or "a one nation NHS" (DH, 1997, para. 7.1), "so that two-tierism becomes a thing of the past" (DH, 1997, para. 5.29). The second was concerned with evidence-based policy or "what works," so that "services and treatment that patients receive across the NHS should be based on the best evidence of what does and does not work and what provides best value for money, clinical and cost-effectiveness" (DH, 1997, para. 7.5).

"What works" was to be decided through the rational technocratic process of "evidence-based policy" and "evidence-based medicine," and implemented via a series of inter-related supporting initiatives, most notably the introduction of a formal system of clinical governance across NHS trusts, the promulgation of national service frameworks, and by the creation of a new institution, the National Institute for Clinical Excellence (NICE), which would "give a strong lead on clinical and cost-effectiveness, drawing up new guidelines and ensuring they reach all parts of the health service" (DH, 1997, para. 3.5).

Evolution of NICE

NICE was later renamed the National Institute for Health and Clinical Excellence and then the National Institute for Health and Care Excellence, however the acronym NICE has been retained. These name changes reflect an expansion of the NICE's role and remit to include evidence-based reviews of public health and social care interventions. Following the most recent NHS reforms, NICE has been granted the status of an "independent" or "arms-length" non-departmental public body.

NICE's implicit political goal was to screen ministers from decisions about rationing resources, although the government and NICE itself tended to use terms such as *hard choices, prioritization*, and that other "R" word, *rational*, rather than *rationing*. "If in the past politicians had sheltered behind the doctrine of clinical autonomy ... in future they would shelter behind the dictates of evidence-based medicine" (Klein, 2013: 202). However, sometimes, ministers asked NICE to reconsider its views, or they ignored its guidance. For example, despite a decision from NICE in 2005 that Herceptin, an expensive drug for early-stage breast cancer, was not cost-effective, Health Secretary Patricia Hewitt nevertheless encouraged purchasing organizations to fund it (Klein, 2013).

NICE's original role was essentially advisory, with its guidance not being legally binding on health authorities purchasing treatments or on clinicians prescribing them. However, the quality improvement role of NICE is now part of primary legislation, as set out in the Health and Social Care Bill 2012, enacted in April 2013. Consequently, it is now mandatory for purchasers to provide funds to give effect to NICE's recommendations, and government ministers themselves are also obliged by law to give due regard to NICE. NICE guidance officially applies only to England, but it is contracted to provide certain products and services to Wales, Scotland, and Northern Ireland.

NICE has indicated that it is inclined to "accept as cost-effective" those interventions with an incremental cost-effectiveness ratio of less than £20,000 (US$25,570) per quality-adjusted life year (QALY). However, the House of Commons Health Select Committee (2007: 7) argued that this threshold was not based on empirical research and is not directly related to the NHS budget.

Approach and Activity

The DH for England and NHS England decide which topics NICE will look at. NICE divides its guidance into five main areas:

1. Health technology: specific medicines, treatments, and procedures
2. Clinical practice: how doctors and healthcare professionals should treat diseases and conditions
3. Public health: preventing illness and facilitating health promotion
4. Social care: services to help people with daily life at home, in care homes, or day centers
5. Quality standards: statements designed to drive quality improvements within a particular area of care

NICE's decisions are made by independent committees or groups. These include patient or public members (lay members), academics, and researchers. NICE makes decisions on whether a drug or treatment should be available, based on

- Evidence: NICE reviews each treatment or new technique
- Cost-effectiveness: including QALY
- Contributions from patient organizations, health professionals, experts, and other interested parties

The self-declared "core principles" of NICE include: independence, methodological robustness, using the best available evidence on clinical and cost-effectiveness, using expert opinion, public involvement, transparency, review, and the application of social values and equity considerations (Ruiz and Breckon, 2014).

From 1 March 2000 to 30 September 2015, NICE published 189 single technology appraisals and 167 multiple technology appraisals; 356 appraisals in total, containing 596 individual recommendations. Overall, 81% of decisions made by NICE (457 of 567) were "recommended" or "optimized" (i.e., recommended for a smaller subset of patients than originally stated by the marketing authorization). Since 2000, when NICE started to produce cancer guidelines, NICE has published 170 individual recommendations on cancer drugs in 124 technology appraisals. Overall, 64% of all recommendations stated that the NHS should use these drugs in line with their marketing authorization ("recommended"), or in specific circumstances ("optimized recommendation") (National Institute for Health and Clinical Excellence [NICE], n.d.).

Successes

NICE has increased the volume and quality of evidence used to support key economic decisions in the NHS and has helped to reduce geographical variation in the allocation of scarce healthcare resources (Williams, 2016).

Williams (2016) points out that the survival of NICE for 14 years, and for the foreseeable future, might itself be regarded as something of an achievement. Despite repeated reform of virtually every other aspect of the system, successive governments have concluded that NICE's work is not just necessary but should be expanded in terms of both the volume and range of guidance it produces. Indeed, interest in NICE's processes and programs has been extraordinary. In 2008, the average number of visits to NICE's website was 486,246 per month. A systematic review identified more than 2000 reports in peer-reviewed journals that included NICE in the title. Countries seeking advice from NICE's policy unit include Bahrain, Colombia, Estonia, Jordan, Saudi Arabia, South Korea, Thailand, and Turkey (Rawlins, 2009).

NICE claims that it has established a worldwide reputation for producing authoritative, evidence-based advice and guidelines. (NICE, n.d.). Moreover, as Danni Mason, head of the What Works team, United Kingdom Cabinet Office, observed, NICE is now regarded as "the go-to organization and not just nationally but internationally" (Ruiz and Breckon, 2014: 16).

Transferability of NICE Methods to Other Countries and Regions

NICE International, which operates on a strict non-profit basis, has been set up as a specific initiative to raise standards of healthcare around the world by providing advice and support to encourage the use of clinically and cost-effective treatments. It also undertakes important research activities, such as generating case studies, preparing tools to help data analysis, and encouraging shared learning through international meetings.

Indeed, the success of NICE has led many governments to explore ways of examining the effectiveness and cost-effectiveness of interventions within their health systems. The evidence required for such assessment has encouraged them to engage in comparative effectiveness research (CER), health technology assessment (HTA), and cost-effectiveness analysis (CEA). Increasingly, the supply of such evidence in many Organization for Economic Cooperation and Development (OECD) healthcare systems is along similar principles to NICE, namely through specially created guidance-producing bodies set up as advisers to health ministries. However, the governance arrangements of these bodies differ substantially, with attendant implications for both the policy formation process and the implementation of this into practice (Williams, 2016).

Chalkidou et al. (2009) point out that many countries now use terms such as *comparative effectiveness research, health technology assessment*, or *evidence-informed policymaking* to describe essentially the same activity. For example, they examined four national-level models created to evaluate health technologies and broader management strategies to inform healthcare policy decisions: NICE (UK), *Haute Autorite de Sante* or HAS (France), Pharmaceutical Benefits Scheme or PBS (Australia), and *Institut fur Qualitat und Wirtschaftlichkeit im Gesundheitswesen* or IQWiG (Germany). According to Williams (2016), in the United States, Medicare, Medicaid, the Children's Health Insurance Program, the Department of Veterans Affairs, as well as private insurance and managed care organizations all have some responsibility for making decisions about what the healthcare "menu" covers. Systems with a stronger central planning function than others, such as the United Kingdom's, assign greater responsibility to statutory bodies, whereas non-profit insurance agencies carry prime responsibility in countries such as Germany and the Netherlands.

Furthermore, again according to Chalkidou et al. (2009), a number of core principles emerged as necessary, and often conflicting, requirements for the operation of CER entities in their four countries. These are

- Independence from central government, insurance agencies, and industries
- Transparency in the way the topics are selected, the evidence is synthesized and assessed, and the final decision is made
- Inclusiveness, achieved through broad and repeated consultation and dialogue with all relevant parties
- Scientific rigor
- Contestability, made possible through a mechanism for reconsidering or appealing a decision
- Timeliness, gained by issuing advice while the technology or practice is still at an early stage of diffusion

Although NICE is not an easily replicable model that can be exported to other countries and contexts, many elements of its methodology, process, evidence base, and products can be adapted to other countries' local realities (Ruiz and Breckon, 2014).

While in many respects NICE is regarded as a success and its operating procedures are worthy of being adopted in other countries and regions, a number of operational problems have been highlighted. For example, a House of Commons Select Committee (2007) report criticized the delay in access to treatments due to the lengthy nature of the appraisals process, and there have been criticisms that NICE has not provided effective guidance when it comes to disinvestment and the commissioning of services (Williams, 2016). There have been suggestions that the tendency to direct resources away from those interventions that do not have NICE guidance may distort clinical priorities and impair both access and quality.

Conclusion

NICE has been a rock of stability during a period of rapid change in the NHS and has established a worldwide reputation as an example of good practice in healthcare decision-making. It has been hailed as an innovation in healthcare decision-making in that its scope and position within the health system make it unique as a mechanism for assessing new technologies and managing their introduction into clinical practice (Syrett, 2003).

According to Britnell (2015: 124), former director general at the DH, one of the three questions* he has been asked most frequently during visits to 60 countries is "How can we establish NICE?" Notwithstanding the limitations previously outlined, it would appear that NICE's approach has much to offer other healthcare systems as they grapple with providing high-quality, cost-effective services in an era of austerity.

---

* The other questions are "What happened to the failed IT program, Connecting for Health?" and "Why do you repeatedly reorganize your health system?"

19

Estonia

Primary Healthcare Reform as a Promoter of Quality in the Estonian Healthcare System

Kaja Põlluste, Ruth Kalda, and Margus Lember

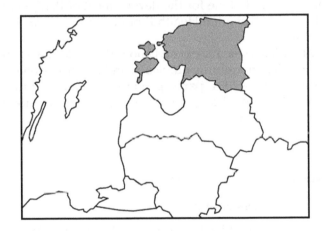

CONTENTS

Background

Estonia is the smallest of the Baltic countries, covering an area of 45,227 square kilometers. In January 2016, the population of Estonia was 1,311,759; of this, the urban population accounts for 68%. In the late 1980s and early 1990s, Estonia, like all Central and Eastern European countries, experienced great changes in its political and economic systems. The regaining of Estonia's independence in 1991 opened the door to new opportunities for the whole society, including the health sector. Dissatisfaction with the previous healthcare system among both providers and users, along with the evident decline in the health of the population, led to reforms in the early 1990s (Lember, 1998).

Beginning with the introduction of national health insurance in 1992, the reform process covered all areas of the health system. One of the most comprehensive reforms in the Estonian health system focused on the strengthening of the primary healthcare system (PHC) (Põlluste et al., 2013). However, attention has also been paid to quality improvement (QI) of healthcare services, and since the late 1990s, many regulations have been established at the national level to ensure quality and to protect patients' rights (Põlluste et al., 2006). An important milestone for the development of PHC and QI was the implementation of the Estonian Health Project (EHP) in 1995–1998 (Põlluste et al., 2006, 2013).

Estonia's admission to the European Union (EU) in 2004 was instrumental to reforms of legislation, training curricula, and the provision of services in the health system. Since 2004, participation in several EU-funded projects has stimulated international cooperation and led to further modifications to the Estonian health system.

Details of the Success Story

Improving the provision of health services in Estonia has required a three-pronged approach: the establishment of a legal framework, the restructuring of the health system with a focus on the development of a modern PHC system, and the development of human resources (Põlluste et al., 2013).

Out of several examples of "success stories," we aimed to find the one that

- Was implemented according to clearly defined objectives
- Has been sufficiently evaluated
- Had an input in the QI of the health system
- Provides a good example for other sectors of the health system in Estonia as well as other countries

We have therefore chosen to describe the implementation of Estonia's PHC reform, which incorporated all the main components of health reform: it looked toward changes in policy objectives followed by institutional change, it was developed through a purposeful and sustained long-term process, and it was led as a political process by the government (Cassels, 1995). Moreover, since 2006, the implementation of reform has been accompanied by the implementation of the QI system within the PHC.

The first step in the reorganization of the existing PHC system involved the training of staff. Prior to the reforms, medical education focused on early undergraduate specialization with one-year postgraduate internships, and the PHC doctors did not have the knowledge and skills required for modern family medicine (FM). In 1991, a group of university FM teachers and scientists established the Estonian Society of Family Doctors (ESFD), which was one of the initiators of a new training curriculum for PHC doctors. The training of family doctors (FDs) in Estonia was organized in two ways. An individually tailored 3-year in-service retraining course was made available to practicing doctors as a first option from 1991 (Põlluste et al., 2013). The 3-year full-time residency training in FM began in 1995 and has become one of the most popular options for medical graduates. By 2004, all practicing PHC doctors were certified as FDs; thus, since 2005, the retraining course has no longer been available (Maaroos, 2004).

The ESFD has been a partner of the Ministry of Social Affairs (MoSA) and the National Health Insurance Fund (EHIF) in the further development of the new PHC system, and the next stages of PHC reform—the formulation of tasks and objectives as well as drafts of new legislative acts—were developed in close collaboration.

The basic tasks of the reform were formulated in 1997 as follows (Lember, 2002):

- To create a list system so that the population could register with a primary care doctor
- To introduce a partial gate-keeping system
- To introduce a combined payment system for FDs
- To give the FDs the status of independent contractors

These reforms, including the educational requirements for FDs and family nurses, were legislated in 1998 (Lember, 1998). Additionally, a number of voluntary QI activities were introduced and implemented in PHC. In 2001, the EFSD introduced a voluntary certification system for FDs, and since 2009, the EFSD has run a voluntary annual accreditation program for family practices. The standards, criteria, and indicators cover the following areas: accessibility to and organization of practices, the quality of medical treatment, and determining whether the practices can provide a learning environment for students as well as serve as a base for conducting scientific work (World Bank, 2015). A number of EHIF-funded clinical guidelines have been produced by FDs, family nurses, and other medical specialists.

An important step in improving the performance of family practices was the implementation of the FD quality bonus system (QBS) in 2006. This joint initiative of the EHIF and the EFSD aims to increase the quality and effectiveness of preventive services and to improve the monitoring of chronic diseases. The results of recent studies demonstrated that FDs who participate in the QBS provide more preventive activities as well as systematic monitoring of chronic illnesses, such as hypertension and type 2 diabetes mellitus (Kalda and Västra, 2013; Merilind et al., 2015).

Patient perspectives on the success of the PHC reform (see Figures 19.1 and 19.2) have been evaluated since 1998 (Estonian Health Insurance Fund, 2016).

Other factors are also indicative of improvement. The results of a study from 1997 showed that 95% of the newly trained FDs were satisfied, and that a well-organized practice, high-quality equipment, and the opportunity to learn new things were the most valued aspects of the work (Kalda et al., 2000). Setting a national standard in 1997 improved the quality of FDs' practice equipment substantially, and with the reorganization of the PHC, the work of the FDs became more comprehensive (Kalda and Lember, 2000; Maaroos and Meiesaar, 2004). The combined system of financing means that the provision of resources in PHC is financially sustainable (Meiesaar and Lember, 2004).

Details of the Impact of the Success Story

Strong leadership, collaboration, and early investment in training were key components of success. Moreover, the reform was initiated at the grassroots level by scientists, university teachers, and practicing physicians.

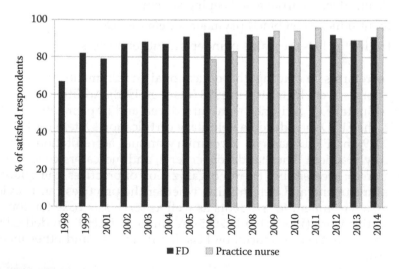

FIGURE 19.1
Satisfaction with the FD and practice nurse.

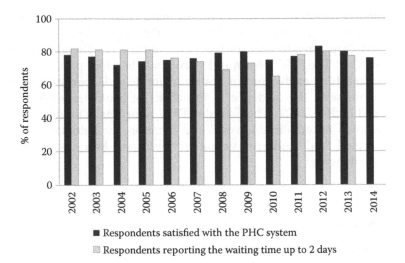

FIGURE 19.2
Satisfaction with and access to PHC services.

Another factor in the success of the reforms was effective planning. The objectives formulated were realistic and achievable, the process was implemented step-by-step, and the transition period was long enough to train staff and to create the infrastructure and legal framework for the changes.

The establishment of relatively simple payment systems and contracts led to the early institutionalization of FM and the use of contracting as a key instrument of change (Atun et al., 2006). PHC funding has been stable since 2003, with an allocation of 13–14% of total EHIF expenditure on health services.

In the initial transition period, healthcare was not "high-politics." This created a window of opportunity for policymakers to introduce health reforms with minimal opposition from politicians (Atun et al., 2006). The reforms therefore had the benefit of both government and popular support.

Implementation: Transferability of the Example

The PHC reform has been the most successful initiative in the Estonian health system. The first step in the process was the development of human resources: a well-trained and highly motivated staff was an important precondition for these particular changes. The involvement of professionals is an important factor that might be transferred to any other initiative within the country. A good example is the implementation of voluntary QI mechanisms in PHC, which can be transferred to the other health sectors as well.

As in many countries in transition, the reform was supported by external funding through the EHP in 1995–1998. This support promoted the initiatives that had already been introduced, and the reform continued after the end of EHP. The PHC reform in Estonia has therefore provided a model for other countries of the former Soviet Union (e.g., Uzbekistan, Moldova, Latvia). Until now, the evidence of the effect of health reforms is sparse (Rechel and McKee, 2009). The Estonian PHC reform is definitely one of the most evaluated reforms in the world and therefore the Estonian experience of multifaceted health reform evaluation could also be transferred to any country in the world.

Prospects for Further Success and Next Steps

There are, however, still some areas that need further improvement. One of the greatest challenges to the Estonian healthcare system is the increasing number of people with chronic diseases. The results of a recent evaluation show that the coordination of patient management between healthcare providers as well as across the health and social service systems could be improved. A number of visits to specialists could be avoided by more effective treatment coordination of patients with chronic diseases and through the provision of more preventive services. Thus, the continuous strengthening of the PHC and the introduction of chronic disease management systems and models based on PHC will be the focus of future developments in healthcare (Kurowski et al., 2015; Lai et al., 2015; Rechel and McKee, 2009).

Conclusion

The implementation of PHC reform in Estonia demonstrates that success depends on many factors. Setting clear objectives and developing human resources, infrastructure, and legal frameworks are essential preconditions for success. Consistent QI will ensure that improvements continue to be made, and that the needs of the population are met.

20

Finland

Evidence-Based Medicine and Health Information Technology: Transforming Clinical Practices in Finland

Persephone Doupi, Jorma Komulainen, Minna Kaila, and Ilkka Kunnamo

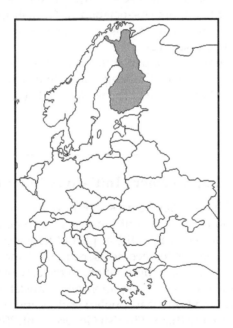

CONTENTS

Background

Finland is a sparsely populated country of 5.5 million inhabitants (Statistics Finland, 2015). Persons residing in Finland are entitled to universal health coverage provided by the Finnish public health and social care system. Three hundred and thirteen municipalities, over half with fewer than 6000 inhabitants, either produce primary healthcare services (individually or in cooperation) or purchase them from private or public providers (Association of Finnish Local and Regional Authorities, 2017b). Specialized care is offered through 21 hospital districts, whose serving populations vary from about 44,000 to 1,580,000 inhabitants (Association of Finnish Local and Regional Authorities, 2017a). Some private hospitals also exist, primarily offering ambulatory or short-stay services.

Finland, just like many developed countries across the globe, is anxiously seeking solutions to a range of challenges threatening the operations of the healthcare system and the future of the welfare state (Lang, 2011).

Current Systems Improvement Initiatives in Finland

Reforms of the health and social care sector have been under discussion by several administrations. The current Finnish government intends to enact a radical reform of the sector by 2019, as part of its wider structural reform program. Public services are to become user-oriented and achieve the necessary productivity leap through digitization. In the case of social welfare and healthcare, the reform aims at integration and translates to utilizing joint resources and improving both basic public services and the information systems employed to provide them (Finnish Government, 2015).

Details of the Success Story

Finland has been among the pioneers of eHealth adoption and implementation in the EU and, in some respects, even globally. The first national strategy for implementation of health information technology (HIT), published in

1995, focused on the principle of citizen-centered and seamless service structures (Work Group Report, 1995). The in-principle decision by the Council of State on Securing the Future of Health Care (Ministry of Social Affairs and Health [Finland], 2002) paved the way toward the widespread uptake of electronic health records, as well as the support and development of health technology assessment (HTA) (Ministry of Social Affairs and Health [Finland], 2002). At present, both the national electronic patient records archive, Kanta, and the service providing citizens' access to their health data, Omakanta, are fully operational, while the development of a social care records archive has begun. The implementation of the new eHealth and eSocial care strategy is set to continue until 2020 (Kallio, 2015).

The eHealth Infrastructure

Electronic patient records (EPRs) and filmless picture archiving and communications systems (PACS) cover 100% of both primary and specialized care and are the exclusive source of patient information in almost all healthcare centers and hospitals, as well as the large majority of private units. Documentation takes place increasingly through the use of structured core data, national classifications, and coding systems. Linking of local systems to the Kanta national archive is advancing steadily. Most physicians use electronic prescribing (mandatory for all, as of 2017), whereby prescriptions are forwarded from the local systems to the national e-prescription repository and can be accessed by any pharmacy for dispensing (Hyppönen et al., 2015).

Tools for All Stakeholders

The health portal, Terveysportti, offers Finnish healthcare professionals a single access point to a variety of electronic tools and resources essential for their everyday work, including timely clinical practice guidelines and access to various scientific databases. The service is available throughout the country's healthcare system and receives about 50 million searches annually. At the core of the portal is the Doctor's Manual or (in its English version) Evidence-Based Medicine Guidelines (EBMG), a collection of almost 1000 clinical guidelines (see www.ebm-guidelines.com). The guidelines are linked to the best available evidence and designed for use at the point of care.

Current Care Guidelines are independent, evidence-based clinical practice guidelines, covering important issues related to health, medical care, and disease prevention in Finland (see www.kaypahoito.fi/web/english).

They are developed and regularly updated by the Finnish Medical Society, Duodecim, in collaboration with various medical specialist societies. The guidelines, which are available in a variety of formats, are intended as a basis for treatment and care decisions, and they can be used by doctors, healthcare professionals, and the general public. Current Care Guidelines are extensively used as references in developing national recommendations on care pathways and acceptable waiting periods for access to treatment.

The closest integration of health information technology and evidence-based medicine (EBM) is to be found in the Evidence-Based Medicine Electronic Decision Support (EBMeDS) system (see www.ebmeds.org). EBMeDS links evidence and clinical practice through the provision of context-sensitive guidance at the point of care. Upon certain "trigger events," such as prescribing a drug or adding a diagnosis, EBMeDS receives structured patient data from EPRs or personal health records (PHRs) and returns reminders, therapeutic suggestions, a comprehensive medication review, and a diagnosis-specific overview containing guidance relevant to each patient.

As a platform-independent service, EBMeDS can be integrated into any system containing structured patient data. It uses simple but efficient technology, and both installation and system updating are easy. It can also be used to channel patient data to electronic forms and calculators. In addition to real-time use, the EBMeDS decision support rules can be applied to patient populations in a process known as "virtual health checks," in order to identify people who would benefit from interventions and to generate clinical quality reports.

Duodecim seeks to ensure that the general public also has access to a wide range of reliable medical information. The channels it uses for this purpose include books, freely accessible online material, services integrated into healthcare systems, and study materials for schools. One of the best known and widely used resources is the health library, Terveyskirjasto.

The health library service (Terveyskirjasto.fi) contains an extensive range of materials. The service provides basic information on medical conditions and diseases, as well as advice on how to get treatment and care. Its articles are accessed more than 50 million times a year. The patient versions of Current Care Guidelines are also published in the health library. The EBMeDS service also provides guidance directly to citizens and patients.

Promotion of EMB principles and practices also targets policymakers. The work of the Finnish Office for HTA (FinOHTA) is focused on addressing the fragmented decision-making relating to health technologies, through practical tools for implementing HTA findings. In addition to full HTA reports, additional services include the Ohtanen database, which provides Finnish-language summaries of assessments of other international members and the European Network for HTA (EUnetHTA), where the Finnish team has coordinated the development of a joint model for context-independent HTA (WHO, n.d.b.).

The Managed Uptake of Medical Methods (MUMM) is a joint program between FinOHTA and public sector specialized medical care, meant to encourage healthcare decision makers' commitment to evidence-based practices (National Institute for Health and Welfare [Finland], n.d.). MUMM has developed a structure for critical appraisal and joint decisions in uptake of new methods before their wide implementation. Since its launch in 2006, the MUMM program has given 60 recommendations on new hospital technologies.

Details of the Impact of the Success Story

The successful synergy and coexistence of EBM and HIT presented in this chapter are the fruit of persistent commitment to a vision and achievement of goals set almost 3 decades ago (Figure 20.1). While changes and adaptations have been driven by a variety of factors, the key objectives have remained unaltered. Effective alignment of policy, funding, research and development, implementation, and multidisciplinary and cross-sectoral collaboration have been essential to progress, as has the successful engagement and involvement of professional societies, individual practitioners, and service providers.

What's the Nature of the Success?

The effects of the effort described here can be observed in three areas: infrastructure, practice, and culture. A variable, expanding, and evolving

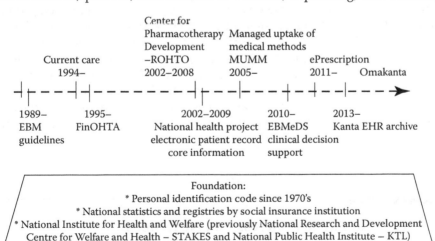

FIGURE 20.1
EBM and HIT in Finland.

collection of tools, infrastructure, and services has been made available to health and social care professionals, as well as decision makers and the general public. As a result, the culture and ways of practicing have changed both at the individual and the organizational level, with the evidence-based approach to decision-making, planning, and assessment becoming the norm. Client empowerment, as well as the integration of health and social care, are both on the horizon (Rigby et al., 2011).

Implementation: Transferability of the Exemplar

The work undertaken thus far will need to be expanded to include the domains of social care and biomedicine. For the former, much can be learned from the errors and setbacks of implementing information technology (IT) in the healthcare sector. Similarly, positive lessons and achievements can also be adopted and adapted as needed. The Finnish biomedical sector is held in high regard internationally and has been duly recognized as a field of strategic importance (Ministry of Employment and the Economy [Finland], 2016). Despite its heavily IT-dependent profile and the acknowledged need for data and services to merge in practice as well as for research, the respective infrastructure in Finland has largely developed without alignment to that of the health and social care sector at large (Commission Expert Group on Rare Diseases, 2016). Activating most of the elements behind the success thus far will be essential to bridging the gap and achieving further progress.

Countries around the globe are making considerable investments in IT, generally driven by the same desire to reduce costs while improving quality and efficiency (Adler-Milstein et al., 2014). Although the integration of verified knowledge in clinical practice is one of the few proven benefits of eHealth, and despite evidence highlighting the importance of engaging users of technology in its planning and roll out, neither has been widely adopted in large-scale implementations (WHO, 2012). Moreover, even in countries with a strong tradition in HTA, alignment and collaboration with eHealth initiatives is rare. The Finnish example can thereby provide a roadmap and concrete examples for achieving valuable synergies.

Prospects for Further Success and Next Steps

Recent economic pressures in Finland have reduced the resources available particularly for EBM and HTA related work—a paradoxical effect, since the need actually increases in times of austerity. Long-term success will require sustaining what has been achieved, while supporting the expansion and creation of links and collaborations to both fields of social care and biomedicine. Ensuring the true engagement of patients and citizens is a challenge that is still to be won. Equally critical will be the ability to stay in the mainstream of international developments.

Conclusions

The significant restructuring of health and social care operations that is currently underway in Finland would not have been feasible without the long-standing commitment and concurrent development of eHealth and EBM. The success of the reform remains to be proven, and several aspects of it have already been heavily criticized nationally. Nevertheless, gains in terms of improved quality of clinical practice and streamlined services have been largely achieved. The challenge will be to not jeopardize future progress by failing to sustain the elements and structures that have made such improvement possible.

21

France

The French Healthcare System and Its Alternative Approach to Patient Safety

René Amalberti and Thomas le Leduc

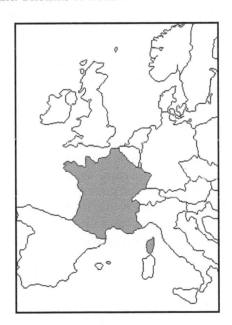

CONTENTS

Background

When it comes to addressing safety in a complex system, there are two main strategies. The first, which involves adopting a "global vision system," prioritizes the development of proactive strategies such as high levels of access to care. Alternatively, a "care-centered vision" may be adopted, focusing largely on reactive strategies, such as mitigation and the lessons learned through mistakes, seeking to strengthen professional obligations. While many Western countries follow a care-centered approach, the French healthcare system is structured around a "global vision system." While this means that the national government very rarely imposes formal national safety initiatives, French patients, paradoxically, still "feel safe" and have high levels of satisfaction.

The French healthcare system's traditional prioritization of this strategy is a legacy of the French conception of public law, public sphere, and public good, and is related to the French embrace of social solidarity as an important value. The concept of solidarity has its roots in the fraternal ideals of the French Revolution, as articulated in the motto "liberty, equality, and fraternity." After World War II, France built its social security system, which includes health insurance, on principles of social solidarity.

Patient safety has never captured the public imagination as an important issue in France. While citizens and politicians frequently complain about the health system—for instance the failure to reimburse the cost of certain drugs or the downsizing of hospitals in rural areas—complaints about adverse events (AEs) are not a major part of the public conversation. The regional press might write about AEs that are the result of medical errors here and there, but these articles are written and understood as general news; very few articles are interested in offering system-wide critiques, and they rarely look beyond the local and anecdotal.

Nor has patient safety ever been on the agenda of any political party, whether left or right. There has been very little political debate on such issues for several decades; even the new National Program for Patient Safety (PNSP 2014–2017), under the authority of the French Ministry, was established without controversy, and it remains little known among professionals, the general public, and the press.

Despite this lack of awareness and interest in the issue, French medical safety figures are similar to other comparable countries (Michel et al., 2008).

Care-Centered versus System-Centered Approach

A care-centered safety approach to improving patient safety focuses on the reduction, and ideally the avoidance, of preventable AEs, reassuring the public by apportioning blame, and then making efforts to find a solution—whether through system-wide reform or individual professional development. In such a configuration, the link between the rate of AEs and safety is unambiguous, supposedly easy to measure, and derives clearly from the classic industrial approach.

An alternative approach places more emphasis on system-centered services (Degos et al., 2008; Rodwin, 2003). It focuses on the broader dimensions of the healthcare system: access to quality healthcare services and patients' rights, for example. This includes clinical prevention and primary care, appropriate referral, and receipt of specialty services ranging from state-of-the-art medical care to new technologies, as well as timely arrival to the emergency room, intensive care unit (ICU), and inpatient hospital services. These dimensions also provide a framework to assess the extent to which a nation succeeds in providing its citizens with a health system that assures patients life-long access to complex healthcare services, both in hospitals and within the community. System-centered services focus on minimizing hospitalization for conditions requiring ambulatory care and reducing unnecessary deaths. These are both areas where France has increasingly been acknowledged as a leader (Nolte and McKee, 2008).

The French National Health Insurance (NHI) system is based on the principle that reducing financial barriers to healthcare access is a good investment for society. Ready access to good primary healthcare and hospital emergency rooms facilitates early diagnosis and treatment, which may, in turn, avert the progression of disease and delay exposure to what can be a potentially dangerous hospital milieu. Instead of placing disproportionate faith in the hypothetical ideal of total safety in hospitals, a system-centered approach emphasizes the importance of delaying and even averting the exposure of vulnerable patients to the hospitals.

All French residents can choose their doctors and specialists; they also have access to both public and private hospitals anywhere, and as frequently as required. France also has one of the best emergency medical assistance systems (the SAMU), providing citizens 24-hour, on-call tele-coordination, home visits by hospital doctors, and direct transfer to ICUs when needed. In order to improve care coordination, a soft gate-keeper mechanism was introduced as part of the French healthcare reforms of 2005. In practice, this means that if patients change their primary care doctor without informing their NHI fund, they are reimbursed at a lower rate. Nonetheless, access to primary care is widely available and waiting times for specialty services are among the shortest in the world.

That the annual number of patients' malpractice claims remains stable and relatively low may be attributed to the relative efficiency of the French system, along with a historical consideration for patients' rights (as described in the next section), and the creation, in 2005, of a national fund providing a no-fault compensation system for aggrieved patients.

Improving the System: Legislating Patients' Rights

In 2002, the Patients' Rights and Quality of Care Act, also known as the Kouchner Act, was passed. This act, which had been actively promoted by patients' associations, amended the Public Health Code and the Civil Code, improving both the rights of patients and the quality of the health system. The Kouchner Act represented a radical redefinition of government priorities, placing "the individual, the person, in other words the patient or the user, as the focus of concerns, at the center of legislation," and thereby moving "from a system of professionals to a system directed toward the individual" (Europatientrights.org, n.d.).

The main emphasis of the act is on patient rights; indeed, a preliminary chapter in the Public Health Code is entitled "Rights of the Individual." The words of article 1111-1 of the Public Health Code could not be more clear: "There can be no democratic health system without a corresponding legal framework of rights accorded to sick people and users." The act itself has three objectives. The first objective is to enhance patients' ability to use their "voice" in the healthcare system. The second objective is to improve the quality of care and to develop continuing education for healthcare professionals and the evaluation of professional practice. A third objective concerns protection against the risks related to diagnostic and therapeutic procedures.

In April 2005, Act No. 2005-370 (Leonetti's law) concerning the rights of patients and the end of life came into force. This new law prohibited unreasonable obstinacy in investigations or therapeutics and authorized the withholding or withdrawal of treatments when they appear "useless, disproportionate, or having no other effect than solely the artificial preservation of life." Relief from pain is a fundamental right of patients (Baumann et al., 2009).

In combination, these two acts and associated amendments mean that France now has extensively developed patients' rights legislation, as well as a no-fault compensation system that is administered by several bodies (for more detail, see Thouvenin, 2011).

A campaign encouraging nurses and doctors to apologize to patients and families following AEs was undertaken by the French National Authority of Health (*Haute Autorite de Sante* [HAS]) in late 2008, and apologies have been included as "best practice" in the accreditation process. Attention has also been paid to giving the public greater access to information about the healthcare system. The French system is not inclined to use patient safety indicators (PSIs) or mortality rates, as is common practice in many countries, as these are considered to be subject to scientific bias. Rather, details of specific healthcare system performance are reviewed and made available to the public; for example, comparisons across regions regarding treatment and access to care may be made, along with specific risks and social indicators relating to equity.

Impact

It may be that the accepted method of measuring patient safety by calculating AEs is not as effective as we think. Recent research has suggested that this approach cannot correctly gauge safety levels (Shojania and Marangvan de Mheen, 2015; Vincent et al., 2014). The French approach shows us that what seems to matter most to patients are far more immediate issues: access to care 24/7, with the right doctor, in the right place, and at the right moment, along with an assurance that citizens' rights are guaranteed, and that apologies and compensation for any errors will be forthcoming.

France has encouraged citizens to place their confidence in the healthcare system, not by trying to ensure that no problems will occur, but by guaranteeing that, regardless of their requirements, the system will provide them with a full range of medical services, and that it is fully accountable for any rupture in this moral contract.

Transferability

France leads the world when it comes to a system-centered approach to healthcare. However, countries such as New Zealand and Denmark and more recently the United States are now considering adopting aspects of the French system to complement their primarily care-centered approaches (including the legal enforcement of patients' rights, showcasing the benefits of recovery, and reaching final good medical results despite AEs). Conversely, France has adopted many, if not most of the universal safety solutions and intervention strategies of the care-centered approach at a local level.

Conclusion

Despite their contrasting emphases, all nations, France included, are working in similar ways to improve patient safety.

While there are some local successes, the global count of AEs is resistant to change. This may be because the parameters of patient safety are in a continual state of flux, with demands in care increasing and protocols changing as treatments become more complex. There will always be some failures in systems that accept some risks for the ultimate benefit of patients; after all, no human activity can be error free, especially across a system with open access 24 hours a day, 7 days a week.

One way to ensure that the system continues to be trusted by patients despite such errors, is to ensure that professionals are transparent about possible risks, and that these risks are managed as well as they can be.

The success of the French health system suggests that the first priority for making medical risk acceptable to the population is not necessarily to tally problems, reduce AEs, and transform the culture of blamelessness, although these are all are legitimate goals. Rather, an alternative priority might be to improve the social contract and partnership between carers and citizens, thereby ensuring equitable and immediate access to treatment, the acknowledgment of citizen rights, the empowering of citizens to become major partners in their own treatment, and guaranteeing that adequate compensation is made when required.

However, due to growing financial constraints in France, some of the advantages of the medical system-centered vision could be reduced, which could in turn have a negative impact on the standard of care. This could lead to France adopting a more care-centered model in the future.

22

Germany

Scaling Up a Population-Based Integrated Healthcare System: The Case of "Healthy Kinzigtal" in Germany

Oliver Groene, Holger Pfaff, and Helmut Hildebrandt

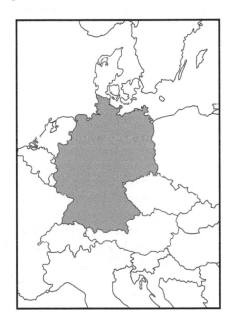

CONTENTS

Introduction

"Healthy Kinzigtal" (HK) is the flagship model of an integrated health-care system and the only fully population-based system in Germany that has been subject to rigorous external evaluation. Based on the Institute for Healthcare Improvement (IHI) "Triple-Aim" model, it simultaneously attempts to improve patient experience of care, increase population health, and reduce the per capita cost of healthcare. Various external evaluations have demonstrated the success of HK in improving quality and care experience, while reducing costs. The general approach, interventions, and evaluation frameworks are widely applicable and deeply rooted in the scientific literature and in models that have proved effective elsewhere. However, a number of conditions need to be met to ensure that the results can be scaled up and successfully replicated elsewhere.

Background

International comparisons demonstrate that the German health system provides high-quality health services for all citizens. However, the German health system is also among the most expensive in the Organization for Economic Cooperation and Development (OECD) (the German national health expenditure was 11.0% of GDP in 2013, compared with the OECD average of 8.9%) and the system does not perform above average when overall population health indicators are compared with similar high-income countries (OECD, 2015a). The reasons for average performance are largely seen in the disincentives embodied in the organization of health services that are not fit to cater to the needs of chronically ill patients.

These problems of care coordination are ongoing and have been addressed by German healthcare legislation in the last 15 years. The 2000 Healthcare Reform Act and the 2004 Modernization Act were pivotal to setting up integrated care systems in Germany. Following these acts, between 2004 and 2008, some 6400 integrated care contracts were set up under this scheme, covering approximately 4 million insured patients and requiring a healthcare expenditure of €811 million (US$869 million). The HK contract is the only German population-based integrated care contract to organize care across all sectors and disease areas. Established in 2004, the system has been subject to rigorous external evaluation (Amelung et al., 2012).

"Healthy Kinzigtal": Germany's Population-Based Integrated Healthcare System

The HK model is based on the "Triple-Aim" approach, according to which three aims are pursued simultaneously:

1. Improving the patient experience of care (including quality and satisfaction)
2. Improving the health of populations
3. Reducing the per capita cost of healthcare (Berwick et al., 2008)

The innovative nature of the program, with its strong reference to theoretical models and up-to-date scientific literature and its rigorous evaluation, means that the HK model is a useful model for other countries to adapt and expand.

The valley of Kinzigtal has about 71,000 inhabitants. Of these, around 33,000 are insured by two major social health insurance (SHI) companies (AOK-BW and LKK-BW), both of which typically have a less favorable risk pool due to their focus on blue collar workers and farmers. Nearly 10,500 of this subset are registered members of HK. However, a key (and frequently misunderstood) characteristic of the model is that HK is financially accountable for all people in the population served, not just for those who are registered members or who receive care from affiliated physicians.

The population-based, fully integrated healthcare system is coordinated by Healthy Kinzigtal Ltd., a regional integrated care management company founded in 2005 by the existing physician network MQNK and OptiMedis AG, a German healthcare management company. OptiMedis AG provides the management know-how, investment capacity, public health and health economics knowledge, and state-of-the art data-warehouse and health analytics. Organizations that cooperate with HK currently include 27 general practitioners, 24 specialists, one pediatrician, five psychotherapists, six hospitals, 10 physiotherapists, 11 nursing homes, five home care services, 16 pharmacies, 38 sports clubs and associations, and six gyms.

The business model of HK has some distinguishing characteristics: at its core is the value-oriented, population-based, shared savings contract based on the "Triple-Aim" approach. Crucial components of this approach include

- The fact that a specific population, representative of a typical risk pool and covered by the integrated care system, can be identified—thereby minimizing the risk of adverse selection
- The support of an "integrator" who has the know-how and competencies to guide the development and implementation of population health improvement programs

- The fact that there are economic rewards from the production of the improved health status instead of a mere increase of services

HK maintains existing reimbursement schemes and financial flows, but the integrator (Healthy Kinzigtal Ltd.) assumes responsibility for the development of the so-called "contribution margin"—the difference between the amount the SHI company receives from the central healthcare fund for the expected (risk-adjusted) mean costs of care of all those insured under German statutory health insurance, and the costs that were actually incurred. A positive contribution margin is then shared between the insurance companies and the integrator. Elements and mechanisms of the overall model are illustrated in Figure 22.1.

Evaluating the Impact of "Healthy Kinzigtal"

The patient-centered care approach, which is paramount to the success of HK, is embedded at three levels: at the structural level, in the planning of interventions, and in the interactions between physicians and patients. At the structural level, patients are represented in biannually elected patient-advisory boards, and they are given opportunities to contribute to identifying and developing new programs. At the level of intervention, a strong focus on shared decision-making and supported self-management is embedded in design and development. At the level of individual doctor–patient interactions, patients joining the program first undergo a comprehensive health check (including a self-assessment questionnaire), based on which an offer to participate in any of the programs may be made. Patients are also given the opportunity to establish health-related goals (such as doing more exercise, giving up smoking, reducing alcohol consumption, or losing weight). These goals are discussed with the doctor and then monitored, accompanied by individual support and participation in patient education and self-care programs as needed. In order to support the patient-centered care approach, physicians, other health professionals, and practice staff are offered training. Underlying all these efforts is an understanding of the patient as a co-producer of his health.

The impact of all activities is evaluated in relation to the "Triple-Aim" approach, supported by two central evaluation studies. The first involves a biannual random survey of the insured regarding their perceived health, satisfaction, changes in health behavior, health-related quality-of-life and levels of activation. The results of the survey demonstrate very high levels of overall satisfaction: 92.1% state they would recommend joining HK and 19.7% state that, overall, they live a healthier life than before joining HK (with 0.4% stating the contrary and 79.9% stating no change). Among insured with an agreed health-related goal, however, 45.4% state they live a healthier life (with 0.6% stating the contrary and 54% stating no change, $p > 0.001$).

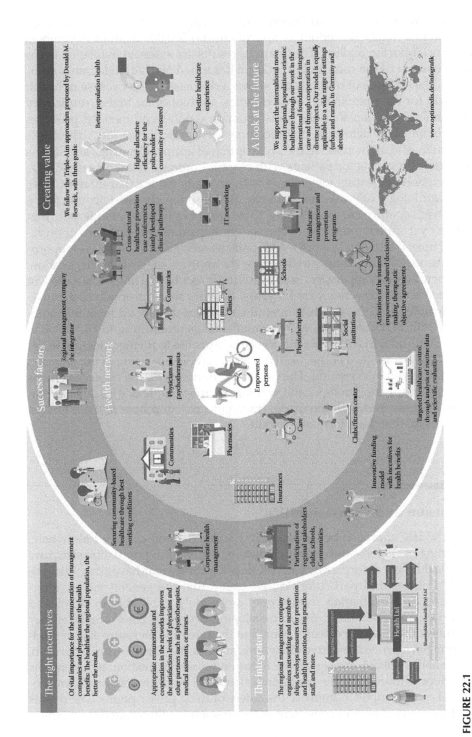

FIGURE 22.1
Infographic: The OptiMedis model for regional integrated healthcare.

The second is a quasi-experimental study comparing the intervention population to a matched random sample of around 500,000 insurance members from neighboring regions. The financial results are assessed in relation to the development of the contribution margin described above (Hildebrandt et al., 2012). The analysis of routine data shows a decrease in the overuse of health services for the prescription of anxiolytics, antibiotics for higher respiratory tract infections, non-steroidal anti-rheumatics, non-recommended prescription for vascular dementia, non-recommended prescription for Alzheimer's dementia, and an increase in the prescription of antiplatelet drugs and statins (where appropriate) for patients with chronic coronary heart disease (CHD), prescriptions of statins for patients with an acute myocardial infarct (AMI), and cardiology referrals for patients diagnosed with heart insufficiency. However, according to routine data, there are also a number of indicators that haven't yet shown a significant change, perhaps due to insufficient observational time. For two indicators—AMI patients on beta blockers and osteoporosis patients with indicated medication—the analysis suggests a deterioration.

Generally, a propensity score–matched control group suggests an increase in life expectancy by 1.4 years, 10 years since inception of the project (Schulte et al., 2014), while overall costs have developed favorably compared with expected costs, with annual savings amounting to €5.5 million (US$5.8 million) in 2013. This difference is expected to further increase in the coming years as some of the health programs will only start paying off years after the initial intervention. The causal mechanisms for the observed effects are not yet fully understood, and whether secular trends or diffuse interventions, as compared with the model interventions, contribute to these effects, requires further, long-term evaluation.

Diffusion and Transferability

Can the HK approach be successfully transferred and achieved elsewhere, including in regions and countries that are different in population structure and health service organization? While all settings will have their idiosyncratic features and particularities, we argue that the general model, interventions, and evaluation frameworks are widely applicable in developed countries, and potentially also in developing countries. For example, all key aspects of the model are deeply rooted in the scientific literature and in models that have proved effective elsewhere, such as the "Triple-Aim" approach, audit, and feedback strategies, the focus on patient activation, interventions to reduce unnecessary hospital admissions and readmission, or pharmacological consultations to improve the safety of drug prescriptions. The results of HK are based on and consistent with the scientific literature (Busse, 2014).

However, a number of conditions need to be met to successfully transfer the model:

- A regionally based company, partly owned by local providers, and familiar with local (health) services issues, is required to plan and deliver local intervention and maintain communications with all stakeholders.
- Because there is a delay between intervention and successful health improvement, start-up investment is needed to set up the companies, engage stakeholders, and design interventions, until earnings are enough for the return-on-investment.
- A vision to go beyond traditional institutional boundaries in the planning of health interventions is needed; in particular, interventions that focus on improving the population's health status.
- The size of the population needs to be appropriate to ensure networking among providers, the identification of local solutions, and the exchange of ideas among all stakeholders (population sizes around 100,000 appear ideal).
- A comprehensive information-technology package (including shared patient records) and competencies for advanced health data analytics to inform intervention planning, feedback reports to providers, and internal evaluation are crucial in order to ensure seamless care and monitor performance.
- An approach focusing on "coopetition" (a portmanteau of cooperation and competition) through transparency and benchmarking is needed to support the continuous striving toward improvement and facilitate effective knowledge-sharing in cross-functional teams.
- A balanced payment system oriented toward achieving the "Triple-Aim," and which allows providers to make decisions about how cost savings are (re-)invested, is needed.
- An innovative culture and friendly interactions are essential to harness value from the relationships with all stakeholders.
- And finally, a long-term (10-year) contract with the purchasers is required to provide stability for the planning of health interventions.

Outlook

The contract to take over the accountability for the HK region by Healthy Kinzigtal, Ltd. was initially restricted to 10 years. It has recently been renewed with the participating SHIs, and because of the positive evaluations the contract is now open-ended, thus providing a stable context to pursue long-term health interventions. In addition, discussions are underway regarding expanding the program to other regions in Baden-Württemberg, other parts of Germany, and abroad. As various prerequisites and interventions have already been established, such as quality indicators, evaluation protocols, program outlines, incentive systems, management guidelines, data warehouse and reporting systems, and so on, it is anticipated that implementation in new areas will be considerably streamlined.

The German government's recent decision to provide €1.2 billion (US$1.28 billion) funding over the next 3 years (2017–2019) to support innovative forms of care delivery and health services research, provides a promising context for further development. At the same time, various European settings are considering setting up similar systems with the support of OptiMedis, private investors are screening the potential for scaling up the model, and research funds are being sought to investigate important questions about the transferability and scalability of the model.

23

Ireland

St. James's Hospital National Haemophilia System

Feargal McGroarty

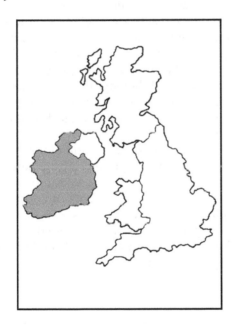

CONTENTS

Background

Hemophilia is an inherited disease caused by the lack of a specific clotting factor in blood, which leads to significant and sometimes life-threatening bleeding. Intravenous infusion of the missing clotting factor is used to treat and prevent bleeds. Regular infusion of clotting factor to prevent bleeding is called "prophylaxis" and is usually self-administered at home by the patient or a family member. Prophylaxis from childhood is proven to prevent the development of severe joint disease and disability. Modern prophylaxis means that people with hemophilia can achieve their full potential, including taking part in sports, education, and the workforce. Effective prophylaxis is tailored to the bleed rate and activity level of each individual patient.

Although the development of clotting factor infusions in the 1970s and 1980s was lifesaving and life changing for people with hemophilia, tragically, contamination of blood products in this period meant that the majority of regularly treated patients with hemophilia were infected with HIV and/or hepatitis. Due to the ineffective manual methods used to record and track and trace the medication, patients were exposed to infection even after a product recall was initiated.

The hemophilia clotting factors used in Ireland now are not derived from blood but are recombinant products, produced by genetic engineering in cell culture-based systems and subject to stringent safety procedures. However, experience has shown that unexpected events can occur, and therefore it is vital that the hemophilia treatment center is able to identify immediately which batch and vial of product has been delivered to and administered to each patient and to be able to immediately locate and recall any vial of product even after delivery to a patient.

Solutions

The complexities surrounding the delivery of a multidisciplinary approach for the management of chronic illness, such as hemophilia, is well documented. Effective chronic illness interventions generally rely on multidisciplinary care teams. Thus, the heart of the chronic care model recognizes that quality care is predicated on productive interactions between patients, their families, and caregivers. Moreover, an informed group of chronically ill patients will, in the general scheme of things, possess a greater understanding of their condition, and know what to expect from the healthcare system. In order for this type of care program to be effective, it is important that the caregivers adopt a prepared and proactive approach founded on evidence-based clinical information and delivered in a manner that optimizes the maximum patient experience and produces better outcomes at both functional and clinical levels (Peyvandi et al., 2016; Schoen, 2009; Wagner et al., 1996).

St. James's Hospital, Dublin (SJH) has therefore developed a comprehensive integrated program based on continuous quality improvement (CQI) to improve patient care (St. James's Hospital, 2015b). The program is composed of four strands: electronic patient record, a cold chain delivery system, the appointment of barcodes (GS1 global standards), and a smartphone scanning app.

Electronic Patient Record

The introduction of the electronic patient record (EPR) replaced the previous hospital chart, which was a paper record and not always available at clinic or at night. The EPR allows hospital staff rapid access to key medical information. It also allows close monitoring of the quality of the service provided by the hospital. Implementation of the EPR ensured easier and quicker navigation through the patient record and standardized care among providers within the organization by ensuring clinical data is easy to read and analyze. This has led to a reduction of paperwork, documentation errors, and filing activities. Other key benefits include

- International Statistical Classification of Diseases and Related Health Problems (ICD)-10 coding to improve efficiency and efficacy of diagnosis classification
- Alerts for the presence of antibodies to the medication (inhibitor status)
- Ability to electronically transmit information to other providers (assessments, history, treatment regime, prescriptions, etc.)
- Electronic prescribing
- Clinic scheduling
- Internal messaging
- Access to patient self-treatment history

Cold Chain Delivery Service

Prior to the implementation of this service, patients who required home treatment received their medication either by collecting it from the local treatment center or having it sent to them by post, courier, or taxi. The combination of ad hoc delivery methods was irregular, inconvenient to the patients, and prone to error. This use of non-validated cold chain delivery along with manual data entry to deliver and record product usage led to both product wastage and documentation delays.

Validated cold chain delivery, whereby medication is delivered direct to patients, was therefore essential for the storage, distribution, and delivery of coagulation factor concentrates (CFC) to patients with hemophilia, within both the home and the hospital environment.

GS1 Global Standards (Medication Barcoding)

The accurate tracking and tracing of CFC using unique (GS1) product barcoding (Figure 23.1) is a critical component in the safe delivery of hemophilia care, as it supports rapid recall, validates optimal product storage, and identifies patients who may have received "at-risk products" by identifying the location of products at all points of the supply chain. The availability of real-time product information also provides important clinical data with respect to individual usage of factor concentrates, both in hospital and in the home environment. In addition, the visibility of all CFC in storage locations nationally, along with their expiry dates, has allowed for stock rotation.

Smartphone Scanning App

The main objective of introducing the app was to harness the power of the barcode to improve patient safety and outcomes by providing real-time data on bleeding episodes to clinicians, to monitor medication recording

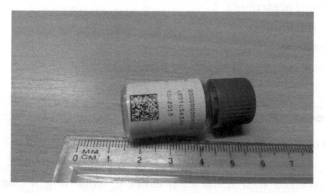

FIGURE 23.1
Medication barcoding.

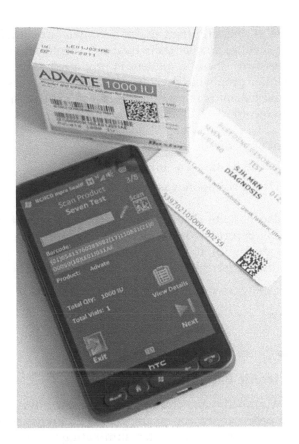

FIGURE 23.2
Smartphone scanning app.

compliance, to identify patients who may have received an "at-risk product", and to facilitate a rapid recall.

Just prior to self-administration, the patient launches the app and scans the barcode on the medication (Figure 23.2). The scanning automates the previously required manual task (medication usage recording), which in turn increases recording compliance and accuracy. In addition, the patient records, via radio buttons and dropdown menus, the reason for infusion of clotting factor, for example prophylaxis or acute bleeding. Using the strategy of "identify, capture, share," all data collected from the app is transferred into both clinical and supply chain information systems in real-time. The three safety checks that take place with the medication scan are

1. A check against the patient's treatment of choice and the medication they are infusing (prescription check)
2. A check that the medication is within date
3. A check that the medication is not on a recall list

If any of these checks fail, then the patient gets an audible and visual warning asking them to contact their treatment center. If all these checks are passed successfully, then the patient is prompted to record the reason for treatment (either prophylactic or on-demand). If the reason selected is "on-demand," the patient is requested to record the bleed site/reason. The patient therefore records

- The amount of medication infused
- The time the medication was taken
- The reason the medication was taken

The patient also has the ability to view their treatment history via a secure web portal. Before the introduction of the app, a treatment record sheet was provided with the medication delivery, and patients were requested to manually record their usage and return the sheet to the treatment center.

National Electronic Patient Record

The EPR has streamlined many clinical and administrative processes, leading to enhanced productivity. For instance, the EPR allows access to patient records instantly at any treatment center, eliminating the need to fax, e-mail, or transport records between the sites. Standardized data entry (ICD-10 coding, questionnaires, patient tracking through their appointment) have been used to drive CQI schemes.

Staff can refer to an instantly accessible, legible, clearly defined summary note with the treating doctor's diagnosis and treatment plan. Medical staff can now access their patients' records from home when on call, greatly improving the quality of care they provide to patients. This aspect of the EPR is especially important for hemophilia patient care, since hemophilia is such a rare condition.

By many measures, the EPR has streamlined and improved the everyday processes that support and enhance delivery of quality care. Clinical and administrative staff cited the following as some of the key features:

- Reminders (personal/discipline/public)
- Alerts (inhibitors)
- Clinic reschedule (bulk)
- Standardized data entry (ICD-10 codes)

- Bespoke functionality (home treatment history)
- Remote access
- One system used by all multi-disciplinary teams
- Reports

Cold Chain Delivery Service and GS1 Barcode Scanning

A pre- and post-service audit was undertaken to assess the impact of the implementation of the validated cold chain delivery service. This audit showed that 221 patients received 30,464 vials of factor concentrate by cold chain delivery between August 2004 and October 2005. Product wastage due to failure of either cold chain conditions or delivery issues reduced from €90,216 (US$102,580) in the July 2003–July 2004 period to zero wastage for the August 2004–August 2005 period, again with the introduction of the efficient, temperature-controlled, door-to-door delivery service. An audit of medication ordering trends by patients (Figure 23.3) showed a substantial decrease in demand, achieving an estimated saving of €5 million (US$5.68 million) per year.

The combination of the cold chain delivery service and barcode scanning has also contributed to greater visibility of all stock, including that held in satellite hospitals around the country. The value of the stock rotated (replacing short-dated stock with longer expiry dates and using the short-dated stock in large treatment centers) was at €600,000 (US$682,200). This represents a potential yearly saving of that amount, as before the introduction of

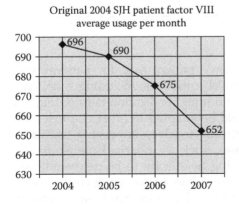
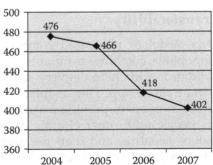

FIGURE 23.3
Patient usage trends.

cold chain delivery and barcode scanning there was no real-time visibility of that stock. In addition, mock recalls can identify the location of 100% of a chosen medication batch within 10 minutes, along with quantities of alternate stock.

Smartphone App and GS1 Barcode Scanning

Because patient infusion data is collected in real-time, clinical staff can view consumption trends and advise the patient if they feel they are treating themselves inappropriately (over-treating or not treating at the appropriate time). This has led to savings of €70,000 (US$79,600) over a 4-month period, based on the first 20 patients using the app (St. James's Hospital, 2015a). The hospital now has over 100 patients using the app.

Medication recording compliance for those using the app is significantly higher (>80%) than those using the paper treatment sheets (<50%). Staff in the clinic are also alerted if a patient (who should be self-administering every 3–4 days) has not used the app to scan their medication for more than 4 days. This helps to monitor and audit compliance rates.

From a patient point of view, the data collected will help improve patient safety by providing important information on their medication status (alerts for prescription errors or out-of-date medication)—and on the patient population as a whole—that has not previously been available to healthcare providers, and other stakeholders involved in the delivery of clinical services to this patient population.

Transferability

This model of integrated comprehensive patient care for patients with hemophilia combines a number of novel initiatives, including a national, validated, cold chain delivery service; unique medication bar coding; and a smartphone app. This template could be adapted in other countries and health systems to provide a systematic approach to improving healthcare for people with other chronic diseases, such as inherited metabolic disorders, hepatitis, and diabetes, allowing healthcare to be delivered more effectively and efficiently to other chronic disease groups. It could also be used in areas such as vaccine distribution, where forecasting and recall are critically important.

Conclusion

Although the delivery of hemophilia care is expensive, the lives of patients and their families can be transformed by high-quality care. Effective prophylaxis and treatment prevents disability, and a need for orthopedic procedures, later in life. A child born today with severe hemophilia can in effect look forward to a normal life expectancy (Franchini and Mannucci, 2012; World Federation of Hemophilia, 2012).

24

Israel

A Nationwide Health Information Exchange Program in Israel: A Unique Case Study

Eyal Zimlichman

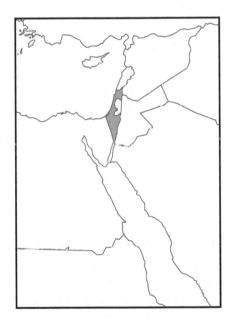

CONTENTS

Background

The healthcare system in Israel is often cited as being efficient, with comparably low national healthcare expenditure (7.5% of GDP in 2013) and continuously improving population health outcomes and high-quality community healthcare services (OECE, 2015a). The reforms that have helped shape this unique system date back to the foundations of the State of Israel, although the last 20 years have seen a new set of reforms centered on equity, patient rights, and patient-centric care. These reforms have implemented national quality measurement programs at the community level and more recently also at the hospital level, with national quality and patient safety initiatives aiming to further improve performance (Zimlichman, 2015).

The Israeli healthcare system is a single-payer system, primarily tax-funded, where universal coverage is provided to all citizens and residents through a national health insurance system that allows those insured to choose one of four competing health plans. The public funds are paid by the National Insurance Agency on a per capita basis, a critical fact that drives competition between the funds. The funds provide all community healthcare services, with hospital care provided mainly by government-owned hospitals, public hospitals, and hospitals owned by the largest health fund (Clalit) (Rosen and Samuel, 2009).

Development and Implementation of the Ofek Program

Healthcare information technology (HIT) use in Israel is more advanced than in many other countries. Since 2005, almost 100% of all encounters in ambulatory settings have been documented on an electronic medical record (EMR), and currently, all hospitals make some use of electronic records, positioning Israel as a leader in EMR uptake (Jha et al., 2008).

Although electronic data proliferated, communication of data between the different EMR systems was not possible as health funds and hospitals had developed their record systems individually. In order to facilitate the sharing of data between organizations, a health information exchange (HIE) program was developed. This program, known as Ofek, was originally led by the Clalit Health Fund (which covers about 50% of the population) as a means of exchanging data between the community and the hospitals. It was expanded as a national program under the leadership of the Ministry of Health in 2014 to include all care providers in Israel. By the end of 2015, the Ofek program included all residents of Israel seen by any provider. Of course, expanding this system as a national program was a complex process, with many technical challenges to be overcome, and a number of legal and ethical issues, including data ownership and opt-out provisions, to be considered.

This inter-operability solution (initially provided by dbMotion Ltd., which was later bought by the U.S. company AllScripts) was enabled through detailed semantic mapping of clinical data that allowed data from disparate systems to be identified and compared. The software allows for a virtual patient record to be created in real-time at place of care. The efficacy of the system is limited by the fact that the data is in display-only form, rather than structured form (as discrete characters). While making clinical information available at the point of care improves decision-making, having the data in display-only form does not enable advanced features, such as decision support and safety alerts. However, the Ofek HIE program appears to have had a positive impact on quality and patient safety for both the ambulatory and the hospital system and has contributed to the lowering of costs.

Impact of the Ofek HIE Program

While HIEs have the potential to improve care and reduce costs of care, the evidence relating to their efficacy is relatively new and patchy, and it tends to focus on the use of HIE systems in an emergency department setting. For example, according to one study, HIE was associated with reduced repeat imaging for emergency back pain evaluations (64% lower utilization of radiographs, CT, and MRI) (Bailey et al., 2013). Another study that looked at an emergency department (ED) setting has found that decisions to hospitalize were reduced by 30% when HIE was used, compared with matched controls for which the system was not used (Vest et al., 2014). The investigators of this study reported considerable cost savings attributed to reduced hospitalization.

Although evidence of the effectiveness of HIE is limited, the Israeli experience could certainly contribute to better understanding as to where and how HIE played a part within the HIT infrastructure and other quality initiatives. During the initial implementation of the Ofek program, the association between use of HIE and the utilization of services and quality of care was examined in both inpatient and outpatient settings. In the context of inpatient services, medical and surgical departments in six hospitals were examined, showing a rapid uptake of the system as measured through entries to the HIE system. However, uptake at medical departments was higher than uptake at surgical units (Nirel et al., 2010). Researchers have found a substantial decrease in use of laboratory testing and some imaging in medical departments, with no significant change in the surgical departments. Regarding outcomes, there was a negative correlation between the use of

HIE and subsequent readmissions or single-day hospitalizations; yet, once again, this too was statistically significant only for the medical departments. The authors concluded that Ofek was a partial success and hypothesized that there is an association between the level of HIE use and the benefits, as seen through resource utilization and some health outcomes.

In their examination of outpatient services, the same research group again found a substantial increase in the use of HIE following the launch of the Ofek program at Clalit (Nirel et al., 2011). When comparing those hospital clinics, in specific catchment areas, extensively using Ofek with those that don't, the researchers found a decrease in utilization of imaging tests, along with a decrease in some laboratory tests. Regarding quality measures within the community, selective improvement was found that could be related to use of HIE, especially when looking at measures involving hospitalization rates. For some other quality metrics, such as mammogram rates, LDL cholesterol levels, and checkup tests for patients with diabetes, no improvement was noted. Again, the authors' conclusions are that use of HIE seems to be associated with lower utilization and selective improvement in common quality metrics. It is clear from these results that further research is needed in order to understand factors that will lead to quality improvement.

In more recent studies, researchers have examined the effect of the Ofek system in more advanced versions (providing more clinical information and from more facilities) on quality metrics, such as readmissions and single-day admissions. In one study, the researchers compared emergency department visits in seven hospitals in which an EMR system as well as an HIE system (Ofek) were used, with departments where neither EMR nor HIT systems were used. The authors found that using both EMR and HIE was associated with an improvement in outcomes (less readmissions and less single-day hospitalization). When analyzing log files of system usage (for both the EMR and the HIE systems), it was evident that these improvements were attributed to the HIE system (Ben-Assuli et al., 2013). The authors also found that these improvements were more significant for some diagnoses (such as gastroenteritis and abdominal pain), but less for others (such as chest pain and pneumonia). This study was the first to compare the benefits of providing physicians with external data through HIE with the benefits of providing local data only through an EMR. The diagnostic disparities also suggest that past clinical history might be a significant factor in the management of patients and in related outcomes, such as readmissions and single-day admissions.

Taking the evidence from the Israeli experience with HIE, it is evident that use of HIE is associated with a reduction in resource utilization (mainly labs and imaging), with an improvement in outcomes as measured through readmissions and single-day admissions, and selective improvement in quality measures. However, any improvement depends on the extent of use by clinicians; across these studies, utilization of the HIE system was around 30% at most. In Israel, at least, where hospitals are chronically understaffed and occupancy rates usually exceed 100%, this low utilization rate can be partially explained by the high workload physicians are encountering. Streamlining access to the HIE system, improving workflows and user interface could improve usability.

Prospects for Further Success, Next Steps, and Transferability

As mentioned, since 2015 the Ofek HIE system has been deployed at all provider sites in Israel as a national program and encompasses all residents. Moving forward, the Ministry of Health intends to launch a second-generation program that will improve the functionality of the system and, more importantly, allow for decision support and alerts that will increase quality and patient safety. The ministry has been attempting to increase utilization of the system, especially within the acute care in-hospital setting, with some success. Bi-monthly usability reports are produced and disseminated to the hospitals and the health plans regularly, showing an upward trend in usability but still demonstrating major variability between hospitals and between services within hospitals.

In terms of the technology, the Ministry of Health initiative to upgrade the system and include critical elements for quality and patient safety, such as alerts and decision support tools, is a step in the right direction. While research into the effectiveness of HIE systems is still in its infancy, studies of other clinical systems suggest that functionality should include medication decision support checks, medication reconciliation, duplicate test alerts, and perhaps also expensive medication/test alerts.

The other challenge for the future, and something that needs to be considered before the system is applied in other countries, is the need to improve implementation so that usability is enhanced. This could be achieved by demonstrating the system's value to physicians, providing continuous reporting to clinical directors on a unit level, and allowing benchmarking to other units—including HIT and HIE specifically—in medical school curriculums. HIE usability should also be improved for other clinical professions such as registered nurses. Of course, maintaining a healthcare system that incentivizes for prevention of readmissions and single-day hospitalizations as well as shortening lengths of stay, would enhance the perceived value of HIE systems.

Conclusion

Israel has achieved a comprehensive level of health information exchange across all levels of care throughout the country. Although research is not conclusive, there is some evidence that the installation of a national HIE system has improved quality and reduced resource utilization in both outpatient and inpatient settings. Future efforts should focus on improving functionality of the national HIE system and improving implementation and usability. The lessons learned from Israel's experience can certainly assist other countries who set out to develop HIE capabilities that will improve quality and patient safety in addition to controlling costs.

25

Italy

Post-Marketing Successful Strategies to Manage Pharmaceutical Innovation

Americo Cicchetti, Silvia Coretti, Valentina Iacopino, Simona Montilla, Entela Xoxi, and Luca Pani

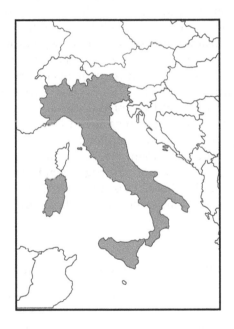

CONTENTS

Background

In order to meet the challenges presented by the current economic crisis, the Italian National Health Service (I-NHS) has recently launched a range of initiatives aimed at containing healthcare expenditure while improving quality and ensuring universality of access to healthcare services. The progressive erosion of the National Healthcare Fund due to the increase of regional financial responsibility for healthcare, along with the normative actions that have been taken to deal with financial deficits in many regions, must be taken into account in any discussion of the economic and political framework characterizing the Italian system. Since 2007, the *Piani di Rientro* (financial recovery plans) have been implemented to restructure and upgrade a number of regional health services, obliging regional decision makers to balance the books in healthcare expenditure annually (Ferrè et al., 2014).

Specific interventions aimed at controlling healthcare expenditure have included the rationalization of hospital care through establishing standards, reducing personnel turnover, reviewing goods and services purchased by the I-NHS (2012–2015), as well as a number of initiatives to contain pharmaceutical expenditure. Pharmaceutical expenditure is of particular public concern, and both national and regional decision makers have made a significant commitment to enforcing measures to control such spending. The monitoring of pharmaceutical consumption has featured in many initiatives. Table 25.1 lists the cost-containment measures implemented in 2014 to contain regional hospital and community drug expenditure. All of these efforts strongly involve the Italian Medicines Agency (AIFA) as the main national authority responsible for pharmaceutical regulation in Italy.

TABLE 25.1

Cost-Containment Measures for Drug Expenditure at a Regional Level

Aim of regional decrees concerning community drug expenditure	Aim of regional decrees concerning hospital drug expenditure
• Incentivizing the use of out-of-patent drugs (42) • Monitoring appropriateness (97) • Promoting direct distribution (36) • Guidelines for prescription (30) • More efficient monitoring of expenditure (53) • Improving distribution • Regulating the copayment	• Update of regional formularies (53) • Identification of prescribing centers for specific drugs (109) • Guidelines for prescription (25) • Centralization of purchase (27) • Rationalizing the prescription of biosimilar drugs (34) • Monitoring the appropriateness of prescriptions along with conditional reimbursement procedures (MEAs) (36)

Source: Elaborated by authors from OsMed data (2015). *Note:* Number of regional decrees issued in 2014 in parentheses, where available. Last update is November 2015. http://www.aifa.gov.it/sites/default/files/Rapporto_OsMed_2015_AIFA-acc.pdf

In 2005, AIFA introduced post-marketing registries in order to

- Improve early access to innovative therapies
- Guarantee the sustainability and affordability of therapies
- Collect epidemiological data
- Monitor the appropriateness and the safety aspects

After the establishment of the Cancer Drugs Registry in 2005, which was the first drugs registry to be developed, the scope of monitoring has progressively been extended to cardiology, dermatology, diabetology, inflammatory diseases, ophthalmology, rheumatology, respiratory, and neurological diseases. The main driver for the implementation of these registries has been the high cost of medicines, many of which are biotech products characterized by a high level of uncertainty regarding effectiveness, safety, appropriate use in real clinical practice, cost-effectiveness, and budget impact issues (Montilla et al., 2015). The scope described above has been extended over time to inform decisions relating to the reassessment of drugs at the national level. Such decisions, which involve the application of management entry agreements (MEAs), are thus taken on the basis of the evidence collected through registries in a real-life context.

Details of the Success Story

This chapter describes the introduction of AIFA registries and MEAs for pharmaceuticals in Italy. Due to their varied nature and their usefulness in informing pricing and reimbursement decisions, these instruments are regarded with great interest in Europe and worldwide (Adamski et al., 2010; Carlson, 2011; Garrison et al., 2013).

Existing literature acknowledges payer–provider agreements as a form of coverage with evidence development. In particular, performance-based risk sharing is expected to produce greater market equilibrium, through the adjustment of price in the post-marketing phase to reflect the outcomes achieved in real life. Indeed, such agreements are often based on a plan whereby the use of the product in the target population is tracked and reimbursement is conditional on performance over a defined time span, after which the level of reimbursement is reassessed. For this reason, these agreements are usually conceived as instruments to address the uncertainty surrounding the pharmaceuticals' performance following market authorization. The financial risk related to uncertainty about drug effectiveness has increased over time due to the rising cost of new treatments. On the supply side, if the payer is reluctant to adopt a new treatment, then the manufacturer

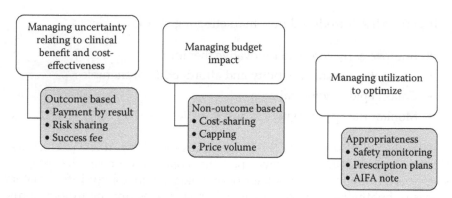

FIGURE 25.1

List of MEAs currently in force in Italy. (Adapted from European Commission, Public Health. Presentation by Italian Medicines Agency at the 4th Meeting of the Commission Expert Group on Safe and Timely Access to Medicines for Patients (STAMP), 2016. Retrieved from http://ec.europa.eu/health/documents/pharmaceutical-committee/stamp/index_en.htm)

bears the risk of reduced revenues for a product that yields value (Garrison et al., 2013; Stafinski et al., 2010; Towse and Garrison, 2010).

Over the last decade, the Italian pricing and reimbursement system has been characterized by the introduction of both financial schemes and performance-based, risk-sharing agreements (MEAs) aimed at fostering access to new medicines with a high level of uncertainty at launch. Figure 25.1 lists the different types of MEAs currently in force in Italy.

Cost-sharing agreements apply a discount to the Italian NHS on the cost of the first cycles of therapy for all eligible patients. While within a risk-sharing approach the discount applies only to those patients who are not responsive to the medication, payment by result provides a full refund from the manufacturer to the Italian NHS for all those who are deemed "non-responders."

Sixty-six percent of monitoring registries currently aim at supporting MEAs. From a data collection perspective, the AIFA registries are divided into drug-product (D-P), drug-product for therapeutic area (DPTA), data collection, and therapeutic plans (see Table 25.2).

Currently, 85 medicines are monitored, corresponding to 77 therapeutic indications; more than 933,000 individual treatments are currently recorded

TABLE 25.2

Types of Data Collection and MEAs (N and %)

Types of data collection and MEAs (%)	N	%
Drug-product therapeutic area registry	30	20
Drug-product registry	108	71
Therapeutic plan	14	9,2
Total	152	100

Source: Update from AIFA registries.

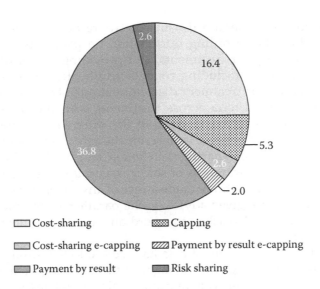

FIGURE 25.2
Types of MEAs (%). (Update from AIFA registries—31/12/2015.)

for a population of about 833,000 patients. Various categories of actors are involved, with different profiles of access to data: AIFA, 21 regions, more than 1500 connected hospitals, over 29,000 clinicians, over 1800 pharmacists, and 48 pharmaceutical companies. Web monitoring is available from https://www.agenziafarmaco.gov.it/registri/ (Figure 25.2).

In 2012, the AIFA monitoring registries system became a structural part of the I-NHS Information Technology (IT) system, and in 2013 an integrated knowledge management system was implemented to optimize the processes through a cross-architecture structure able to improve the quality of data recording and to enhance the quality of data analysis. Information deriving from registries, in terms of consumption (i.e., number of patients treated) and outcomes, must be provided to determine potential re-funding by the I-NHS.

Details of the Impact of the Success Story

The implementation of monitoring registries has been successful in Italy for a number of reasons. First, the registries have supported the development of MEAs, thus simplifying and accelerating patients' access to new treatments. The automated workflow allows the prescriber to track and monitor therapeutic drug indication, adverse reactions, drug interactions, and costs. The main pillar of the web system is the check of eligibility criteria for correct use: whenever these criteria are not met, the data recording is interrupted and a detailed text alert about the inappropriateness of the request is displayed.

Drug-product registries are also an effective resource for gathering real-practice safety data, recording information on patient baseline characteristics, including prior treatments, and providing a longitudinal view of patients' treatment, including route of administration, dose, duration of use, and reason for treatment discontinuation/interruption. The standardized eligibility criteria across treatments with the same therapeutic indication allows for comparison of the different treatment options. Furthermore, it is also possible to describe the actual treatment pattern for certain conditions by comparing different strategies. Additionally, registries help to increase awareness of safety issues: upon registry inception, clinicians and pharmacists are made aware of any adverse events and incidents of note, and are given advice on the parameters and modalities for reporting. Users are also asked to record any adverse events whenever a drug is prescribed.

So far, a significant amount of data has been collected through registries. Also, data collected by registries, along with those coming from the pharmacovigilance flow and other economic information, facilitate the reassessment of pharmaceuticals' value, and allow revisions of pricing and reimbursement decisions after a pre-agreed period (usually 24 months). This activity eventually determines a reconsideration of the original reimbursement and pricing decision (Siviero, 2012).

Implementation: Transferability of the Exemplar

Currently the drug product post-marketing registries are unique within the I-NHS. However, the use of registries to monitor the use and performance of medical devices is now the focus of intense debate within the health technology assessment arena. Law N. 86/2012, which established a national registry for breast implants, provided the first legal imperative to introduce registries for these technologies. This registry has not yet been fully implemented and only some regional and local data are currently being monitored. The complex regulation of pharmaceuticals (which is not as binding for medical devices), along with the increasing push for cost containment, has been the main driver of the registries' success and has strengthened the commitment for a variety of stakeholders.

The Italian experience with monitoring registries could also be transferred to other jurisdictions. Indeed, several countries have already undertaken similar measures with the aim of rationalizing pharmaceutical expenditure, fostering patients' access to innovation, and producing real-world evidence.

Prospects for Further Success and Next Steps

Several measures could potentially be introduced to further improve the system. At a European level, adaptive pathways will become the "regular" market access path for innovative technologies, thus the implementation of European registries will become a strategic requisite to generate relevant evidence. To this end, AIFA is taking part in the European Network for Health Technology Assessment's (EUnetHTA) Joint Action 3, focusing on evidence generation, and is committed to the design and implementation of European registries.

Nationally, registries could become the main source of real-world evidence, representing a starting point for cooperation among patients, academia, regulators, HTA doers, payers, and companies. Evidence generated could also contribute to the design of integrated healthcare approaches and pathways and to be used to develop e-health tools for improving adherence and promoting patients' self-management.

Conclusion

AIFA registries for new drugs can be seen as tools that help to balance the necessity of guaranteeing early access to promising technologies with the need to tackle the uncertainty characterizing the products at launch. While post-marketing registries have different forms and serve different purposes, and further work needs to be done to ensure that evidence is exhaustive and has further applications, they have thus far proved to be a valuable tool to collect real-world data.

26

Malta

Reform of the Medical Profession and Reversal of Brain Drain in Malta: A Success Story

Sandra C. Buttigieg, Kenneth Grech, and Natasha Azzopardi-Muscat

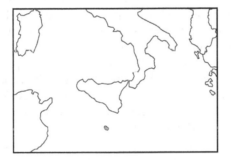

CONTENTS

Background

Malta, which has a 316 km² landmass and a population of 425,384, lies in the middle of the Mediterranean Sea. It is the smallest, yet most densely populated, European Union (EU) member state (National Statistics Office [Malta], 2014). Malta has a universal health system, where care is mainly provided freely by the state to Maltese nationals, although the private sector and church/non-governmental organizations (NGOs) contribute specific complementary services. The Health Ministry, which is directly responsible for the provision and regulation of health services (Azzopardi Muscat and Brand, 2014), recently launched its first national health system performance assessment framework (Grech et al., 2015). Of note, between 1994 and 2007, a new acute general hospital, replacing the main hospital, was constructed and commissioned, thereby increasing pressure on authorities to provide resources from the already-depleted pool of medical professionals. Furthermore, Malta was experiencing rising waiting lists for secondary/tertiary care, primarily due to its aging population.

Accession to the EU and Reform of the Medical Profession in Malta

Medical brain drain depletes healthcare resources in originating countries and widens the gap in health inequities worldwide. Medical brain drain has featured widely in the literature, with its negative effects on health systems being observed for a number of years (Bojanic et al., 2015; Gouda et al., 2015; Nullis-Kapp, 2005; Schnidman, 2012). Since the EU's expansion, and the associated ease of movement between member states, the problem has worsened in Europe (European Union, 2011; García-Pérez et al., 2007). Upon Malta's EU accession in 2004, many foreign naturalized medical doctors left to pursue their careers in the more developed EU countries. Accession also encouraged new Maltese medical graduates to pursue their careers abroad, mostly in the United Kingdom, which at that time began refusing to license non-EU doctors in favor of those from the EU, thereby further encouraging Malta's medical brain drain (*Malta Independent*, 2006). Additionally, Malta's postgraduate medical and specialization training was poorly structured, and salaries of government-employed medical specialists were among the lowest in Europe. Before 2008, for example, doctors in the United Kingdom earned at least four times more than their counterparts in Malta (*Malta Independent*, 2006).

Improvements as a Result of the Reforms

Until the adoption of the Health Care Professions Act in 2003, the 1901 Medical and Kindred Professions Ordinance regulated Malta's medical profession (Ministry for Justice, Culture and Local Government, 2003). Although the need to redesign the medical profession's regulatory and training framework had been on the agenda for decades, successive governments failed to undertake the necessary reforms. As part of Malta's EU accession, an overhaul of the legislative framework was implemented to incorporate the EU Acquis (or body of common rights and obligations) on training, along with the member states' mutual recognition of professional qualifications (Deguara and Azzopardi Muscat, 2002).

This process provided an opportunity for the implementation of other reforms not directly mandated by the EU. For example, due to changes in legislation introduced through the Health Care Professions Act, the Medical Council was, for the first time, governed by a majority of elected medical practitioners. This signified an important step toward autonomous self-regulation. Furthermore, this act also led to the establishment of the Specialist Accreditation Committee and over 40 specialist registers were instituted, each with its own training program. The Postgraduate Medical Training Center (PMTC) was established in 2008 to provide clearly defined, directional and formulated training, as well as career pathways for post-graduate medical trainees and their trainers. PMTC programs emphasized the importance of engaging in stints abroad, which established links with state-of-the-art institutions in the United Kingdom, Italy, and Belgium.

As an ex-British colony, Malta has traditionally depended on the United Kingdom for postgraduate medical training, and indeed, the recent establish-ment of the United Kingdom's Foundation Program in Malta has strength-ened this historical link. As well as retaining Maltese doctors, the Foundation Program has attracted fresh graduates from other countries—making up for those Maltese who prefer to pursue their postgraduate studies in the United Kingdom.

Another milestone in the reform process was the recognition of family medicine as a specialty, with the Malta College of Family Doctors develop-ing a comprehensive specialist-training program (*Malta Independent*, 2010).

Doctors' working conditions have also been reformed. In order to coun-teract the factors driving outward migration, the Maltese government was constrained to improve doctors' remuneration in the public service (Busuttil, 2005). The 2007 collective agreement introduced remuneration on a sessional basis and created incentives for doctors to dedicate themselves fully to the public service. This was tied to the concept of job planning and performance review, which for the first time linked clinical work to key performance indicators. The agreement was reviewed in 2013, with performance mea-surements being extended to the resident specialist grade and general prac-titioners (Azzopardi Muscat et al., 2014).

In-Country Data to Illustrate the Success of the Reform

Data from the UK Foundation School, Malta, provides a clear picture of the reversal of the medical brain drain between 2007 and 2015. Figure 26.1 shows a downward trend from 2007/2008 to 2011. In 2012, there was an inexplicable

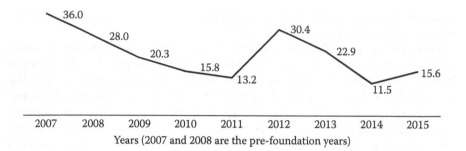

FIGURE 26.1

Percentage of graduates from medical school, University of Malta, who left Malta for further studies. (From C. Galea, UK Foundation Medical School Malta Manager, personal communication, January 20, 2016.)

upward spike of graduates leaving Malta (30.4%). However, this was of minimal concern since the Foundation Program recruited the required number of foundation year doctors from eligible foreign graduates.

Since 2009, the PMTC has enabled 56 trainees to receive training abroad while providing training to a record 500 trainees.

Impact of the Reforms on the Maltese Medical Profession

Through these reforms, the brain drain was reversed, and Malta has now become a net importer of medical doctors, particularly in the foundation years and for junior training posts. The reforms have also been successful in encouraging young medical graduates to consider taking up family medicine, reversing a decades-old trend where hospital posts tended to attract the best talent. Job planning and review has also become an integral aspect of professional medical practice.

The success of the reforms can be attributed in part to a careful and open consultation process, in combination with an explicit attempt to democratize medical regulation. By placing the medical professionals themselves in the driving seat, ownership of the process was achieved. The ability to make use of EU funds, such as the European Social Fund, was a small incentive that facilitated early efforts at implementation. The transition was carefully handled with judicious use of the principle of acquired rights (which guarantees that a vested right cannot be reduced by subsequent legislation) in order to enable a smooth transition from the old to the new regime, thereby safeguarding practitioners who had commenced their training prior to 2004. The specialist training system was established in such a way as to recognize domestic specialist training, foreign specialist training, and hybrid programs, so that doctors could obtain their training both in Malta and abroad. This is an invaluable component of training in a small state setting. The imperative to implement the associated EU directives is considered to have pushed through these substantial reforms within a short period of time (Azzopardi Muscat and Brand, 2014).

Implementation: Transferability of the Exemplar

Malta has always relied upon the proficiency and skills of its human resources to excel and compete, especially when it comes to the training and development of healthcare professionals (Rechel et al., 2006). New initiatives include the conversion of the bachelor degree in radiography to a dual qualification in 2010 (diagnostic and therapy, replacing the earlier diagnostic-specific radiography course), as well as the development of a Master's program in medical physics in 2012. In both examples, training was possible through the collaborative efforts of the Ministry of Health and the University of Malta, together with foreign partners. Both programs included substantial training in centers of excellence in the United Kingdom. Radiographers who have trained in diagnostics and therapy, as well as specialist medical physicists, are now working in Malta, contributing to better quality care, and sustaining local training for future cohorts. A similar initiative is being planned for allied healthcare professionals working in highly specialized and specific clinical areas such as optometry, orthotics, and physiological measurement.

Like Malta, many other European states are facing difficulties in retaining their healthcare workers and stemming the exodus of highly trained specialists. With the assistance and collaboration of foreign partners, Malta's experience in developing local specialist training programs could serve as a model for many of these countries.

Prospects for Further Success and Next Steps

The challenge for Malta is to sustain the success and to further develop strong links with centers of excellence in Europe. The next step will be to build a more robust infrastructure of quality control with both internal and external evaluations of all specialist-training programs.

Currently, the EU is spearheading the development of European Reference Networks. This initiative presents member states with the opportunity to support each other in building and sustaining medical manpower. Collaborative postgraduate medical training in centers of excellence will ensure a critical mass of specialists in different fields across Europe.

Conclusion

An article in the local press entitled "Brain Drain Reversal? UK Doctor Says Better to Work in Malta" (*Times of Malta*, 2015), reflects the success of the medical profession reforms in Malta. Challenges inherent to postgraduate medical training in a small island state, however, still remain. These include limited resources, a small catchment population, limited case mix, and low volume of specific diagnoses. Advances in communication technology ensure that international affiliations are also possible through videoconferencing, telemedicine, virtual reality, e-learning, and e-libraries; however, these require substantial investment.

Despite these challenges, Malta has acquired and maintained an excellent medical reputation and has successfully stemmed the medical brain drain. However, in order to maintain the stabilization of medical manpower and quality of postgraduate training, Malta, being a small state, must be part of the European network. In this way, Malta's healthcare system can provide high quality of care to its citizens, and serve as a center of excellence in specific medical fields within Europe.

27

The Netherlands

Patient Safety in Dutch Hospitals: How Can We Explain Success?

Roland Bal and Cordula Wagner

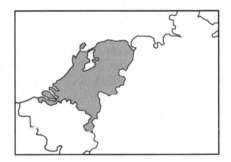

CONTENTS

Background

Ever since the Harvard Medical Practice Study and its endorsement by the U.S. Institute of Medicine in 1999, the identification and reduction of adverse events in hospitals, including preventable mortality, has been a priority in the development of health systems worldwide (Kohn et al.,

2000). Like other countries, the Netherlands followed the United States in taking measures to determine the number of adverse events, including unnecessary deaths, that occur during hospital care. Dutch data from 2004 and 2008 showed an excess of potentially preventable mortality of around 2000 patients per year. Following the release of the 2008 figures, the then minister of health set a target to reduce preventable adverse events and hospital mortality by 50% over the next 4 years. A national patient safety program—the Prevent Harm, Work Safely program—was established to attain this goal. By 2011/2012, there had been a considerable decrease in preventable adverse events—amounting to 30% after multilevel corrections for data clustering and patient mix (Baines et al., 2015). During the same period, potentially preventable mortality rates dropped to just below 1000 patients per annum.

Much of the success in reducing hospital mortality has been credited to the Prevent Harm, Work Safely program (see https://www.youtube.com/watch?v=rkLC1OIJsSM for a video overview of the program and its progress). Indeed, the program's executers—including the Ministry of Health, the Dutch Hospital Association, the National Patient and Consumers Association, the Association of Medical Specialists, and Health Insurers Netherlands—were quick to claim credit for the success of the program. However, research shows that the program was not the only factor in the reduction of adverse events—in fact, not one hospital had completely implemented the program when the figures were released (de Blok et al., 2013).

Theoretical Background

Patient safety is a tough nut to crack, not only in practice, but also in terms of research. More than 10 years ago, Harvard University-based health policy innovator, Lucian Leape, along with other leading patient safety experts, complained that the field was rife with "evidence-bias"; that is, interventions that have proved effective in clinical trials are favored over more complex interventions where such clear evidence is not available—or even possible (Leape et al., 2002). Similarly, as Dixon-Woods et al. (2011) argue, due to a lack of rich descriptions and theoretical understanding of such interventions, there is a marked lack of insight into why patient safety interventions are effective in the first place. For example, in their "Explaining Michigan" paper, Dixon-Woods et al. (2011) propose several social factors that might explain the success of the central line venous infection program in the larger Boston area. These include isomorphic pressures on the hospitals, making them more alike organizationally; the creation of strong networks between hospitals, exerting normative pressures; the reframing of central line infections as a social, rather than solely medical, problem; along with the building of a "grassroots" professional movement (Dixon-Woods et al., 2011). While these factors are only generalizable to other patient safety interventions to some extent, they do exemplify that such interventions, in order to be effective, need to be embedded in a much wider program, and that such programs need to include professional, organizational, and comprehensive system changes.

The Dutch Patient Safety Program

The Prevent Harm, Work Safely program was one in a series of national and local interventions aimed at improving quality and safety in the Dutch hospital sector. While it is outside of the scope of this chapter to detail all these initiatives, one program that needs mentioning is the Better Faster program, as this program set the scene for national patient safety initiatives and included a large number of system stakeholders. The Better Faster program consisted of three pillars:

- The setting of performance indicators by the healthcare inspectorate (which are still in use today)
- A series of inquiries and reports by various captains of industry on quality and safety (including one, by the then CEO of the oil company Shell, entitled "You Work Safely Here, or You Don't")
- A quality collaborative, lasting from 2004 until 2008, including 24 (of a total of 95) hospitals and comprising a broad set of professional and organizational interventions (Berg et al., 2005; Dückers, 2009)

The Prevent Harm, Work Safely program was established directly after the Better Faster program, but followed a different course. Rather than focusing more generally on quality, the program directly targeted patient safety. The program had a truly national reach, with all hospitals participating in the program. In addition, it was largely regionally organized, with regional hospital groups undergoing training programs and setting up patient safety networks to share experiences. The program had two main objectives: the implementation of a safety management system in hospitals, comprising such issues as blame-free reporting, risk analysis, and the development of a proactive patient safety culture; and the introduction of interventions concerning 10 practical clinical themes that were found to be of relevance in preventing adverse events and hospital mortality, such as post-operative wound infections, early detection of critically ill patients, and high-risk medication (Baines et al., 2015).

Explaining Success

How can we explain the success of the safety program? Of course, the program did play a role in lowering the rates of adverse events. For example, many of the interventions were targeted at elderly hospital populations, and there was a significant decrease in the rates of adverse events within this population. Further, a decrease in preventable adverse events was seen in surgical processes, which were also targeted by the program.

While it is important to establish the effectiveness of the program, it also begs the question: how was it effective? This question can be considered from two perspectives. First, it is important to note that programs themselves don't save patients, care does—and local interventions usually and necessarily depart from the exact program guidelines (Wensing et al., 2012). It is therefore necessary to establish what changes were made in the provision of care across the different hospitals to effect this decrease in adverse events. Second—and this will provide the focus for the remainder of this chapter—it is necessary to identify the conditions under which such a program was able to succeed. We propose five factors:

1. Experience in project work
2. Market competition
3. Public pressure
4. Activities of regulatory agencies
5. Public reporting of adverse events and mortality

Experience in Project Work

Quality of care has been on the agenda in the Netherlands since the late 1980s, when, due to an economic crisis, proposals were made to cut expenses and reform the healthcare system. From 1989 onward, several conferences on quality of care were organized that mobilized relevant parties in healthcare to develop quality policies. This resulted in proposals for accreditation and clinical guidelines, based on the idea that healthcare providers themselves were responsible for the quality of care, a principle that was later recognized in the Quality of Care Act of 1996.

In the aftermath of these initiatives, hospitals introduced many quality improvement initiatives, supported by newly created hospital quality managers, as well as by an increasing number of consultancies and semi-public organizations such as CBO, the Dutch Institute for healthcare improvement. As a result, hospitals became increasingly proficient in quality improvement. The

Better Faster program came about as a result of these reforms, and although only 24 hospitals participated, it had a strong effect on non-participating hospitals as well, with many implementing certain features of the program. Moreover, this program ensured that hospital boards became familiar with quality work, thus improving their capacity to perform quality improvement projects.

The commitment of hospital boards, the presence of experienced quality managers, and the involvement of medical specialists all contributed to the success of the Better Faster program. The success of this program meant that essential elements were already in place, paving the way for further safety initiatives such as the Prevent Harm, Work Safely program.

Market Competition

From 2006 onward, regulated competition was gradually introduced into the Dutch healthcare system, making insurers responsible for the procurement of care, with increased levels of pricing freedom. The system of regulated competition introduced a new cost awareness in hospitals, which were incentivized to pay close attention to the efficiency of the care provided (Bal and Zuiderent-Jerak, 2011). Attending to patient safety was an integral part of this, as it became clear that hospitals could save money by attending to safety, for instance by preventing infections. Moreover, insurers, who had until then mainly played an administrative role, became strong external actors interested in quality and safety, and many of them supported quality assurance and improvement.

Public Pressure: Scandals and Inquiries

Over the last 10 years, there have been a number of public scandals involving failing hospital quality and safety. Most notable was the 2008 scandal surrounding the high levels of post-operative mortality rates following cardiac surgery at the Radboud University Hospital (OvV [Dutch Safety Board], 2008). The Radboud case set the scene, not only because the hospital's inadequate safety measures were made public, but also because it was evidence of a wider system failure. Subsequent inquiries reframed quality and safety as being profoundly influenced by the governance of the hospital system (Behr et al., 2015). Cases like the Radboud also increased public and political pressure on the hospital system to improve quality and safety. The media have since focused on hospital safety, which in turn provides a strong incentive to tackle safety issues.

Activities of Regulatory Agencies

Partly in response to such scandals, the healthcare inspectorate has taken a more stringent approach to hospital quality and patient safety in their system reforms. The inspectorate shifted from its conventional focus on *learning* to an *assurance* style when it came to inspections (Robben et al., 2015). This change was also prompted by the inspectorate itself being scrutinized by the media, and shown to be partly responsible for the quality and safety scandals. Consequently, the inspectorate not only became more rigorous, it also put quality and safety on the agenda, with an emphasis on issues of safe surgery, the treatment of frail elderly, and medication safety—all areas in which a reduction in adverse events were seen. The governance of quality within hospitals was also made a priority, strengthening the role of hospital boards.

Public Reporting

A final development that should be mentioned, is that since the early 2000s, hospitals have been put under increasing pressure to publish performance data. Whereas these data were initially focused on process indicators, increasingly they also embody outcome indicators, including hospital mortality. Although the effect of this increased numerical transparency of healthcare quality is unclear, it has helped to ensure that issues of quality and safety remain on the agenda of hospital boards, and has stimulated quality management processes in hospitals (Quartz et al., 2013).

Conclusion

While the classic quality improvement report follows a whodunit logic—focusing on the "active ingredients" that can explain the success of an intervention—we have a followed a *howdunit* logic in this chapter, focusing on how the program could be successful in the first place. Taking as our starting point the argument provided by Dixon-Woods et al. (2011) that rich, contextual analyses are necessary to explain program success, we identified several factors in the Dutch healthcare system that can provide for such a contextual explanation of the success of the patient safety program. These include the gradual building of quality improvement capacity and experience within the hospitals, as well as a series of external incentives that have pushed hospitals further along this path: market competition, public scandals, the changing style of the healthcare inspectorate's supervision, and the public reporting of performance data. It is the alignment of these elements with the patient safety program, we argue, that explains the success of the program.

28

Northern Ireland

Adopting a Collaborative Approach to Improve Care for Women and Their Babies in Northern Ireland

Levette Lamb, Denise Boulter, Ann Hamilton, and Gavin G. Lavery

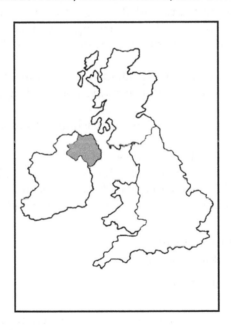

CONTENTS

Background

The health system in Northern Ireland (NI) has been integrated with social care for several decades and delivers services to a population of 1.8 million people via five integrated Health and Social Care (HSC) Trusts and the NI Ambulance Trust. The system, like many others, has used regulation and performance-managed targets as a means to improve standards of care. While this has undoubtedly produced successes, it has also led to behaviors that address targets without leading to improvement. The development of a system-wide body, focused entirely on quality improvement (QI) has helped increase recognition of (1) the contribution that QI can make to improving the processes of care, and (2) the importance of workplace culture to the delivery of high-quality care and the engagement of our workforce. In a time of resource limitation, QI is increasingly seen as the way to improve services for patients by harnessing the training, instincts, and expertise of staff.

Despite these advances, a big challenge remains. How do we move together toward this new way of thinking and working, and away from a system based on inspection and regulation, a system that seems to find itself attributing blame to staff who are increasingly stressed, demotivated, or disengaged?

Improvement across Health and Social Care (HSC) in NI over the next 5 years will continue to follow the 10-year strategic plan formulated in Quality 2020 (Q2020) (Department of Health, Social Services, and Public Safety [Northern Ireland], 2011). Themes in Q2020 include

- Transforming the culture
- Strengthening the workforce
- Measuring the improvement

The HSC Safety Forum (Safety Forum), established in 2007 and now part of the Public Health Agency, provides system-wide leadership in QI and safety, and facilitates the themes mentioned above. This has involved establishing QI collaboratives focused on specific areas of care (maternity, pediatrics, mental health, nursing homes) or specific problems (deteriorating patients, sepsis, acute delirium). In addition, the Safety Forum has grown QI capacity and capability by funding, facilitating, and providing training to both front-line staff and strategic leaders. Some of these trained individuals have led or supported the development of QI training at hospital systems level. This has consequently seen the development of ward-based teams using their QI skills to change how they work and measuring the improvement. This approach has led to an agreed set of attributes, an Attributes Framework (AF) for leading QI across the entire HSC system (Department of Health,

Social Services, and Public Safety [Northern Ireland], 2014). This AF is guiding both undergraduate and postgraduate staff training and development.

The demographic/societal changes common across the developed world mean the demand for management of long-term conditions (e.g., chronic obstructive pulmonary disease, diabetes, obesity, and alcohol-related conditions) is increasing rapidly. Technologically, HSC is relatively well placed, having developed and implemented a generic electronic care record (NIECR) that has widespread clinical engagement. While financial resources are under more strain than ever, paradoxically this has given QI some leverage, since spending our way out of the problem is no longer an option. We must redesign processes to be more reliable and less wasteful.

Other strategic drivers include the need to deliver increasingly complex (often hospital-based) care safely and reliably, and a growing consensus that hospitals will no longer be the hub for the care of long-term conditions. How do we design a system that appropriately balances high quality, safety, and sustainability with the wishes of citizens to have their care close to home?

Details of the Identified Success Story and Its Impact

The Strategy for Maternity Care in Northern Ireland 2012–2018, aims to "provide high-quality, safe, sustainable, and appropriate maternity services to ensure the best outcome for all women and babies" (Department of Health, Social Services, and Public Safety [Northern Ireland], 2012). The strategy emphasizes that safe, effective maternity care that results in good outcomes and experiences should, wherever possible, follow evidence-based best practice.

In recognition of these challenges, the Safety Forum established a system-wide maternity QI breakthrough collaborative supported by a clinically led advisory group. A breakthrough collaborative is designed to help organizations or systems create a structure in which interested parties can easily learn from each other and from recognized experts in topic areas where they want to make improvements (Institute for Healthcare Improvement, 2003). The maternity QI collaborative has representatives from all HSC Trusts (providers), commissioners, Public Health Agency, and the Department of Health, Social Services, and Public Safety (strategy and policy).

It was recognized from the outset that strong clinical leadership was pivotal to engaging front-line teams. Indeed, there is an international body of evidence that demonstrates that strong clinical leadership is an essential component of successful health systems (Ahmed et al., 2015). For this reason, the collaborative is chaired by a front-line senior obstetrician supported by the Safety Forum.

Collaborative learning sessions are focused events that bring together front-line teams to share best practice, learn, and plan future QI activity. The basic tool used by teams is the Model for Improvement. Teams are encouraged to develop aims that are specific, measurable, actionable, realistic, and timely, and to use small tests of change to make improvements to care. The program and content of learning sessions are shaped by the collaborative advisory group.

The collaborative advisory group developed a driver diagram (see Figure 28.1), which was discussed, modified, and agreed to by the collaborative teams. This became the blueprint for the work of the collaborative, and focused on three key areas:

1. Promoting the normalization of pregnancy and childbirth
2. Effective communication (between professionals and with women and families)
3. Safe labor and delivery

Promoting Normalization of Pregnancy and Childbirth

Pregnancy is a normal physiological process and, for the vast majority of women, a safe event. Through the Safety Forum maternity QI collaborative, trusts have adopted a range of approaches to promote normality, including the introduction of birth choice clinics in each trust. These clinics provide an opportunity for women who have previously had a Caesarean section or traumatic birth to explore the birth choices for their current pregnancy. In parallel, multi-professional programs have been provided to ensure midwives and others have the knowledge and confidence to help women in labor achieve a normal birth where possible. Figure 28.2 is a time series plot

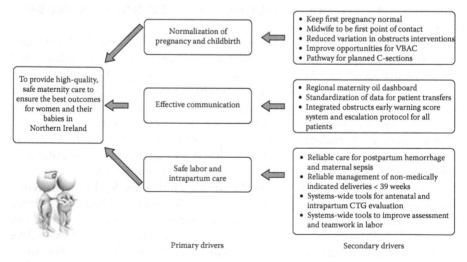

FIGURE 28.1
Maternity QI driver diagram.

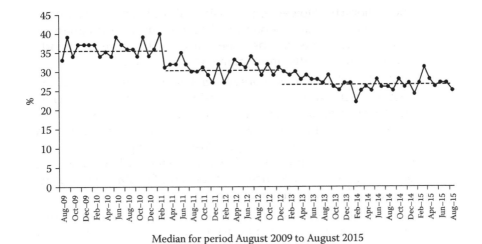

Median for period August 2009 to August 2015

FIGURE 28.2
Caesarean section rate (elective and emergency) 2009–15.

(run-chart) showing Caesarean section rates achieved in the largest maternity unit in NI, which has approximately 6000 births per year.

Effective Communication (Inter-Professional and with Women/Families)

One of the stated desired outcomes for the NI Maternity Strategy is "effective communication and high-quality maternity care" (Department of Health, Social Services, and Public Safety [Northern Ireland], 2012). The maternity collaborative is addressing this goal through a range of initiatives detailed as follows:

- *A regional maternity dashboard:*
  This QI dashboard provides a graphic summary of progress toward key process and outcome metrics that has been developed, tested, and agreed on by all maternity units and staff over a number of years. The dashboard aims to provide data that can facilitate QI, improve decision-making, and influence choice. It allows trusts to monitor changes in their own practices over time, and to benchmark against other similar units with the aim of reducing variation.

- *An integrated early pregnancy/antenatal/postnatal obstetric early warning score system:*
  The early detection of severe illness in pregnant women has been, and remains, a challenge to all clinicians, due to the low frequency of such events and the fact that they can be masked by the normal changes in physiology associated with pregnancy

and childbirth. However, increasing clinical complexity due to rising rates of maternal obesity, diabetes, and later pregnancies means such events can be expected to occur more frequently, and with (potentially) more damaging outcomes.

While early warning score systems for post-natal women have been used in NI for some time, prior to 2014 there was lack of standardization and some units were not using early warning scoring for antenatal women and those in early pregnancy. By implementing an agreed single Obstetric Early Warning Score system across all units in NI, we have standardized a way to detect deterioration, reduce variation, and facilitate the transfer of patients between maternity units.

The system has been trialed and audited using both quantitative and qualitative data derived from responses of front-line staff. This revealed

- >90% of charts had the correct score calculated.
- 83% of respondents felt confident that the chart would help them to identify women who were unwell or who required senior review.
- 86% of respondents were confident that the chart contributed to the effective management of women on the ward.

- *A standardized in-utero inter-hospital transfer protocol:*

  To enhance effective communication between all parties at both the sending and receiving hospitals, a regionally agreed in-utero transfer protocol was developed, piloted, and refined using audit for improvement. The current document is in use in all units across NI. A modified version has also been developed for use in midwifery-led units transferring women in labor to obstetric care.

Safe Labor and Delivery

Pregnancy and labor is a safe event for the vast majority of women. The collaborative has worked to improve the quality and safety of services delivered to women and to reduce variation in practice. Maternity units have undertaken QI initiatives in the reliable management of postpartum hemorrhage, severe sepsis, and non-medically indicated deliveries before 39 weeks' gestation.

There has been significant collaboration in the development of both antenatal and intrapartum cardiotocography (CTG) evaluation stickers, which use a checklist approach to improve reliability and reduce variation in interpretation of CTG data on fetal well-being. This has facilitated a common approach and common terminology among obstetric and midwifery staff when raising concerns or escalating to senior staff. These tools have been revised to reflect changes in national clinical guidance.

Implementation: Transferability of the Exemplar

The NI maternity QI collaborative has been in existence since 2012, and built on work by a previous perinatal improvement group. At the beginning, some organizations were achieving higher levels of performance than others; some had experience of quality improvement; some participants had more to learn, others more to teach. The key to the success of this work has been staff engagement—obstetricians and midwives working and learning together to improve the care delivered to women and their babies. Members of the collaborative have described how the group has fostered a sense of community and increased attention on maternity care within their organizations. Building relationships has also been central and has occurred not only across professions but also across organizations. Over 4 years, teams have progressed from resisting the sharing of data to co-producing a regional dashboard in which all key data are shared. Teams frequently suggest new information to be included in the dashboard.

Is this work transferable? The answer is yes—if the conditions are favorable. This collaborative has a strategic context (the NI Maternity Strategy) and has the support of the Safety Forum to provide focus and drive. There has been buy-in and support from both commissioners and front-line clinicians, and as a result several quick wins have been possible. This has helped build momentum. Establishing ground rules of trust, openness, and support has been essential in making the collaborative a safe environment to share incidents and maximize learning.

Prospects for Further Success and Next Steps

The strategic direction of the NI maternity collaborative is continually under review, and new initiatives are undertaken once they're agreed on by the clinical teams leading the work. The next phase will focus on reducing stillbirths and building on the existing achievements in CTG monitoring. As with all quality improvement work, maintaining enthusiasm and momentum and ensuring that achievements are sustainable remains something of a challenge. However, this improvement community has provided a vehicle through which problems can be addressed, ideas shared and tested, and a culture of improvement can flourish.

Conclusion

The success of the NI maternity QI collaborative can be demonstrated both in terms of (1) cultural change (where quality improvement really is viewed as central), and (2) the development of practical tools, refined by front-line teams, which increase reliability, reduce variation, and make it easier to do the job well. Such outcomes can only occur when front-line teams (clinicians and managers) are engaged, and when there is a shared agenda for commissioners of clinical services, improvers, and front-line clinicians. Building the relationships that underpin this is not easy; it requires careful handling and, most of all, time.

29

Norway

Improving Patient Safety in Norwegian Hospitals through a Standardized Approach toward the Measurement and Monitoring of Adverse Events

Ellen Tveter Deilkås, Geir Bukholm, and Ånen Ringard

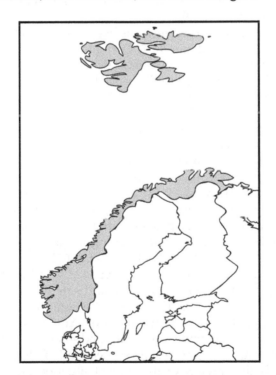

CONTENTS

Background

In Norway, as in most European countries, health coverage is statutory and opting out is not permitted. Patients have no discretion over what is covered, but they are allowed to select their healthcare provider. Healthcare provision is organized at two hierarchical levels: municipal (local) and national. Municipal authorities are responsible for primary care and enjoy a great deal of freedom in organizing health services.

Specialist care is the national government's responsibility. The National Ministry of Health and Care Services owns four regional health authorities (RHAs), which in turn own hospital trusts. The ministry governs through directives, annual budgets, and meetings. Annual directives from the Directorate of Health—a subordinate body of the ministry involved in planning and implementing healthcare policies—supplement the ministry's directives (Ringard et al., 2013).

The Norwegian healthcare system has been through substantial changes in recent decades (Ringard et al., 2013). Currently, several large-scale changes are either being implemented or evaluated by the government. On January 1, 2016, a major reform took place in the central health administration system, merging a number of public agencies into fewer and larger units. A political initiative addressing the relationship between the national government and the RHAs is also underway. Locally, the number of hospital trusts providing acute/emergency surgical care is being re-evaluated, and municipal reform, including a reduction in the number of municipalities, is under consideration.

In addition to these potential structural reforms, there is ongoing debate over service content. There has been discussion about priority setting (i.e., how to best allocate scarce health resources), and initiatives aimed at enhancing patients' choice of hospital provider are being implemented. Increased attention is also being paid to issues relating to quality and patient safety within the public health services (Deilkås et al., 2015b).

Prevention and follow-up of adverse events (AEs) in health and care services are among the most visible quality and safety issues on the health policy agenda. In November 2015, an expert committee, appointed by the ministry in 2013, published a public report on AEs. According to its mandate, the committee was to review how AEs and suspicion of legal violations within the health and care services are subsequently followed up. Thus, the report contains both a review of the current situation on AEs and assessments, as well as policy recommendations (Ministry of Health and Care Services [Norway], 2015).

There are several sources of information for AEs in Norwegian hospitals. Death and severe patient injuries are reported to the National Board of Health Supervision. The board received 1271 reports between June 1, 2010 and December 31, 2014. In 2014, of 414 reported incidents, 303 involved deaths and 63 involved severe injuries. The National Reporting and Learning

System (NRLS), established in 2012, also receives reports from hospital trusts on the number and type of AEs and "near misses." The NRLS received about 9500 reports in 2014, of which almost a fifth were classified as severe injuries or leading to death. The System for Patient Injury Compensation (NPE) also provides information on AEs. In 2014, more than 60% of all individual patient claims came from the four RHAs (total number of claims was 5217) (Ministry of Health and Care Services [Norway], 2015). Since 2005, there has also been a national registry for incidence of surgical site infections.

While all of these systems provide valuable information, it is impossible to obtain an estimate of the national level of AEs based solely upon these sources. However, quantitative and standardized information about AEs and harm in Norwegian hospitals is available through medical record review using the Global Trigger Tool (GTT) (Deilkås et al., 2015a; Griffin and Resar, 2009). Our success story examines the development of Norway's national system for monitoring AEs. The monitoring is based on the GTT method, which the Institute for Healthcare Improvement developed to standardize and streamline medical record reviews. The records of 10 adult patients are randomly selected from hospital discharge lists every fortnight. Records are reviewed with criteria (triggers) indicating risks of AEs. Results are analyzed in time series with statistical process control.

Why Did Norway Choose to Monitor Adverse Events in All Hospitals?

Professor Peter F. Hjort, a founder of Norwegian health services research, became painfully aware of risks related to healthcare after his wife sustained a critical brain injury during a neurosurgical operation in January 1998. The experience motivated him to write a book about AEs and, in 2005, to participate in a national working group set up to give advice on how to increase learning from AEs (Hjort, 2007). The group acknowledged a lack of incentive or capacity to learn from the available AE reports, and considered that "resistance to looking at ways to reduce risks was larger than resistance to report adverse events." It recommended the establishment of a National Center for Patient Safety (Langaas, 2006). In 2007, the National Center for Patient Safety was established to synthesize information from existing AE reporting systems and increase knowledge about risks and ways of reducing AEs. In 2011, the Norwegian Ministry of Health and Care Services started a national campaign to reduce AE rates.

In 2002, the World Health Organization estimated that hospital levels of AEs in Western countries were around 10%, based on medical record reviews from hospitals in several countries (WHO, 2002). International research also showed that systems reporting AEs in healthcare were unreliable when it came to accurately estimating rates, suggesting that medical record reviews could be used to estimate AE rates more accurately (Sari et al., 2007; Vincent, 2007). Documented experiences from a large Norwegian hospital convinced the CEOs in the campaign's steering group that medical record review with the GTT would provide data of adequate consistency for monitoring AE rates nationally (Deilkås and Hofoss, 2008; Griffin and Resar, 2009). Their decision was ratified by the Ministry of Health. Simultaneously, international research recommended GTT for surveillance of AEs in hospitals at a regional level (Sharek et al., 2011).

How the Monitoring Was Mandated and Organized

In January 2011, the Ministry of Health decided that all hospitals in the country were to review randomly selected medical records to map AE rates according to the GTT method. The secretariat of the National Patient Safety Campaign trained GTT teams in all hospitals and coordinated the review through a protocol specifying how the review was to be applied in Norwegian hospitals, and how data were to be reported nationally (The Norwegian Patient Safety Campaign, 2013). Medical records from March 2010 were used to provide a baseline. Data reported nationally had to be unidentifiable to comply with regulations for personal protection. A spreadsheet for reporting AE data annually to national level was provided.

Extranet, a web-based tool created by the Institute for Healthcare Improvement, was provided to facilitate analysis of data at hospital level with statistical process control. This enables hospitals to analyze their own data in run charts. Some hospitals have observed significant AE rate decline (Deilkås, 2015a; Norwegian Directorate of Health, 2016). National rates have been published annually since 2011. Between 2011 and 2013, there was a significant decrease in overall national AE rates, with a smaller decrease in rates of AEs with higher severity (see Figure 29.1) (Deilkås, 2015a). Based on these results, the Ministry of Health and Care Services has required all hospitals to reduce their AE rates by 25% between 2012 and 2019. National AE rates are now published three times a year.

Why Did the Monitoring of Adverse Events Succeed?

To our knowledge, no other country has monitored AEs in all acute care hospitals with a national system for medical record review. The intention was to make government and CEOs more receptive to information regarding

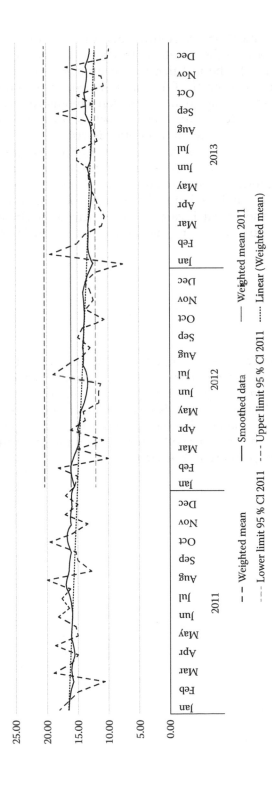

FIGURE 29.1

Estimated percentage of discharges with at least one AE from 2011 to 2013. The dashed black line shows AE rates over time. A black smoothed line shows means of 10 consecutive dots. A gray horizontal line marks the mean level in 2011, with 95% confidence intervals marked with dashed horizontal black and gray lines. The dashed gray line shows the linear trend. (Drawn from Deilkås, E., Bukholm, G., Lindstrøm, J. C., et al. (2015). Monitoring adverse events in Norwegian hospitals from 2010 to 2013, *BMJ Open*, 5(12), e008576.)

risks in patient care. Patient safety culture surveys show that prioritization of patient safety varies substantially both within and across hospitals (Deilkås and Hofoss, 2010). The fact that the government has set national goals for AE reduction based on the GTT measurements proves that it has led to increased leadership engagement. The national monitoring system for AEs and national patient safety culture surveys will show if the combined efforts succeed in reducing AE rates and variation in risk.

To develop the Norwegian AE monitoring system further, medical records could be reviewed across caregiving levels, for instance, by expanding observations to include long-term care in nursing homes, in order to identify AEs that first emerge after hospital discharge. The system could also be adapted to monitor psychiatric and pediatric care, and treatment at the clinical level. Cross-country comparisons would be interesting and would increase our understanding of AEs.

Conclusion

The Norwegian system for monitoring AE rates at the local and national levels is a successful step on the journey toward a comprehensive system of patient safety. The effective partnership between the ministry and the Steering Group of the National Patient Safety Campaign contributed to the program's success, as did the fact that the method was logical to clinicians. Our experience may perhaps inspire other nations to unite governing leaders with clinicians to map and reduce AE rates.

30

Portugal

Reducing Hospital-Acquired Infection in Portuguese Hospitals: A Collaborative Approach toward Quality Improvement

Paulo Sousa and José-Artur Paiva

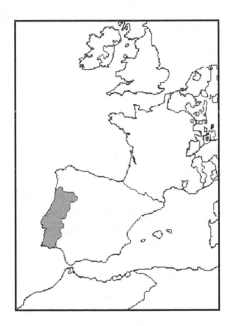

CONTENTS

Background

Despite differences in structure, resources, accountabilities, and priorities, the Portuguese healthcare system shares common goals with other countries in regard to quality and safety improvement.

Portuguese residents have universal access to healthcare provided by the publically funded National Health Service (NHS). Health spending in Portugal (excluding investment expenditure in the health sector) was 9.0% of GDP in 2013, which is slightly higher than the Organization for Economic Cooperation and Development (OECD) average of 8.9%. Health expenditures have decreased by nearly 2% since 2009 (10.7%), mainly due to the country's ongoing economic difficulties.

The Economic, Political, Social/Cultural, and Technological Forces Influencing Improvement Efforts

Notwithstanding economic constraints and the effects of continuous political changes, Portugal has a strong culture of health quality improvement that is reflected in the high-quality level of healthcare professionals, innovative hospitals (in terms of structure and management), and the use of cutting-edge technology.

A number of remarkable health quality initiatives involving evaluation and improvement have been implemented. These include clinical audits; the use of a set of quality indicators to monitor specific areas longitudinally; accreditation of hospitals and primary care centers; development and publication of clinical guidelines and systems for auditing their implementation; and patient satisfaction surveys.

At the political level, and as a reflection of this shift in philosophy, the Health Ministry created the Department of Quality in Health (DoQH) in 2009. One of the first steps of the DoQH was to define a 10-year strategy for quality improvement initiatives. More recently, the Health Ministry launched the Patient Safety National Plan for 2015–2020.

As a full member of the European Union (EU), Portugal is fully aligned with EU directives. This means that Portugal is party to the provisions governing the free movement of persons, which guarantee the rights of all European citizens to receive safe, high-quality healthcare services throughout Europe.

Hospital-Acquired Infection: A Safety Issue That Keeps Us Awake at Night

Improving the safety of patient care is a significant challenge for the Portuguese healthcare system, as it is for many health services around the world. While it may be impossible to build a completely fail-safe system, the creation of a healthcare system that is aware and systematically reflects, learns, and acts to reduce unintended patient harm is a reasonable and achievable aim.

Many countries, like Portugal, have taken initiatives over the past years to address quality and safety issues in healthcare. In the aftermath of the U.S. report, *To Err Is Human* (Kohn et al., 2000), patient safety has gained momentum among healthcare policymakers as well as healthcare professionals and managers. Although the safety problems should not be underestimated, it should also be recognized that healthcare systems have been addressing issues like hospital infections, falls, and bedsores over a long period of time. There is, however, little consistency in data, and measurements may be quantified differently in different contexts without adequate understanding or explanation of the same.

As one of the most common sources of preventable harm, hospital-acquired infections (HAI) represent a major threat to patient safety. However, there is a robust body of evidence detailing interventions that can substantially reduce the incidence of HAI; indeed, recent analyses indicate that at least 50% are preventable.

HAI are a matter of great concern to patient safety, and they affect both the quality of care received and costs incurred during treatment. According to the point of prevalence survey of healthcare-associated infections and antimicrobial use (2011–2012), developed by the European Center for Disease Control (ECDC), Portugal's infection rate—10.5%—is significantly higher than those of most other European countries and almost double that of the European average of 5.7%. Antimicrobial use (45.3% in Portugal; 38.5% in Europe) is also relatively high.

Portugal has made efforts to reduce the rate of hospital infections over the past years. Infection control activities in Portugal date from the late 1980s, and in 1996 a national infection control program was set up. An ongoing infection surveillance program in intensive care units (ICUs), bloodstream, surgical sites, and neonatal infections has been running since 2002, and in 2008, a national program for the prevention of antimicrobial resistance was established. Because the results of these programs were less than satisfactory, in 2013, the two programs were merged into a single national priority program (Program for the Prevention and Control of Infection and Antimicrobial Resistance), which was integrated into the National Strategy for Quality in Healthcare. Subsequently, activities have focused on two main areas: the reduction of infection rates and the promotion of the rational use of antimicrobial drugs. Although it is too early to know whether the observed improvements will be sustained in the long-term, the initial results are promising.

In 2013, The Gulbenkian Foundation, a private non-profit organization with cultural, educational, social, and scientific interests, and a mission to improve the lives of the most vulnerable, commissioned a group of international experts to analyze the Portuguese healthcare system. This analysis involved looking forward 25 years, in an effort to "create a new vision for health and healthcare in Portugal," describing what this would mean in practice and setting out how it might be achieved and sustained (Crisp, 2015). The recommendations of this report identified three major areas for improvement to be implemented by the Gulbenkian Foundation with the support of the health ministry. The high rate of HAIs was one of the identified areas, and an immediate and short-term challenge was to reduce HAIs by 50%, for a group of 12 NHS centers—a total of 19 hospitals—over a period of 3 years. This initiative, Stop *Infeção Hospitalar!* (SIH), commenced in late 2015.

Stop *Infeção Hospitalar!*: A Model and a Way to Improve Care

To respond to this ambitious challenge, the Gulbenkian Foundation invited the Institute for Healthcare Improvement (IHI) to become a program partner, on account of its expertise in running large-scale collaborative improvement projects and its persistent focus on execution, measurement, and results.

The SIH initiative focuses on four main types of HAI:

1. Catheter-associated urinary tract infection (CAUTI)
2. Central line–associated bloodstream infection (CLABSI)
3. Surgical site infection (SSI), namely hip and knee replacement, colorectal, and gallbladder
4. Ventilator-associated pneumonia (VAP)

The pilot sites include general wards (CAUTI and CLABSI), intensive care units (CLABSI and VAP), and orthopedic and general surgery (SSI) departments.

A Breakthrough Series Collaborative methodology (see Figure 30.1) has been utilized as a means of reliably implementing and spreading

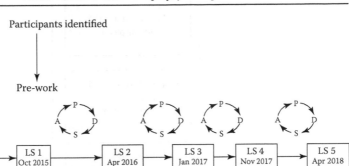

Action Plan for 3 Years – Stop *Infeção Hospitalar!*

FIGURE 30.1
Schematic representation of the breakthrough series collaborative SIH.

evidence-based practices that are known to substantially reduce the incidence of HAI across the set of 12 centers, including 19 hospitals, and representing around 25% to 30% of all inpatient episodes in Portuguese NHS hospitals.

One key function of the SIH quality improvement (QI) initiative is to build a learning community and system capable of future ongoing sustainable improvement. The program aims to build improvement capability and improve organization cultures over time. Multidisciplinary front-line teams have been supported to design, test, and implement improved work processes designed to deliver safer and more reliable care to patients. A large number of teams from hospitals or clinics seeking improvement in a focused area come together in a working environment where all members learn and all members teach. Teams are taught improvement methodology including The Model for Improvement (see Figure 30.2) (Institute for Healthcare Improvement, 2003). Leadership commitment is a prerequisite for participation. Interventions include participation at learning sessions, educational interventions, and discussion of activities and progress at coaching conversations by telephone, WebEx calls, and face-to-face meetings. Other key elements of the SIH program include

- An evidence-based change package (e.g., bundles for insertion and maintenance of urinary catheter and central line catheters)

- A robust measurement and data collection system (e.g., outcome, process, and balancing measures)

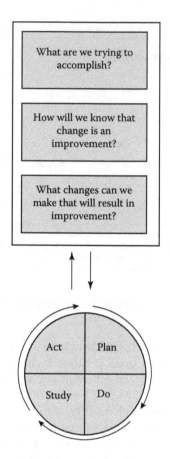

FIGURE 30.2
The Model for Improvement (IHI). (From Institute for Healthcare Improvement. (2003). The breakthrough series: IHI's collaborative model for achieving breakthrough improvement, IHI Innovation Series white paper, Boston.)

- A strategy for building capacity (creation of a sustainable infrastructure for healthcare improvement, implemented first at the 19 participating hospitals and then at other hospitals throughout the country)
- An evaluation plan to measure the success of the QI initiative and to identify areas for improvement along with a dissemination plan to publish and share practices and results achieved

Data Collected and Preliminary Results: Safety Culture and Contextual Factors

Data on patient safety culture and contextual factors (e.g., improvement capability, and leadership) that might affect outcomes has been collected. For safety culture evaluation, the Agency for Healthcare Research and Quality (AHRQ) patient safety culture survey will be conducted on three separate occasions—in March 2016, March 2017, and April 2018—thus facilitating evaluation of the potential change in this data over the course of the project. The data collected thus far (March 2016), arises from a response rate of around 85% and is currently being analyzed. Regarding improvement capability, leadership, and other contextual factors, the Model for Understanding Success in Quality (MUSIQ) survey (applied in October 2015 and at the end of the collaborative) and the Project Progress Score (PPS), reported monthly, were applied. The MUSIQ score reported in October 2015 varied from 119.08 to 151.25 (mean 130.17), showing a hospital readiness for adopting innovative initiatives. PPS scores varied from 1.5 to 2.5 at the beginning of the project, which is in line with expectations. All teams are expected to have reached a score of 4–4.5 by May 2018.

Process Measures for CAUTI

Teams are supported to measure and improve key care processes. Figure 30.3 shows the reduction in the number of urinary catheter insertions (bundle element 1) in one hospital. Catheter use dropped from an average of seven patients to 2.67 in the 12-month period.

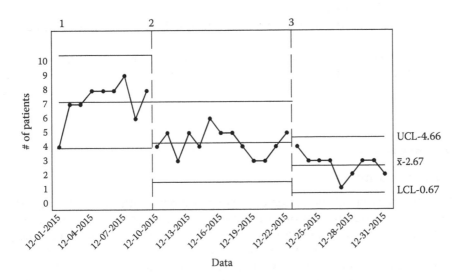

FIGURE 30.3
Number of urinary catheters used in one participating hospital.

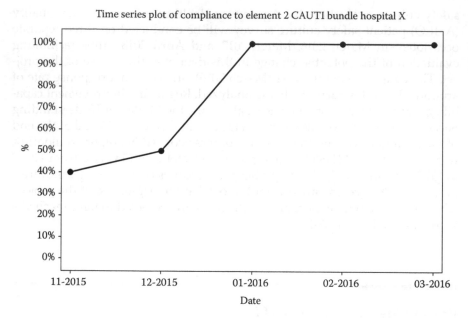

FIGURE 30.4
Compliance in use of aseptic technique when performing urinary catheter insertion.

Figure 30.4 shows levels of increased compliance in use of aseptic technique when performing urinary catheter insertion (bundle element 2). The bundle compliance was 40% at the beginning of the project and rose to 100% over a period of 2 months.

Similar results are found across the hospitals that are part of this QI initiative.

If these results are maintained and improved, as it is expected, there will be a very positive impact on the main outcome indicator—reduction of HAI rates.

Economic Impact

An economic impact evaluation of the improvement initiative is planned. We believe that better evaluation of the costs of HAIs, in particular the savings that can be made when instances are reduced and/or prevented, could help providers and payers justify investing in this area. In addition, sound estimates of the potential system-wide cost savings could mobilize policymakers to invest the resources needed to enable progress, and thereby improve care while simultaneously restraining rising healthcare costs. According to an estimate from the Portuguese Health Ministry, a reduction of 50% in HAI rates in the hospitals of the NHS could save €280 million (US$299 million) per year (Crisp, 2015).

Transferability Scale and Spread within Portugal

The SIH initiative will systematically spread knowledge regarding safety interventions that have already been tested and implemented on prototype units in each participating hospital, and that have been shown to be both reliable and effective. The monthly collection and analysis of data will allow real-time learning and improvement. Best practices will be gathered and shared through the collaborative learning system, through the website and WebEx calls, in addition to face-to-face meetings. Over time, it is anticipated that SIH results will influence department/hospital/health policies and other healthcare institutions throughout Portugal, which will learn from the initiative and be "infected" by its underling methodology, practices, and "philosophy."

Conclusion

The SIH initiative focuses on an issue that is at the forefront of the healthcare agenda in Portugal. This is the first time that a "structured collaborative" initiative in Portugal has united doctors, surgeons, nurses, and pharmacists, as well as management from different hospitals, with the aim of sharing best practices and results, overcoming barriers, and changing safety culture, in an environment of transparency where all teach and all learn.

While preliminary results do not yet show a sustainable improvement, we are optimistic that the commitment, expertise and energy of healthcare professionals and hospital management will ensure that the SIH initiative achieves its objective of halving HAI, with obvious clinical, economic, and social gains.

31

Russia

Progress in Healthcare Quality in Russia

Vasiliy V. Vlassov and Alexander L. Lindenbraten

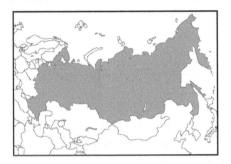

CONTENTS

Background

The Russian Federation, the largest and most populous republic of the USSR, declared independence in 1991, inheriting from the USSR both debts and assets, from state property to a massive army. In addition, the national system of healthcare—the first entirely state-owned and funded system in the world—was inherited. This system was significantly underfunded: by law, the Soviet system mandated unlimited care, but in practice, the possibility of receiving world-class care was very limited. Only hospitals reserved for the party elite had reasonable amenities and access to pharmaceuticals; these were managed by the special KGB-controlled service and were not accessible to the general population. During perestroika (the period of reform under Gorbachev), the system was described as funded "on a residue

principle,"—that is, by the money that remained after all other state requirements, like defense or industry, were accounted for (Cassileth et al., 1995).

During the first 10 years of post-Soviet development, the healthcare system was severely underfunded, and it wasn't until 2006 that total funding
from all sources approached even the relatively low levels of 1991. No actual
healthcare reform was implemented, however, other than the introduction
of compulsory medical insurance (CMI). Even Soviet medical provisions for
the presidential administration, with their exclusive healthcare facilities and
resorts, were retained. However, there were important developments relating to aspects of healthcare regulation, the system of incentives, and medical
guidelines. The object of this chapter is to present the major developments in
the current system of quality management in the Russian healthcare system,
and to consider the lessons learned.

Move to Quality

Compulsory medical insurance (CMI) was introduced in 1993 to increase
the funding of the healthcare system through the imposition of additional
taxes (Supreme Council, Russian Soviet Federative Socialist Republic, 1993).
Subsequently, however, the government reduced the healthcare budget,
effectively maintaining the same low level of funding. New basic healthcare
legislation (1993), together with the introduction of CMI and a number of
other new acts, encouraged discussion of treatment options, access, and coverage. In a short time, the first simple Russian "standards of care" (similar to
technical standards in industry) were created to satisfy the requirements of
the new insurance industry (Russian Federation, 1993; Shishkin and Vlassov,
2009).

A number of foreign sponsors and international organizations were
involved in efforts to transform Russian healthcare. One of the important
initiatives in these projects was the development of evidence-based clinical practice guidelines (EBCPG). The National Program of Standardization
was introduced in 1996, at a time when the necessity of establishing EBCPG
was gaining currency all around the world (Ollenschlager, 2003). The initial
idea of the National Program of Standardization was to create an array of
national prescriptive documents, not only EBCPG, but also classifications of
medical procedures for payment purposes and so forth. Crucially, evidence-
based guidelines, which prescribed treatments and provided advice about
what should be covered by CMI, thereby helped to reduce the prevalence of
unnecessary treatments (Cassileth et al., 1995).

The introduction of CMI also necessitated the development of quality control in the interactions between patients, hospitals, and healthcare administrations. The provision of such guidelines has meant that hospitals and

practitioners are now clearly accountable when it comes to medical malpractice, and the number of medical cases taken to court by insurance companies as well as by citizens has risen since the 1990s.

Unfortunately, the financial situation in the country has only improved slowly. Small additional sums of money directed to healthcare have been spent on vertical projects, such as purchasing expensive equipment for major hospitals, or complex upgrades of equipment for ambulatory care facilities. Only after 2005 did the financing of the system begin to improve, but since 2013, a new raft of problems in the national economy have taken their toll on the healthcare budget. Since the late 1990s, the healthcare system has been systematically reduced. Of particular concern is the ongoing reduction of access to healthcare in rural areas, which has worsened since 2013.

Both insurers and the Ministry of Health were convinced that the introduction of EBCPG could be an effective way to improve quality of care despite the lack of funding. It was proposed that EBCPG should prescribe minimum requirements of evidence-based care that would be covered by government- and insurance-provided funding, while the shortfall would come from other sources. This idea was not implemented, primarily because national regulations have no provision to formally limit care. Additionally, current funding levels in some regions meant that the minimal package would be of an unacceptably low standard, particularly when compared with the standard of care provided in developed countries. As a result, the rationing continues to be implicit. Currently, only the Russian Society of Clinical Oncologists differentiates between "minimal" and "optimal" therapies in their EBCPG: the "optimal" representing best current practice and "minimal" the cheaper alternative.

As of 2000, the National Program of Standardization delivered dozens of EBCPG and created the first Russian methodology for the development of such documents. In 2003, the National Program of Standardization was abandoned, and as a part of government reforms, the National Service for Surveillance in Healthcare (http://roszdravnadzor.ru) was established to oversee the quality of healthcare independently of the Ministry of Health and the regional healthcare administrations. While a comprehensive system of healthcare quality control has not yet been firmly established, there are now mechanisms in place for the benefit of both professionals and patients.

First, in 2011, all these reforms were ratified in new healthcare legislation (Russian Federation, 2011). Following the first post-Soviet laws, the new regulations included a range of mechanisms to guarantee quality. Additionally, a new kind of regulation, "orders of the provision of healthcare," was introduced. Initially designed to provide a template for the patient journey within the system, these documents also defined the criteria of eligibility for the provision of specialist care, along with a recommended structure and staffing of the healthcare facilities.

Second, a new type of prescriptive document or "standard" was introduced, stipulating the required average treatments for common conditions.

These standards became the subject of intense national debate, and they were ultimately taken to the Supreme Court. While the Ministry of Health insisted that these standards were planning documents only, proposing levels of funding and volume of care, the Supreme Court understood them to be firm recommendations for the content and volume of care that patients were eligible to receive.

Third, the new law recognized the EBCPG as documents that must be produced by medical professional associations for the purpose of advancing the quality of medical care. The Ministry of Health manages the process, and as reported in 2015, in only 2 years, more than 1200 EBCPG have been developed. Unfortunately, however, the EBCPG are prepared without explicit methodology, and overall quality cannot be guaranteed. The Ministry of Health is planning to use the EBCPG to create new instruments of quality control in healthcare (Vlassov, 2016).

Fourth, for the first time in its long history, the Russian healthcare system has introduced an external quality control system. This has been implemented nationally in the form of patient service evaluations; however, it is still too early to say whether it has been effective. External mechanisms of quality assurance have never been welcome in the Russian system, and indicators relating to the functioning of hospitals are still not available either to the public or health practitioners.

Fifth, the "pay-for-performance" contracts (effective contract) were introduced in 2012 in order to pay doctors. However, this mechanism appears to have failed. Part of the problem was that they were introduced before the objective EBCPG-based indicators were available.

Stimulated by global developments and international cooperation, as well as changes to national legislation, many hospitals, both private and state-owned, have begun implementing quality management systems. A number of hospitals have received accreditation, including certification from the U.S. Joint Commission.

Transferability: Lessons Learned

The current economic crisis has resulted in the mass closure of hospitals, putting the hospital system under enormous pressure. Not only have doctors and nurses become overstretched, they have been put under the additional pressure of performance evaluations and quality demands. Unless such multi-directional pressures are factored in, it is impossible to properly evaluate the success of the quality assurance program. Thus far, the implementation of a quality management system has been highly advantageous to the Russian healthcare system despite the continuing underfunding, and hopefully efforts on the quality management front will continue to mitigate the effect of shortages in the system.

While there have been some improvements, it is impossible to judge the extent to which the introduction of international EBCPG to the resource-poor system has been a success. Without assurance that the best care will be provided and covered, substandard healthcare will continue to damage the morale of both patients and practitioners. We believe that it is better to develop the EBCPG oriented to the resources available, but the methodology for the preparation of such guidelines is yet to be created.

Conclusion: Prospects

Despite shortages in the financing of healthcare, the health of the population in Russia is improving, as are processes for quality management in healthcare.

32

Scotland

Partnership and Collaboration as the Hallmark of Scottish Healthcare Improvement

Andrew Thompson and David Steel

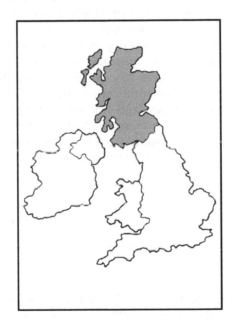

CONTENTS

Introduction

> Effective partnership working with people, staff, and partners across the
> public, third, and private sectors and industry will continue to be the
> hallmark of our approach.
>
> (Scottish Government, 2015, p. 6).

Partnerships, which can take many forms, feature increasingly in policy statements in health systems that are making the transition from centralized and hierarchical government-provided services to networked systems of governance, involving state and non-state actors (Richards and Smith, 2002). The drivers for these changes include the increasing complexity of problems and the incapacity of government alone to resolve them. The need for joint working is enhanced during times of rapid change, such as the recent implementation of austerity measures (Wildridge et al., 2004). Effective partnerships rely on meaningful collaboration between the various stakeholders, and critical success factors include a shared vision, trust, clear and consistent communication, shared decision-making and accountability, a focus on process and outcomes, and people who can work across boundaries (Carnwell and Carson, 2009). Collaborative governance, as it has become known, is a formal public agency-led arrangement that is deliberative and aims to promote consensual public policy (Ansell and Gash, 2008).

Background

Partnership and collaboration have been the dominant motif of strategic policy for NHSScotland since 1997. The break with the "market-style" approach of the previous decade was signaled in the White Paper "Designed to Care," which identified four main partnerships: between government and citizens; patients and professionals; different parts of NHSScotland; and NHSScotland and other organizations that could help improve health and service quality (Scottish Office, 1997). Following a change of government in 2007, this approach was confirmed in Better Health, Better Care, which emphasized shared ownership and accountability with the Scottish people and NHSScotland staff, and then reinforced in the Healthcare Quality Strategy for NHSScotland and Achieving Sustainable Quality in Scotland's Healthcare: A 20:20 Vision (Scottish Government, 2007; 2010; 2011a). This emphasis, described as mutuality, is in stark contrast to the neoliberal reforms based on markets and competition, which have elsewhere led to a high degree of organizational fragmentation and increased transaction costs (Thompson and Steel, 2015).

Examples of Partnership Working

The impact of this approach upon the improvement and reform agenda in Scotland at macro, meso, and micro levels, for example on quality and safety and on health and social care integration, has been extensively analyzed by ourselves and others, most recently by the Organization for Economic Cooperation and Development (Ham et al., 2013; McDermott et al., 2015; OECD, 2013; Thompson and Steel, 2015). In this chapter, we draw upon this analysis and highlight three further examples: vertical partnerships between service providers, or managed clinical networks (MCNs), that focus on particular services or health conditions, such as diabetes; and two service partnerships around staff governance and public involvement.

1. Managed Clinical Networks

MCNs were the most important strategic development emerging from the Acute Services Review of 1998, which defined them as: "Linked groups of health professionals and organizations from primary, secondary, and tertiary care, working in a coordinated manner, unconstrained by existing professional and health board boundaries, to ensure equitable provision of high-quality, clinically effective services throughout Scotland" (Scottish Office, 1998). Subsequent guidance stressed the importance of patient and carer involvement in MCNs and of collaboration with social care. While there are over 130 MCNs in existence, we will focus on the example of diabetes care as a particularly well-established partnership.

Each health board was mandated to develop a MCN for diabetes by the end of 2003 (Scottish Executive Health Department, 2001). Building upon preexisting informal networks, shared care—involving hospital doctors, specialist nurses, general practitioners (GPs), podiatrists, and ophthalmologists—is now universal, underpinned by a real-time information system that enables individual patients to be tracked along the care pathway.

Early evaluation of one MCN (Tayside) identified improvements in clinical outcomes between 1998 and 2005, significantly for type 2 diabetes and to a lesser degree among type 1 patients, which was largely due to enthusiastic leadership, shared vision, and commitment by primary care and specialist clinicians. The next priority was seen to be greater patient and managerial engagement (Greene et al., 2009). Achievements nationally include a reduction of over 40% in diabetes-related amputations and early introduction of comprehensive diabetic retinopathy screening (Kennon et al., 2012). The latest Diabetes Improvement Plan highlights considerable progress in many areas of diabetes care as well as continuing challenges, for example in glycemic control for type 1 diabetes; and it emphasizes the need to work with patients to help them self-manage in a safe and effective way through educational initiatives and mutually agreed, individualized care plans (McKnight, 2015).

More generally, healthcare professionals attribute MCNs' success to the cultural change they have engendered, facilitating greater collaboration, shared vision, and inclusion (Guthrie et al., 2010). Patients tend to highlight improvements to coordination, communication between professionals, and systematic follow-up, while not necessarily improved access. Influence and persuasion, rather than contract and control, are seen as enabling MCNs to resolve some of the difficult policy challenges.

2. Partnership with Staff

Since 1998, the concept of partnership working has been developed as the approach to employee relations in NHSScotland. Partnership structures—involving trade unions, managers, and, at the national level, government—have been put in place to involve staff in key decisions on strategic, workforce, and operational issues. Nationally, the Scottish Partnership Forum (SPF), co-chaired by the chief executive of NHSScotland and a leading trade unionist, is a strategic body contributing to setting the overall direction of the service. In addition, two committees comprising staff and management representatives develop detailed policies for managing staff. These policies are then introduced at local-board level through Area Partnership Forums and an elected employee director serves as a non-executive on each board.

These developments are underpinned by "staff governance," a system of corporate accountability for the fair and effective management of staff, and which, uniquely, is enshrined in legislation. All boards are expected to meet the staff governance standard to demonstrate that staff are well informed, appropriately trained, involved in decisions that affect them, treated fairly and consistently, and provided with a safe working environment (Scottish Government, 2012). A staff governance committee, chaired by a non-executive, provides assurance that this is happening.

In contrast to the difficult industrial relations in the NHS during the 1980s and 1990s, there is no question that these arrangements have led to a much more harmonious climate—one that retains the confidence of both "sides." In this respect, Scotland's record stands in stark contrast to greater turbulence in England. For a time, partnership worked effectively on wider strategic issues also, with the SPF having real ownership of the policies that were produced; but its influence has waned in recent years, with its meetings becoming more a forum for information-sharing. Nonetheless, an independent evaluation covering the years up to 2011 concluded that, although not unique, the partnership agreements in NHSScotland had "matured into probably the most ambitious and important contemporary innovation in British public sector relations" (Bacon and Samuel, 2012).

3. Public Involvement

In recognition of the need to work in partnership with people rather than doing things to them, a framework was developed for involving citizens in NHSScotland: Patient Focus and Public Involvement (Scottish Executive, 2001). Its aim was to ensure services are patient-centered and to enable public involvement in their design and delivery. Since 2005, the Scottish Health Council (SHC) has had the statutory responsibility for ensuring that all health boards deliver on this strategy, through the provision of advice and support. Recent developments include a collaborative tool of engagement, Our Voice, to bring together health and social care services with the general public to enable purposeful engagement coupled with feedback on their impact or how their views have been considered (Scottish Health Council, 2016).

As part of the mutuality agenda in Better Health, Better Care, citizens are defined as partners and owners of NHSScotland. Patient experience forms an integral part of the Better Together program, and a participation standard against which health boards are judged has also been developed (Scottish Government, 2007). Where major service changes are planned, health boards are assessed against national standards on how well they engage local communities (Scottish Health Council, 2015).

The Patient Rights (Scotland) Act of 2011 aims to improve patient experiences and support greater involvement in their health and healthcare (Scottish Parliament, 2011). As an example of collaboration between the voluntary sector and NHSScotland, recent evaluation of Chest, Heart and Stroke Scotland's Voices Scotland program concluded that it has made significant progress in relation to the production of materials, facilitation, and support, with patient self-management and co-production central to its aims (Scottish Health Council, 2014).

While there has been no formal evaluation of the impact of the mutuality agenda, there are many signs of commitment and genuine collaboration across statutory and non-statutory organizations, with citizen involvement evident across NHSScotland.

Transferability

Various factors have been posited as enablers of partnership in Scotland: the relatively small population and strong networks that facilitate brokerage between government, healthcare professionals, and managers; relative organizational stability; and the high degree of political consensus among political parties and civil society that provides policy continuity and support (Ham et al., 2013; McDermott et al., 2015). There is wide international interest in Scotland's approach, but without further exploration of the precise influence of factors such as these, it is difficult to gauge how far it is transferable to other countries.

Prospects for Further Success

These brief examples, in tandem with earlier publications on quality and safety and on health and social care integration, illustrate that the partnership rhetoric has been a major driver of policy and service improvement over the last 20 years. There is also clear evidence that collaborative working is contributing to the achievement of desired outcomes. Further evaluative research is needed, however, to demonstrate this conclusively, including comparing its relative effectiveness with systems that rely on markets and competition to generate improvement. This will also help to address doubts that have been expressed about the sustainability of this approach in the face of the unprecedented challenges currently confronting all healthcare systems.

What is clear is that, culturally and politically, partnership is deeply embedded and will be a hallmark of improvement in the public sector in Scotland for the foreseeable future (Scottish Government, 2011b). Moreover, as Innes and Booher have argued, this style of working can be self-reinforcing:

> Many of the most valued outcomes of collaborations are of the systemic variety—that is, they not only produce specific outcomes, but they also affect the system by changing attitudes, relationships, and capabilities of players.

> (Innes and Booher, 2010, p. 35)

33

Serbia

Using Data to Protect Vulnerable Children

Mirjana Živković Šulović, Ivan Ivanovic, and Milena Vasic

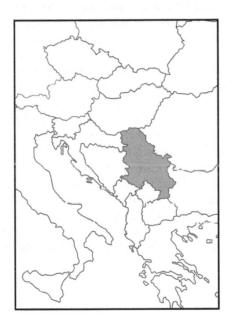

CONTENTS

Background

Violence against children is a problem that affects all societies, cultures, and regions worldwide. Although violence against a child constitutes a gross violation of that child's rights, millions of children are subjected to everyday violence. Violence causes suffering and trauma, which may have detrimental effects on the child's subsequent development and well-being.

During the last quarter century, children in the Republic of Serbia living in unfavorable environments have been exposed to an increased risk of violence (Government of Republic of Serbia, 2005). Current data indicate a trend of growing family and peer violence among children and youth.

Article 19 of the United Nations (UN) Convention on the Rights of the Child, which came into force in 1990, enshrined the fundamental right of all children to protection from all forms of violence (United Nations General Assembly, 1990). The convention was ratified by the Council of Europe (CoE), of which the Republic of Serbia is a member state, and in line with the UN Secretary-General's recommendations, the CoE have developed integrated national strategies for the protection of children against violence (Council of Europe, 2009; United Nations General Assembly, 2006).

As a response to these international recommendations and guidelines, the Republic of Serbia has developed national policies to define the goals, tasks, procedures, and responsibilities of both the system and individuals in an effort to protect children from abuse, neglect, and all forms of exploitation. A number of plans that prioritize the protection of children from violence have been implemented, including the National Plan of Action for Children (2004), the National Millennium Development Goals in the Republic of Serbia (2007), and the National Strategy for Youth (2008). The General Protocol on Protection of Children from Abuse and Neglect (2005), which targets the problem of child abuse and neglect specifically, is now mandatory for every individual and all institutions in the country (Ministry of Labour, Employment and Social Policy [Republic of Serbia], 2005).

Details of the Identified Success Story

The need for an efficient and cooperative interdepartmental network was satisfied by the creation and gradual implementation of Special Protocols for the Protection of Children from Abuse and Neglect, which were adopted by the social welfare system and the police in 2006, by the education sector in 2007, and by the healthcare system and legal institutions in 2009.

The healthcare protocols, which were developed for healthcare institutions and healthcare workers, provide guidelines that help to protect children against abuse and neglect within healthcare institutions at all levels (Ministry of Labour, Employment and Social Policy [Republic of Serbia], 2005). Due to their close and continuous contact with the general population, primary healthcare services play an exceptionally important role, not only in prevention, but in early detection, registration, and treatment of such cases.

Primary care workers are also responsible for referring cases to secondary and tertiary institutions (Ministry of Health [Republic of Serbia], 2009). The protocol ensures that all healthcare workers are obligated to report suspected cases of abuse to specialist teams, which have been established within each catchment area, based on the specific character of the institution and its social environment. The role of such teams is to recognize and report cases of child abuse and neglect; to assess the risks, needs, and existing condition of the child and the family; and to plan protective and treatment interventions (Pejovic-Milovancevic et al., 2012).

While the regular reporting of statistics in the Republic of Serbia ensures that the number of children whose death is the result of violence is monitored, the healthcare system has, until recently, had no established reporting method that would enable the ongoing effects of violence on a child's health to be monitored. Data show that while 12 children died as a consequence of violence in 2000, the number had decreased to four by 2006 (Government of Republic of Serbia, 2005).

Although many individual health institutions have established professional teams for data collection, this has not yet been translated to the national level. As detection and registration is the significant first step leading to further interventions, the system of data collection and processing at national level has recently been expanded with the support of The United Nations Children's Fund (UNICEF).

During 2013–2014, a joint European Union and UNICEF project, Protecting Children from Violence in Southeast Europe, was implemented (UNICEF, n.d.). As a part of this project, and in order to establish an adequate, modern, and sustainable system for nationwide data collection and reporting, the Institute of Public Health of Serbia has developed a database for the protection of children from abuse and neglect in the health system. During the first phase, in 2013, 13 health institutions were given access to the database, with teams specializing in child protection able to utilize this technologically advanced system. In the second phase, in 2014, the system was implemented in an additional 60 health institutions.

So far, one-third of Serbian health institutions have connected to the online recording system. According to 2014 data, 37 institutions responded by inputting 476 questionnaires and registering 451 instances of suspected abuse and neglect (Sulović, 2016).

The highest rate of exposure to abuse and/or neglect—25% of all cases—involved children between the age of 12–14 years (Figure 33.1). Among those children who had suffered abuse specifically, 30% were aged 12–14 years (Figure 33.2). Two-thirds of the reported children had suffered physical abuse (62.8%), more than half emotional abuse (54.5%), almost one-quarter sexual abuse (22.9%), and one in 13 children (7.7%) had witnessed domestic violence. Boys between the ages of 9 and 11 (40%) and girls between the ages of 12 and 14 years (35%) were most likely to have been exposed to sexual violence. Boys aged 12–14 (27%) and girls aged 15–17 (33%) were most likely to be subjected to emotional violence.

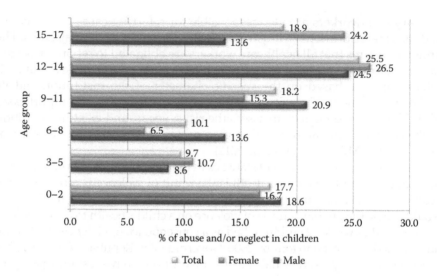

FIGURE 33.1
Distribution of reports on child abuse and/or neglect, by gender and age, Serbia, 2014.

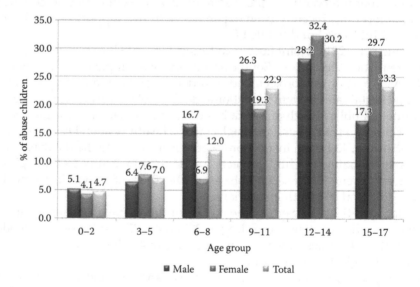

FIGURE 33.2
Distribution of reports on child abuse by gender and age, Serbia, 2014.

The number of children reported suffering from neglect was 216. Of these, 52.8% were boys and 47.2% girls. Almost one-third of the neglected children were aged 0–2 years (32%).

From a total of 216 reported instances of neglect, more than half of the children suffered medical neglect (51.8%), 46.3% emotional neglect, 38.4% physical neglect, and 26.9% educational neglect.

Among all reported cases, a total number of 22 children had been exploited—with nine cases of non-sexual exploitation, and 13 cases of sexual exploitation. Children older than 12 were more likely to have been exploited.

Of the cases recorded, more than half (57%) were exposed to various forms of abuse in a family environment, while 20% were abused in the local community, and around 12% had been exposed to abuse in an educational institution (Table 33.1).

In more than a fifth of reported cases, children were at high risk of abuse and neglect (22%), while almost one-half (47%) were estimated to be at moderate risk.

After the registration of cases of abuse and neglect, health workers report to the relevant institutions and plan health interventions for each individual case. According to these individual plans, specified interventions are undertaken (Table 33.2).

Data analysis for 2015 is underway, with the total number of instances of suspected abuse and neglect (as reported by 67 participating institutions) rising to 842.

TABLE 33.1

Distribution of Reports by Environment of Abuse, Serbia, 2014

Environment of abuse	Distribution (in %)
Family	57.4
Educational institutions	12.4
Social institutions	1.3
Other institutions	9.0
Local community	20.0
Total	100.0

TABLE 33.2

Distribution of Interventions Provided to Abused and Neglected Children, Serbia, 2014

Intervention	Distribution (in %)
Medical treatment and psychological support in health institution	48.5
Referral to other health institution	12.6
Hospitalization	18.7
Other	20.2
Total	100.0

Details of the Impact of the Success Story

The main objective of the data-reporting application is to ensure that information is continually updated so that health institutions are able to analyze and respond to any instances of child abuse and/or neglect.

The analysis is designed to enable relevant institutions (social, educational, juridical, police, local self-governments) to develop specific programs, activities, and interventions in order to

- Identify, refer, and act upon cases of violence against children
- Strengthen the child protection services response to violence against children
- Create programs to reduce violence against children
- Develop and improve working protocols for professionals, and so on

Analyses of collected data have allowed experts to begin developing ways to improve the special health service protocol for the protection of children from abuse and neglect. The introduction of specific medical evidence and documentation on registration of instances of child abuse and/or neglect is also a priority.

Implementation: Transferability of the Exemplar

In accordance with the recently adopted Serbian Law on Health Documentation and Healthcare Records, from the 1st of January 2017, all healthcare institutions will be obliged to use this system to report any suspected violence against children (Republic of Serbia, 2014).

The database stores information relating to the characteristics of each child, details of the examination, treatment, risk assessment, type of abuse, neglect or exploitation, as well as any diagnoses. In addition, information pertaining to suspected perpetrators and details of any planned interventions on behalf of the child and family, and/or in cooperation with other services, is also recorded.

The International Classification of Diseases (ICD-10) was used in the development of the database. This enables a comparison of data at both national (between Serbian institutions and districts) and international levels (among Serbia and other countries).

The system has applications in other areas such as education. Several Balkan states, that is, Bosnia and Herzegovina and the Republic of Macedonia (FYRM), have already expressed interest in using this data system.

Prospects for Further Success, Next Steps, and Conclusion

Child victims are no longer invisible: every year health professionals are better able to detect and treat the consequences of abuse and to report each instance to the relevant system.

The implementation of these applications in healthcare institutions in the Republic of Serbia has increased the availability of nationally significant medical information to analysts, planners, and professionals, in addition to decision makers at all levels.

All relevant healthcare institutions have been advised of the reporting obligations and database/monitoring system, however, in order to extend this reporting system to all health professionals/institutions, Internet connectivity is required. Further development of the reporting system thus needs to be coordinated at both the national and local level.

34

Spain

Organ Donation and Transplantation: ONT's Success Story

Rafael Matesanz, Elisabeth Coll Torres, and Rosa Suñol

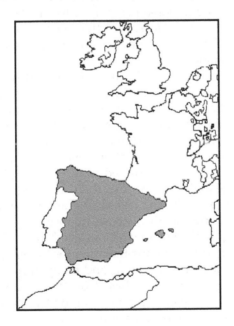

CONTENTS

Background

Transplantation is the best option for those patients with terminal organ failure, both in terms of survival and quality of life. The increased likelihood of successful transplants has led to the steady increase in the demand for organs for transplantation all over the world. While donations cannot keep up with demand anywhere, there are significant differences between countries. Deceased donors may be nonexistent in many countries, but can exceed 30 donors per million population (pmp) in others (Report of the Global Observatory on Donation and Transplantation, 2013).

Numerous efforts have been undertaken by countries to increase donation and consequently transplant rates. Classic measures of dealing with organ shortage range from promotional campaigns to legislative changes, including the development of tools to record the donation wishes of the living. Nevertheless, none of these strategies has proven effective in maintaining an increase in organ donation.

The European Commission has been working hard since 2007 to improve the quality and safety of organs, increase organ availability, and make national transplantation systems more efficient and accessible. The European Commission proposed a dual mechanism of action. In the first instance, an action plan encouraging active coordination and cooperation between member states has been developed. A set of priority actions in the form of a large number of projects has been co-funded with the aim of helping countries with low organ availability to improve their availability rates, identifying the most efficient systems, sharing experience, and promoting best practices. In addition, a legal ruling containing basic quality and safety principles was formulated, resulting in the European Directive 2010/53/EU on standards of quality and safety of human organs intended for transplantation.

These policy measures, the directive, and many of the actions of the plan itself have, to a large extent, been based on the Spanish Model of organ donation and transplantation, a system based on two basic principles: organizational measures and continuous adaptation to change. This model has been shown to be the world's most effective in achieving high rates in organ donation in a sustained way for more than 20 years (Matesanz et al., 2011).

Details of the Identified Success Story

Measures similar to those proposed by the European Commission were initially adopted in Spain after the Spanish National Transplant Organization (ONT) was created in 1989. The ONT was conceived as a technical agency of the Ministry of Health in charge of overseeing donation and transplantation activities in the country. The basic legal, organizational, and technical framework necessary to ensure successful implementation of the measures was already in place: Spanish transplantation law contains the basic elements of any transplantation law, and the Spanish healthcare system is a public one with a universal coverage and is technically dependent on prepared, innovative, and motivated transplant teams and other healthcare professionals (Matesanz et al., 1998).

The Spanish Model takes a systematic and organizational approach to the process of deceased donation, and encompasses the following elements:

- The coordination of donation activities has been structured at three distinct, but interlinked levels: national (ONT), regional (17 regional coordinations), and in each procurement hospital. The first two levels act as an interface between the technical and the political strata and support the process of deceased donation. Health competencies in Spain are transferred to 17 autonomous regions, so any national decision on donation and transplantation activities is agreed upon by the Regional Transplantation Commission, which comprises the ONT as chair along with the 17 regional coordinators. The hospital level of coordination is represented by a network of officially authorized procurement hospitals that are directly in charge of developing the deceased donation process. This network has grown from less than 20 hospitals in 1989 to 189 in 2015, an evolution that reflects the significant efforts made by the system and the political support received during this period.
- The transplant coordinator (TC) is considered the key figure in our model. TCs in Spain have a unique profile, conceived to facilitate the early identification and referral of possible donors. TCs are in-house professionals and members of staff of the procurement hospital concerned. They are nominated by and report to the medical director of the hospital, and therefore do not report to the transplantation team. Most of the TCs are employed on a part-time basis, which enables them to be appointed even at hospitals with low deceased donor potential. Importantly, a majority of TCs are also critical care physicians, so their daily work is carried out in those units where 12% of deaths occur in persons with a clinical condition compatible with a brain death diagnosis (de la Rosa et al., 2012).
- The ONT acts as a supporting agency to the network of procurement hospitals, but is not exclusively an organ-sharing office; it manages waiting lists, transplant registries, statistics, and provides general and specialized information and actions to improve the whole process of organ donation and transplantation.
- The Quality Assurance Program in the Deceased Donation Process, in place since 1998, is based on a continuous clinical chart review of

all deaths occurring in critical care units of procurement (de la Rosa et al., 2012). The program, which has thus far focused on brain death donation, aims to monitor deceased organ donation potential, evaluate performance, and identify key areas for improvement.

- Since 1991, over 15,000 professionals in Spain have done training in organ donation. These courses are aimed not only at TCs, but health professionals in general, especially those who work in areas that are likely to be associated with organ donation: intensive care, emergency departments, stroke units, and so on.
- A positive and trusting public attitude toward organ donation has been achieved by working closely with the mass media and through the ONT network's development of a solid and open communications policy (Matesanz and Miranda, 1996).
- Finally, as with any other medical activity performed within the public healthcare system, hospitals are reimbursed for their donation and transplantation activities. The corresponding regional health authorities allocate a specific budget to cover both human and material resources needed for the effective development of these activities at every hospital.

Details of the Impact of the Success Story

At the end of the 1980s, the rate of Spanish organ deceased donation was mid-low in contrast to other European countries, with around 14 donors pmp. Since then, Spanish rates have been steadily growing and now occupy the highest deceased donation rates ever recorded for a large country (46.77 million citizens). The Spanish donor rate has been maintained at 35–36 pmp in the last years (Figure 34.1), which is well above the 19.7 or the 26.6 donors pmp reached by the European Union and the United States respectively in 2014.

Along with this increase in the number of organs available for transplantation every year, the number of patients who have received transplants, always following strict principles of clinical priority, quality, and safety, has grown steadily from around 1300 procedures in 1989 to over 4000 from 2011.

Implementation: Transferability of the Exemplar

The features of the Spanish Model can be reproduced in other settings as long as a set of conditions are fulfilled (Matesanz, 2013). Results will be influenced

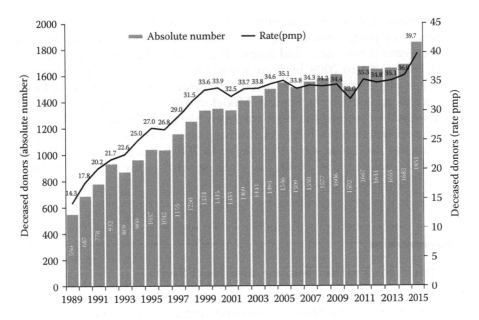

FIGURE 34.1

Deceased donation activity in Spain. Absolute number and rate (donors pmp), 1989–2015. (From Organización Nacional de Trasplantes database.)

by the preexisting structural conditions, such as the legal, organizational, and technical factors mentioned earlier.

The existence of a national public health system with full coverage of the population is virtually a *sine qua non* of the Spanish Model. The development of a national program like the Spanish one needs a public health network, which can be difficult to find in countries without a strong national health system. Certain elements of this model can be implemented in selected hospitals or regions, but a full-scale adoption of the model requires a national system. Although adequate finances are clearly necessary and there is a minimum level under which it is not possible to develop such a system, transplantation medicine cannot be considered a luxury restricted to the richest countries. Additionally, it is important to remember that there are many examples showing that renal transplantation produces huge savings compared with the cost of dialysis for end-stage renal disease.

Other factors that influence organ donation, such as the number of available doctors and nurses, acute beds, and intensive care unit facilities, should also be considered. In summary, the Spanish Model can be partially or totally adapted to other countries or regions if basic conditions are guaranteed.

This organizational approach has been adopted outside Spain with variable results. The region of Tuscany, in Northern Italy, successfully adapted the Spanish Model some years back, resulting in a sustained increase in deceased donation activity, reaching levels of over 40 donors pmp (Simini, 2000). More recently, Croatia and Portugal have adopted the model in part, establishing a national transplant agency, a network of procurement hospitals, and employing resident TCs in hospitals. As a result, from 2006 to 2009, both countries increased their deceased donation rates by 37% and 54% respectively. Efforts are underway in Latin America to implement the Spanish Model in a manner that adapts to local circumstances through the Iberoamerican Network/Council of Donation and Transplantation (RCIDT). As a consequence of these initiatives, organ donation has increased since the start of RCIDT by an average of 52%, the highest increase in the world, for a region with more than 500 million people (Matesanz et al., 2015).

Prospects for Further Success and Next Steps

The system will face a number of new challenges in coming years: the transplantation needs of the Spanish population are expected to increase, while the potential of brain death donation has decreased in recent years. Novel strategies to adapt to the changing demographics have been explored and are being implemented in Spain through a strategic plan: the 40 pmp Donors Plan (Matesanz et al., 2009). With the assistance of a number of experts, ONT identified, carefully analyzed, and selected several areas of improvement. Specific areas of action include

- Detection and management of brain-dead donors, with four specific sub-areas: access to intensive care units, new forms of hospital management, foreigners and ethnic minorities, and evaluation/maintenance of thoracic organ donors
- Expanded criteria donors/no standard risk donors
- Special surgical and perfusion techniques
- Donation after cardiac death, considering both type II and III of Maastricht

Conclusion

Spain is the only large country in the world that has experienced a continuous improvement in deceased organ donation over a 25-year period. The Spanish Model shows that organ shortage is not due to a lack of potential donors, but rather to a failure to establish organizational measures that help convert many potential donors into actual donors. The Spanish Model can be partially or totally adapted to other countries or regions if basic conditions are guaranteed. The key point is to know the strengths and weaknesses of each system and to continue to work to improve the system where necessary, to ensure that organs are available to patients in need.

35

Sweden

Sweden Mines the Gold in Clinical Data for Research and Better Patient Care

John Øvretveit and Mats Brommels

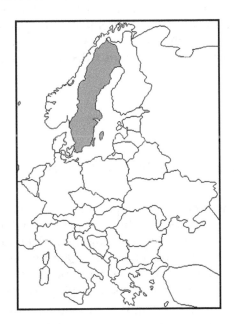

CONTENTS

Background

Sweden has built over 100 databases and systems that collect, store, and enable the use of clinical data for the benefit of patients. This chapter describes how these systems were developed and utilized, and explores their future role. The global digital healthcare revolution means that these databases and systems will be increasingly important for healthcare and illness prevention: each technological development adds to the value of the data collected and provides new and more efficient ways to collect and use digital data. This chapter provides lessons about the value of such databases in the digital era, and describes how to build, finance, and regulate the collection of the data, as well as how to best use such data to improve information analysis and presentation. The Swedish quality registries provide an example of an organized implementation system and governance structure that emphasizes the use of the registers for quality improvement, and enables providers to develop shared decision-making practices using registry data.

Definitions of Terms Used in This Chapter

- Clinical database or register: a repository, now usually electronic, for storing clinical data about individual patients, which may include some or all of the following—demographic data about the patient, diagnosis, treatment, and outcome. "Quality registries" are the name given to clinical databases developed in Sweden, originally for research purposes but now for multiple purposes.

- Information system: a system that turns data into usable information involving software and hardware for collecting, analyzing, and presenting analyzed data to inform the actions of patients, providers, managers, and others for research purposes.

Details of the Success Story

The Swedish National Quality Registers play an increasingly important role for many different stakeholders: they have become a strategically important asset in Sweden's quest to become a knowledge-based economy and a center of global medical innovation. They have already proved their success in enabling research that would not otherwise have been possible, and in their everyday value to patients, clinicians, and managers. As other countries seek to develop clinical databases, the Swedish experience of building the most comprehensive and sophisticated national registers in the world provides a valuable example of how to develop these registers and make use of them. This analysis is based on our independent research into the governing organization of the registries and an in-depth study of one advanced registry (Øvretveit and Keel, 2014; Øvretveit et al., 2013).

Sweden has been developing quality registers for more than 35 years, and there are now over 100, mostly disease-based, registers (http://kvalitetsregister.se/). The registers were developed initially by clinicians for medical research and operated by host clinical departments in different medical research centers. While the databases rely on clinicians voluntarily updating information during their "free time," they are now funded by government, both directly, with county healthcare personnel inputting data, and indirectly, by ensuring that health information technology supports the registers. A new generation of "smart registers" is emerging, uploading data from electronic health records using specified protocols, and giving patients and clinicians the information they need at the time and place they need it. The systems that make this possible are one element of a learning health system (Institute of Medicine [IOM], 2014).

The Swedish Rheumatology Quality Register (SRQ) is one such "smart register," and is illustrative of the system's success (Swedish Rheumatology Quality Register, n.d.). The SRQ, which is linked to other databases and utilizes state-of-the-art software that works in real-time, enables patients to track and self-manage their conditions, and allows quicker and more fact-based decisions for clinical practice, public reporting, and research, as well as for clinical process improvement. Using this system, patients report symptoms, health, and quality of life before visiting a clinician. The system is designed to take this self-reported data and combine it with other data to create a graphical display of the patient's health status, along with their personal health and treatment trends. The clinician also inputs clinical examination and laboratory data. The patient and clinician, together or separately, can then view these data and this helps the patient and clinician work to optimize health according to what matters to the patient. The structured data from each visit is exported to the national register, which builds data sets that can be analyzed to contribute to improving patient population health and for research.

The Swedish Hip Arthroplasty Register also provides a useful example of a successful registry. Established in 1979, this National Quality Register records and monitors all total hip replacements carried out in Sweden. All follow-up operations are also registered, an important element in improving quality of care (Svenska Höftprotesregistret, n.d.).

Clinical data about patients can be used to improve care and maintain health over short, medium, and longer terms:

- Short-term: showing patients the history of their treatments and outcomes enables them to provide better self-care, and helps providers give more effective care, which can reduce service utilization.
- Medium-term: providing data on performance for improvement of management and quality project teams.
- Longer-term: enables faster and lower cost research, and research not otherwise possible through clinical data collection, analysis, and linkage of data between databases.

Details of the Impact of the Success Story

The clinical practice improvements made possible by the SRQ include patients self-managing their diseases. Rather than regular checkups, patients can schedule a doctor or nurse appointment when needed, significantly reducing wait times. Avoidable use of services is minimized, and the confidence of patients to manage single or co-existing chronic diseases is increased. Both short-term and long-term savings are likely, as well as improved quality of life. Patients reported that using their own data increased their confidence in the time-trend visual displays of changes over time. Physicians also reported that they had confidence that the comparisons across physicians and practices were valid (Hvitfeldt et al., 2009).

The introduction of expensive biologic drugs in 2000 led to some funding for the SRQ from the drugs industry, as the registry agreed to include a reporting facility to allow physicians to report specific drug events (Essen and Lindblad, 2013).

The Swedish Hip Arthroplasty Register has facilitated both clinical improvements and research. Orthopedic surgeons' use of patient data to select the most effective and long-lasting hip procedures and prostheses has reduced the revision rate by 80% over 10 years (Herberts and Malchau, 2000). A report to the Swedish government by the Boston Consulting Group calculated a 10:1 payback for the cost of these publicly funded registries, and estimated that the United States could save $2 billion of $24 billion costs for hip replacement repair by funding and using such a register (Larsson et al., 2012).

There have, however, been challenges that need to be borne in mind by others seeking to follow these examples. During the early days, when data-entry was manual, some physicians were resistant to the additional time and cost burden, and dubious about the likely benefits to the individual clinician or department (Essen and Lindblad, 2013). More recently there have been increasing concerns about the privacy and security of patient data, and issues about linking patient data across databases. The systems necessary to address these concerns add costs and take time to develop. There are also concerns that patients whose health levels are lower and who have poor computer literacy may not receive the same benefits, and this may increase health inequalities.

Individuals with the skills and capability to design and implement the systems are scarce in Sweden and elsewhere, but their expertise is necessary to enable data capture and to turn the data into actionable information for daily use. There is also a shortage of skilled researchers able to understand the data and use it to answer traditional and new research questions. Finally, as the county health systems and government increase their funding for the systems, physicians may become more concerned about the use of the data for physician performance management: it is already possible using linked registry data to compare physicians' "value performance" in terms of the cost of a patient's care relative to the outcomes achieved.

Implementation: Transferability of the Exemplar

Others who are considering developing local or national registers or a smart register similar to those described in this chapter would be wise to consult Gliklich and Dreyer's *Users Guide* (2010) and consider the following:

- Whether and how to develop a stand-alone smart register system of this type with a view to later integration into a larger, digitally enabled learning health system. The two examples, the hip and arthritic registers, were initially developed by clinicians in stand-alone PCs, and later integrated in various ways into larger digital systems.

- Does the increased understanding and more effective treatment and co-care justify the extra time needed by the patient and physician to input and use the information? In earlier designs, a few physicians and patients questioned whether it was worth it (Hvitfeldt et al., 2009). But as the data is also used for other purposes, the total value of this system needs to be considered.

- It is important that patients and clinicians share design and ownership of such systems, but it can be difficult to find the time and energy, as well as the appropriate skills, to develop such a system. Others may be able to find already-developed systems, such as those described above, which they can then adapt to their needs, rather than doing all the development work themselves.

- While the system encourages physicians to engage in practices that are more patient-centric, or that involve "co-care," some physicians need training to use the system in this way.
- Data security involves many costs and challenges.
- There is some risk that health inequalities will be increased.

Conclusion

The Swedish quality registries demonstrate the value of digital data, appropriately collected, analyzed, and presented, for better-informed, real-time clinical decisions. The systems not only collect and store the data, but also analyze and present the data as required by users in an actionable form. In addition, the data and the system can then be utilized for many other purposes. These registers are sub-systems of a larger learning health system that "generates and applies the best evidence for the collaborative healthcare choices of each patient and provider; driving the process of discovery as a natural outgrowth of patient care" (IOM, 2007, 37).

36

Switzerland

Switzerland's Use of Breakthrough Collaboratives to Improve Patient Safety

Anthony Staines, Patricia Albisetti, and Paula Bezzola

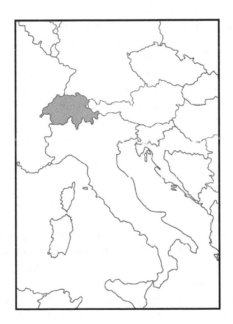

CONTENTS

Quality and Governance in the Swiss Health System

International comparisons of healthcare systems show that the Swiss health system is considered high performing (OECD and WHO, 2011). It offers a choice of healthcare providers, and medical and nursing professionals are well trained. Facilities are equipped with up-to-date technology, and the Swiss population benefits from universal healthcare coverage that allows quick access to care.

Ensuring high standards of care is one of the main goals of the Federal Law on Health Insurance (1996). This defines quality in terms of outcomes, appropriateness of care, and patient satisfaction. Systems for quality control and improvement, however, remain weak. In particular, there is no overview of the current quality of healthcare provision.

With a few exceptions, healthcare policy and its implementation are the responsibility of the 26 states (cantons). This decentralization makes it difficult to develop national standards for healthcare quality, as every state legislates to its own agenda and time frame. The Swiss Confederation has tried to develop a steering role in quality and safety of care and to secure funding for improvement projects. A law defining roles, responsibilities, funding, and coordination between confederation, states, insurers, providers, and patients is currently being discussed in the national parliament.

Although it is proving difficult for Switzerland to establish a national framework to measure and assess quality of care, a number of patient safety initiatives are already under way. The Swiss Patient Safety Foundation (SPSF), i.e., the national reference center, develops and implements national programs in line with the Swiss Confederation's quality strategy and is active in research, education, and other projects. Measurement is provided by the National Association for Quality in Healthcare (ANQ), which publishes a few national indicators that are compulsory for hospitals.

Numerous providers have launched projects to improve quality and safety of care. We believe, however, that national and regional coordination will be key to future success. One such approach to lead and coordinate learning and improvement is the Breakthrough Collaborative model.

Breakthrough Collaboratives in Swiss Healthcare

The Breakthrough Collaborative model, developed by the Institute for Healthcare Improvement (IHI), is a structured approach in which multidisciplinary teams from various facilities, working in parallel, join in applying evidence-based best practice through a multimodal change concept in a defined area of care. These teams meet for periodic learning sessions where they share results measured along a set of agreed indicators, as well as experience about best ideas for implementation within periodic learning sessions (Franco, 2011). An organizing body provides the design of the program, including the improvement package, the indicators, the data collection tools, the training, and the structure for shared learning. The model has been used by the Hospital Federation of Vaud (FHV) and the SPSF to spread best practice among hospitals who have volunteered to participate in the program.

The SPSF has used this model in combination with theoretical models to implement national patient safety programs (Goeschel et al., 2012). Additionally, these programs combine widespread dissemination of recommendations in German, French, and Italian; basic information on best practice; and practical implementation tools within a national campaign, together with a comprehensive 2-year Breakthrough Collaborative involving 7–10 selected hospitals. The FHV has used the model as a methodology for shared learning and improvement between its legally autonomous member hospitals.

These entities have each launched three collaboratives. This chapter, however, focuses on each entity's initial collaborative, as these have been completed and assessed. For the SPSF, this was the safe surgery collaborative; and for the FHV, it was a collaborative on preventing adverse drug events. Table 36.1 shows the key success factors and the weaknesses and barriers of these two collaboratives. The next sections provide an overview of the programs and their most salient results. More detailed information is available in previous publications (Mascherek et al., 2016; Staines et al., 2015).

National Safe Surgery Program of the Swiss Patient Safety Foundation

The goal of the Safe Surgery Program, conducted between 2012 and 2015, was systematic implementation of the surgical checklist, improving the quality of implementation, the safety climate, and team communication. The key elements of the implementation package involved improving leadership, building multi-professional project teams, developing local champions, adapting the checklist by defining the items and the exact procedure, reflecting/redefining the upstream processes, and coordinating practical training in standardized use of the checklist. In the 2 years of the Breakthrough Collaborative, four workshops were held and data were collected twice. The collaborative's design was based on two axes, including a national campaign, and the Breakthrough Collaborative (Figure 36.1).

The participating hospitals showed significant improvement (standardized difference with Cohen's d) in frequency (1.2), satisfaction with use (0.3),

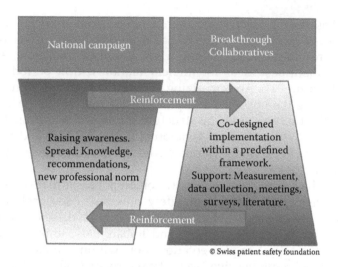

© Swiss patient safety foundation

FIGURE 36.1
Biaxial design of the national programs.

subjective knowledge (0.8), and perception of checklist use as a norm (0.3) (Mascherek et al., 2016). Users also found the checklist more familiar (0.6) and easier to use (0.4). The safety climate and team communication improved significantly, but the size of the improvement remains small and can only be interpreted within a cluster of results. The national survey of surgical professionals in 2015 found that subjective knowledge and regarding checklist use as the norm had improved over 2012, and 90% indicated that more was done for patient safety than in the previous year.

Adverse Drug Event Prevention Collaborative from the Hospital Federation of Vaud

The adverse drug event (ADE) collaborative took place over 2011 and 2012, with post-implementation measurement for 12 months in five hospitals. It aimed to reduce drug events, and featured seven one-day workshops during implementation and three more post-implementation to facilitate cross-learning between professions and hospitals, and to provide input from experts (Figure 36.2).

Pill box discrepancies were reduced from 6.5% ($n = 4846$ doses) in 2011 to 4.4% ($n = 7355$) in 2012 ($P < 0.001$) to 3.0% for the first 3 months of 2013 ($n = 2251$) ($P = 0.004$). The rate of ADEs/1000 doses decreased across time (1.8 in 2010, 1.1 in 2011, and 0.6 in 2012/13 [$P = 0.008$ for 2010–2011, and $P < 0.001$ for 2011–2012/2013]) (for further discussion of these results and their limitations, see Staines et al., 2015).

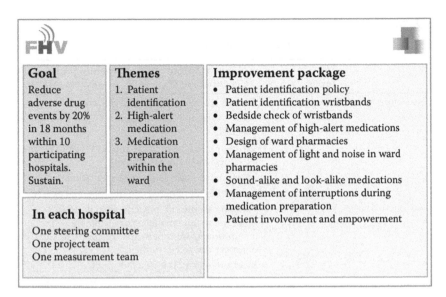

FIGURE 36.2
Key features of the ADE collaborative.

Implementation Success Factors and Transferability of the Exemplar

Despite differences in scope and subject, there are many similarities between the two programs (see Table 36.1), and the same could be said about the other collaboratives. The key contributing factors for success seem to be the capacity of the collaboratives to stimulate learning and communication across professions and hospitals, and to influence culture within the participating teams. The team members have, in most cases, learned from the experience, and have become passionate and motivated champions within their organizations. This is in line with the literature and appears to be an important factor when designing for sustainability (Øvretveit, 2002).

Both organizations are currently making the Breakthrough Collaborative model part of their core strategy. Topics of further ongoing collaboratives are: medication reconciliation and safer use of urinary catheters (for SPSF), and hand hygiene compliance and pressure ulcer prevention (for FHV). The model, which is supported by the Federal Office of Public Health, is also attracting interest from elsewhere in Switzerland. One Swiss hospital is testing it internally, with teams from different wards, to improve the reliability of handoffs.

The Breakthrough Collaborative model can be applied to any aspect of healthcare where there is evidence that best practice needs to be implemented

TABLE 36.1

Success Factors and Barriers in the Collaboratives

	Topic	Surgical Safety Checklist (SPSF)	Preventing Adverse Drug Events (FHV)
Success factors	Design	• Convincing level of scientific evidence to start from • Required signed commitments of participating hospitals • Cross-professional approach workshops to facilitate exchange and common training • Measurement alongside implementation • Availability of national and international experts • Theoretical concept, procedures, milestones, time-line requirements for participation, commitments from participating hospitals clearly defined prior to recruitment • Ready-to-use tools for the hospitals	
		• Nationwide recommendations defined before starting • Two axes with "cross-fertilization" concerning dissemination of knowledge and raising awareness • Champions on hospital and national level	• Ability to measure outcome • Monthly reporting and feedback of data
	Implementation	• Emulation between participating hospitals; learning organization • Leadership and management skills from hospital project leaders	
		• Local adaptation of checklist • Practical trainings and observations for standardized use of checklist • Executive support	• Local adaptation of interventions through improvement cycles • Visibility of some interventions such as improving light in ward pharmacies
Weaknesses and barriers	Design	• Unavailability of outcome measures and data proving effectiveness of project activities • Impossibility of including all interested hospitals in project	• Allowed participating hospital to involve only some departments • Allowed two hospitals to join 6 months after the official start. • Post implementation measurement for only 12 months
	Implementation	• Tight schedule during some phases of the project	• Resources not fully allocated by participating hospitals

or spread. The two-axis design of the safe surgery initiative, including a national campaign, contributed to the success of the national program and enabled awareness to be raised widely. Coordination of the different activities at national, state, and regional level could lead to further improvements and foster the spread of knowledge and change, as well as supporting regional improvement projects. Some of the features of these case studies depend on the ability to invest significant resources, but the core process of the collaborative model does not, and could therefore be used in low-resource environments.

Prospects for Further Success and Next Steps

There is a great need in Switzerland and worldwide for the implementation of evidence-based practice. Too often, there is a gap between best practice as described in the literature and what is reliably implemented at the bedside and within organizations. The Breakthrough Collaborative model has much to offer in closing this gap. The challenge is to overcome the classical barriers to implementing evidence-based practice, such as lack of knowledge, skepticism toward the evidence, belief that one's patients are different, want of user-friendly guidelines, lack of tools, and insufficient time for implementation. The collaborative model, as illustrated in our case studies, can help to reduce almost all of these barriers. The most important challenge is the active engagement of executive boards and the integration of patient safety improvement goals into the strategy of healthcare organizations. Additional research and project evaluation is needed to assess the applicability and the effectiveness of the model in primary care, long-term care, and for large-scale change versus local use.

To develop the collaborative model further and to boost the transferability of improvements, it is important to keep track of the implementation of improvement interventions within participating institutions, and to assess the relative contribution of all interventions. Mixed methods research should be systematically coupled to collaboratives, to understand the quantitative elements, but also the importance of the context, culture, and organizational readiness: all are important aspects of implementation science.

Conclusion

Many Swiss citizens, healthcare professionals, and politicians believe that they have the best healthcare system in the world. There is, however, no evidence that Swiss healthcare is superior to that of other high-income countries. In such an environment, improvement of care is a challenge and has lagged behind other countries.

Breakthrough Collaboratives have supplied a model that integrates awareness-raising, knowledge-sharing, fostering of cultural change, and the development of champions who have become organizational change agents. The model has had convincing results in Switzerland and is gaining momentum. However, further research is needed to measure results and to assess specific as well as system-wide contributing factors.

37

Turkey

Establishment of a National Healthcare Accreditation System

Mustafa Berktaş and İbrahim H. Kayral

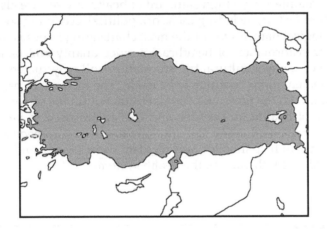

CONTENTS

Background

In today's Turkey, diversified healthcare services are being provided for a population of nearly 80 million people within more than 1500 healthcare facilities and by almost 800,000 healthcare staff. Given limited and diminishing resources, programs will need to be critically transformed to increase the efficiency of the administration of such large-scale healthcare services. In 2003, the Republic of Turkey's Ministry of Health (MoH) declared a new Health Transformation Program (Ministry of Health [Turkey], 2003). In addition to principles of human centrism, sustainability, participation, and competition, one of the main principles of the program is continuous quality improvement in healthcare. "Quality and accreditation for qualified and effective health services" is an essential component of the program.

At a macro level, government commitment is needed to maintain the quality of healthcare services. MoH has enacted multiple legislative regulations to improve patient safety and satisfaction, helping to ensure health quality and patient safety on a national basis. Efforts have been made to minimize a number of risks, such as those associated with severe malpractice problems, surgical errors, and so on.

However, maintaining a high standard of healthcare service also depends on many other factors, including those of a political, economic, sociocultural, and technological nature. One of the most challenging issues is the need for an overall transformation of healthcare service quality and patient safety. However, such a major cultural transformation will only succeed if the necessary implementations continue to be made. The increase in patient expectations, along with the pressure of competition within the sector, means that both quality of healthcare services and cost issues need to be considered simultaneously (Kayral, 2014). The development of a comprehensive accreditation system will help monitor and regulate these factors, and thus ensure the continued strengthening of the health system.

Details of the Turkish Success Story

Many macro policies have been implemented in Turkey's health sector over the last 2 decades, but there is still much potential for further structural transformation. Each policy can bring important changes and innovative modifications to the sector. In this context, the most important challenge we face today is to develop an accreditation system on a national basis, which is to be built according to principles of the International Society for Quality in Healthcare (ISQua) for generating quality service and creating a culture of patient safety. This system should conform to international standards, and as such will require major transformations at both micro and macro levels, incorporating changes both practical and theoretical. The development of such infrastructure changes in response to quality, and accreditation concerns within the health sector will prove beneficial to all tributaries of the system.

There are 866 public, 556 private, and 69 university hospitals in Turkey. Total beds number 206,836, and total operating rooms number 5682. Under this structure, 644 million patient admissions occurred during 2014. According to the Organisation for Economic Co-operation and Development's (OECD, 2015b) health data, the average of doctor admissions is above the OECD average. At any one time, an average of 70% of hospital beds are occupied. Health staff consists of 760,000 employees, 135,000 of whom are medical doctors. Maintaining qualified healthcare services on such a large scale requires systematic efforts to ensure the success of the whole system (Ministry of Health [Turkey], 2015c).

Improvements to the Turkish healthcare system began with the issuing of 100 quality standards by the MoH in 2005 (Ministry of Health [Turkey], 2011). Over the following years, the standards have undergone modifications in both quantity and extent, increasing to 150 in 2007, 354 in 2008, 388 in 2009, and to 621 standards with the final revision in 2011. The common point of all the issued standard sets was to develop and maintain a quality culture at a basic level in all healthcare facilities, and to ensure systematic improvement. It is now mandatory to implement these standards in every hospital within the borders of the country.

These efforts were designed to produce a high level of quality within healthcare institutions. As a result of these improvements, healthcare is now designed in accordance with the national accreditation system and, since 2012, conforms with international guidelines. Since 2013, a series of studies have taken place, culminating in the issuing of ISQua-endorsed Standards of Accreditation in Health–Hospital by MoH. Some hospitals, accredited by ISQua since 2014, have also established ISQua-accredited Surveyor Training Programs. Between 2014 and 2016, a number of other accreditation initiatives were also launched; these include setting standards for dental health, dialysis, and medical laboratories (Ministry of Health [Turkey], 2015a).

Details of the Impact of the National Accreditation System

Initiatives involving more than 1500 hospitals have been created since 2012, and all are important to the continuing improvement and patient-safety culture in the country. In addition, they have ensured that Turkey has achieved ISQua accreditation and alignment with international standards. Predetermined quality targets that simultaneously support Turkish requirements and adhere to ISQua principles have broadened the extent and qualification of these standards. Surveyor Training Programs have provided a background for the MoH to train surveyors who can assess performance against standards and to prepare systematic assessments according to internationally valid benchmarks.

These measures, which have been instituted across the whole health system, have a dual purpose. The first objective of these initiatives is to improve the quality culture in healthcare by involving all 760,000 healthcare staff. The MoH has conducted 18 symposiums in different Turkish cities in order to facilitate the creation of a safety culture. In order to support a scientific approach and encourage further discussion in this field, five congress meetings have been conducted, and the initiative has published 30 books and eight peer-reviewed journal articles. As recently as 2014, 1200 healthcare facilities have been evaluated according to healthcare quality standards (Ministry of Health [Turkey], 2015b).

The second objective is to ensure that the Turkish healthcare system conforms to international standards. In order to achieve this, healthcare facilities involved in quality system implementation have been encouraged to create their own solutions and promote innovation. This includes educating and involving staff in the development of the accreditation standards. Thus far, improvements have been accomplished in accordance with international and national studies, which have been conducted in conjunction with the World Health Organization (WHO) and with the imprimatur of ISQua.

In addition, legally binding regulations, crucial to the legislative infrastructure of the national accreditation system, have been prepared and implemented. Thus, Turkey's Institute for Quality and Accreditation in Healthcare has been established to support healthcare accreditation in Turkey. The first accreditation assessments are scheduled to begin 2017. In accordance with the goals of the scientific boards that comprise the institute, the main objective is to provide guidance and support for quality and accreditation studies in a range of healthcare services (Müezzinoğlu, 2014).

Implementation: Transferability of the Exemplar

Besides the accreditation system, which has been established for all healthcare services in Turkey, additional accreditation and regulatory systems are being created within the overarching initiatives of the Health Transformation Program. These include systems of accreditation for undergraduate and graduate medical training, provision of nursing care, and clinic-based national accreditation systems. The regulation of medical tourism along with related healthcare facilities for medical tourism is also being considered.

Turkey has close religious and cultural ties with much of the Muslim world, including Northern Cyprus, Macedonia, Kosovo, and Azerbaijan. Collaboration with countries such as Kazakhstan, Kirghizstan, Turkmenistan, Ukraine, and Moldova, are also possible, as Turkish is spoken in these countries. Indonesia, Kuwait, Saudi Arabia, Oman, Lebanon, and many other Muslim countries are also potential partners, and it is likely that various cooperative studies will be possible. Developments, protocols, and advances can be shared, and joint investments made. If these countries are linked more closely, the transfer of accreditation system designs and experience can be made across these different countries.

Prospects for Further Success and Next Steps

The Turkish national accreditation system for healthcare services plans to be fully in action in 2017. It is expected to begin with the assessment of hospitals around the country, with the aim of achieving accreditation by the Turkish Institute for Quality and Accreditation from that year. For that purpose, the institute, whose legal and structural formations have now been finalized, is expected to accelerate the accreditation of hospitals throughout Turkey. Additionally, the institute also aims to apply for ISQua organizational accreditation. In support of this, a web-based measurement and evaluation system is being established to monitor the outcomes of the accreditation system on a regular and objective basis, and to foresee and implement all necessary improvements.

The accreditation system is aiming to be an international benchmark for excellence. It will support the development of a safety culture for Turkey, with the potential for transfer of these benefits to the countries mentioned above. Clearly, this national system needs to be supported by regional cooperation and innovative research. Increasing patient-oriented implementation activities and focusing on the sharing of know-how and good practice will accompany the use of health technologies in the most effective ways possible.

Conclusion

The Turkish MoH has declared the components of the Health Transformation Program as a core initiative in support of "the continuous quality improvement in healthcare" principle. When all the studies and work underpinning the program are taken together with WHO involvement and other systematic efforts by member countries of ISQua, it is clear that the Turkish reforms are important not only in the national context, but that they also have international ramifications. In this regard, establishing Turkey's Institute for Quality and Accreditation in Healthcare and the underlying studies relating to its development, represents a huge step which is designed to involve over 1500 hospital administrations and all healthcare staff in Turkey. The overarching goal is to improve patient satisfaction, productivity, and efficiency, and create a strong platform of qualified staff providing better healthcare services for patients.

38

Wales

Implementing Shared Decision-Making in Practice: Demonstrating Strategic Improvement

Adrian Edwards

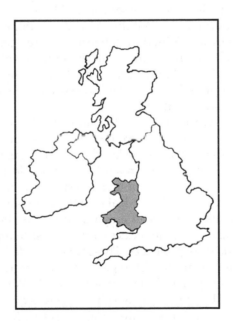

CONTENTS

Background

The Welsh National Health System (NHS) is a publicly funded health system, modeled on the English NHS, and servicing a population of around 3 million people. Under the responsibility of the devolved Welsh government, health services are delivered through seven health (delivery) boards and an additional three strategic organizations.

In recent years, the Welsh NHS has been the subject of bitter partisan wrangling in the United Kingdom, with Tory Prime Minister David Cameron claiming that problems in the Welsh system—in particular, longer waiting times for treatment—were due to the Welsh Labour government's mismanagement. Beyond the oversimplifications of party politics, however, these problems are more likely to be a consequence of Wales' unique demographic profile: the Welsh population contains a greater number of elderly people than the rest of the United Kingdom (almost 20% are aged 65 or over, while the UK average is 17%), with commensurately higher levels of chronic illness (Welsh Government, 2015; World Bank, n.d.). Many people live in relatively isolated rural and deprived regions, and access to care is more complex and expensive than in more populated areas.

Wales has struggled with cuts in funding under the UK government's austerity measures, which have amounted to an 8% budget decrease since 2010. Health spending in Wales has fallen over the last decade, and seems set to continue to fall: according to recent projections made by the Nuffield Trust, the 2015–2016 Welsh NHS budget will be 3.6% lower (in real terms) than in 2010–2011 (Roberts and Charlesworth, 2014). In order to deal with these budgetary constraints, the Welsh health system has put greater emphasis on prevention, social care, and public health, looking for ways to reduce costs while still improving healthcare outcomes and healthcare experiences. These have included a number of public health campaigns, including the Change 4 Life campaign, which promotes a healthy and active lifestyle, and the Choosing Wisely Wales campaign, modeled on the successful U.S. program, which encourages doctors to avoid unnecessary tests, treatments, and procedures (Malhotra et al., 2015). Such procedures are not only costly, but in some cases, can be actively harmful (McCaffery et al., 2016). Wales has also established an opt-out system for organ donation—which is expected to increase organ availability by 25% (Welsh Government, n.d.).

Summary of Current Efforts to Enhance Care

The Minister for Health and Social Care in Wales, Professor Mark Drakeford, called 2014 the "Year of prudent healthcare." He described prudent healthcare as "healthcare that fits the needs and circumstances of patients and actively avoids wasteful care that is not to the patient's benefit" (Drakeford, 2014). The core principles of such an approach require that any service or individual providing a service should

- Achieve health and well-being, with the public, patients, and professionals as equal partners through co-production.
- Care for those with the greatest health need first, making the most effective use of all skills and resources.
- Do only what is needed, no more, no less; and do no harm.
- Reduce inappropriate variation using evidence-based practices consistently and transparently (Welsh Government, 2016).

Prudent healthcare aims to create and embed a patient-centered system, with patients receiving the most appropriate and agreed treatments. This also reflects the contribution individuals can make to their own health and well-being. Since the prudent healthcare agenda was introduced in 2014, the NHS in Wales is now shifting from engaging in discussions about what prudent healthcare means, to embedding the principles into everyday practice (Welsh Government, 2016).

The national improvement program, 1000 Lives Improvement, is one such practical application of prudent healthcare principles. First introduced from 2008–2010, the program was developed to help organizations and individuals deliver the highest quality and safest healthcare for the people of Wales. Through engagement with NHS boards and strategic organizations across Wales, the 1000 Lives program sought to save an additional 1000 lives and prevent 50,000 episodes of harm.

Following the success of the initial campaign, the program was expanded into 1000 Lives Plus in 2010, with all seven health boards in Wales now working to extend the initiative's quality improvement methodology into new areas, thereby making a visible and tangible impact on services for patients and the public.

Our story will detail the progress made in addressing the challenges of improving patient-centered care, a particularly fraught area—through the process of shared decision-making. This process was promoted, disseminated, and embedded through a collaborative effort between the 1000 Lives initiative and the support of a regional health board. This provides an example of prudent healthcare in practice, as well as illustrating the ways in which culture and structure may impact on strategic change.

Details of the Identified Success Story

Shared decision-making is "a process in which clinicians and patients work together to select tests, treatments, management, or support packages, based on clinical evidence and the patient's informed preferences. It involves the provision of evidence-based information about options and possible outcomes, together with decision support counseling and a system for recording and implementing patients' informed preferences" (Coulter and Collins, 2011, vii). When decision-making is shared between healthcare professionals and patients, decision quality and patient satisfaction are improved and, in some cases, result in more cost-effective care.

Since 2010, Cardiff University, in partnership with an equivalent implementation project in Newcastle upon Tyne, England, has been undertaking a program of work on the translation of earlier research on shared decision-making into routine practice (The MAGIC program—Making Good Decisions in Collaboration, funded by the Health Foundation) (Lloyd et al., 2013; The Health Foundation, n.d.). In Phase 1 (2010–2012), implementation efforts were led by university researchers and focused on specific teams (breast cancer, ENT, primary care practices). The MAGIC program fostered shared decision-making by initiating a range of interventions, including providing training workshops; facilitating development of brief decision support tools, such as Option Grids (see www.optiongrid.org); initiating a patient activation campaign (Ask 3 Questions); gathering feedback using decision quality measures; providing clinical leads meetings, learning events, and feedback sessions; and obtaining executive board-level support.

Phase 2 (2013–2014) was led by the health board itself, rolling out the training and other program elements to 10 clinical teams, including pharmacy, with input across the health board. A further research phase—Phase 3 (2015–2016)—has examined where, when, why and, how shared decision-making works best in selected teams, such as breast cancer and renal cancer, where culture and experience are supportive to making it happen routinely.

Following these translational implementation projects, 1000 Lives Plus has been seeking to transfer this learning to other areas and health boards. For example, a generic and inter-professional training program in shared decision-making has been developed and provided for other South Wales districts, with national learning events and local training workshops.

The initiative has had considerable impact on patient care and experience, with work currently being undertaken to improve the management of referrals to orthopedics in the Aneurin Bevan University Health Board, Gwent. In the usual care setting, this service is characterized by high demand and resource-pressured environments, with long waiting times for both consultations and surgery, and doubts about whether the most appropriate treatment is typically provided to the most appropriate patients. The service has been substantially redesigned, and now features a "surgical interface clinic" in which physiotherapists or clinical nurse specialists see patients referred with osteoarthritis of the knee. Using shared decision-making principles and decision aids, coaching, and peer support from other patients in similar situations, patients are made aware of and can access a range of conservative treatment options (physiotherapy, pain relief, weight loss services, joint injections) to address their priorities, which also enables the surgical services to provide for patients with the greatest need.

Details of the Impact of the Success Story

We believe the Shared Decision Making Project, in the context of prudent healthcare policies and principles, has been successful for several reasons. In line with the principles of the Triple Aim framework, it addresses key needs: resource efficiency, patient experience, and healthcare choices that are potentially transferable to the entire population. The strategy has been disseminated across Wales, and is multidisciplinary and based on inter-professional learning where possible.

It is also particularly timely, as patient involvement, autonomy, and shared decision-making are becoming the legislated "standard of care" in the NHS. In this way, it is becoming normalized into practice, and patient expectations of the process of care to achieve the best health outcomes are also raised.

There is considerable interest in looking for new or wider contexts in which the same model of translation, transfer, and impact could be achieved. One example of a successful translation can be found in the establishment of chronic pain clinics in Pembrokeshire.

Implementation: Transferability of the Exemplar

From the experience gained to date, and the interest in further transfer and impact for patients and public, there seems every prospect of further development of the Shared Decision Making Project in Wales' NHS. Legislation, policy support, enthusiasm from national and regional bodies, and evidence of successful implementation and transfer all support this.

Our experience does indicate that there is a continuing need to maintain these system-wide and local improvements—fatigue can and does set in, even in this favorable environment, and staff turnover means that new team members may require support. Continuing training provision, signposting of decision support resources, promotion of patient activation, board- and management-level interventions all require constant reinvigoration and continued availability.

However, we believe this exemplar case study offers insight and cause for optimism. We believe it should be easily transferrable to other countries, especially those with publicly funded systems, and particularly in countries where healthcare systems are smaller, potentially more agile, and readily able to adopt change. The lessons are still likely to be relevant to all countries and types of systems: it is possible to start small, and grow upward and outward to achieve successful implementation of system-wide improvements that address patient-centered and prudent healthcare.

Prospects for Further Success and Next Steps

The imperatives behind prudent healthcare will endure as pressures on constrained healthcare budgets and the healthcare needs of a growing aged population become increasingly the norm. Framing the principles of prudent healthcare as a way to address these issues provides support for a range of improvement measures in the NHS in Wales. These measures have government- and policy-level support, organizational and managerial priority, and buy-in from both the public and clinicians at the front-line of healthcare delivery. This is an essential context for and enabler of further change and improvement. Evidence of change and benefits will be the next prerequisite, and should be demonstrated by the continued dissemination of the practices promoted in Choosing Wisely Wales and the Shared Decision Making Project, among others, to reinforce the drive to continual improvement and healthcare quality.

Part IV

Eastern Mediterranean

Samir Al-Adawi

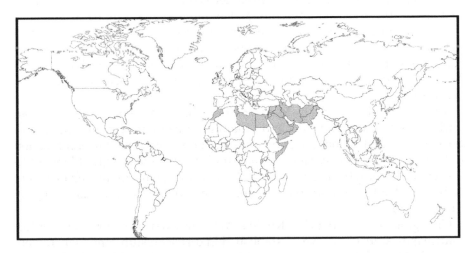

We turn now to our penultimate section. The World Health Organization's (WHO) region of Eastern Mediterranean consists of 21 countries that extend from Afghanistan in the north, to Djibouti in the south, and Morocco in the west. The majority of people living across the Eastern Mediterranean are Muslims, but with significant minorities subscribing to other religious denominations. Considered by many to be the cradle of civilization, the region has a rich and diverse sociocultural heritage.

Like the beautiful and distinctive mosaics for which it is famous, this region has widely contrasting demographics, and varying levels of social, political, and economic stability. Some countries of the region still endure sociopolitical instability, socioeconomic insecurity, factionalism, and population displacement. Despite such challenges, there are many successful healthcare initiatives that should be acknowledged and applauded. The stories presented in this compendium originate from 12 of the 21 countries included in WHO's Eastern Mediterranean region.

Despite decades-long social and political unrest, Afghanistan has leaped forward in meeting the healthcare needs of its citizens. Omarzaman Sayedi, Edward Chappy, Lauren Archer, and Nafiullah Pirzad discuss how Afghanistan has launched mechanisms to audit its healthcare services. Thus, the standard of healthcare services has improved despite all the difficulties the country has been experiencing.

Salma Jaouni Araj and Edward Chappy write of another successful initiative forged under challenging circumstances. Jordan's success story began with the instigation of the Health Care Accreditation Council (HCAC). The ultimate quest of HCAC has been to nurture quality and safety standards for healthcare facilities. Due to this initiative, the majority of healthcare institutions in Jordan have been subject to accreditation audits and are now aligned with international best practice.

Iran has been operating with three-tier healthcare (public-governmental, private sector, and non-governmental organizations). Empirical evidence ostensibly suggests that such a system fails to provide for the healthcare needs of those who are most economically vulnerable. Under the banner of reform initiatives known as the Health Transformation Plan, Ali Mohammad Mosadeghrad discusses how Iran reduced accelerating health expenditure with stunning success.

Meanwhile, Nasser Yassin, Maysa Baroud, Reem Talhouk, Sandra Mesmar, and Sara Kaddoura from Lebanon highlight imaginative social media initiatives to solicit blood donations via the non-governmental organization (NGO) known as *Donner Sang Compter*, under the motto "to give blood without expecting anything in return." As a result, many more Lebanese are willing and able to donate blood—improving what was previously a highly uncertain process.

Changing topic and pace, Khaled Al-Surimi narrates how key performance indicators (KPIs) were established in district health centers in Yemen. An individual dubbed as *Sadiq*, or friend, was employed to liaise between the health authority and district health centers. Al-Surimi noted adherence to KPIs was high; and this constituted a success story not just for Yemen, but for other regions grappling with the implementation of KPIs.

Other countries of the Arabian Peninsula that are a part of WHO's Eastern Mediterranean region, namely Saudi Arabia, Kuwait, the United Arab Emirates (UAE), Qatar, Bahrain, and Oman, belong to a political and economic entity known as the Gulf Cooperation Council (GCC). GCC countries have relatively small populations and high income, due to their successful exploitation of hydrocarbon in recent decades. Despite its affluence, the GCC lacks some important success markers in healthcare delivery. However, the GCC's unified procurement system for pharmaceuticals and medical supplies, has been a great success. As the executive board of the Health Ministers' Council for Cooperation Council States reports, unified procurement has reduced the cost of healthcare as well as laying groundwork for unified cross-border pharmaceutical policies.

Some individual GCC countries have also embarked on worthy and successful initiatives. In the case of the UAE, Subashnie Devkaran discusses how the once chaotic health insurance policy arrangements were transformed by implementing a single payment system. Now the country has mandatory insurance for all, something many other countries would like to replicate.

Across in Qatar, David Vaughan, Mylai Guerrero, Yousef Al Maslamani, and Charles Pain focus on the successful implementation of an "early warning system" (EWS), designed to detect the severity of patients presenting with complaints, which, in turn, determines the course of action to be taken. The implementation of the EWS resulted in 40% reduction of adverse medical outcomes. Such an achievement constitutes a success story for Qatar, and also paves the way for another version of this system from the case presented in Australia in Section V.

Ahmed Al-Mandhari, Abdullah Al-Raqadi, and Badar Awladthani from Oman narrate how a computerized medical database system for all patients has created a network of primary, secondary, and tertiary healthcare facilities—a system that is the envy of many. This network allows doctors to review all patient visits to clinics and hospitals in Oman, send electronic referrals, and view various prescriptions. This provides an efficient and reliable repository of patient histories and assists with future referral plans.

Finally, Syed Shahabuddin and Usman Iqbal from Pakistan explain how a cardiac surgery database was developed for the first time at the Agha Khan hospital. Such a database can be used as a model to study other diseases and assess the allocation of resources. Shahbuddin and Iqbal predict that this sort of database, if adopted elsewhere, will improve the efficiency of the healthcare system overall.

39

Afghanistan

Improving Afghanistan's Hospital Services: Implementation of Minimum Required Standards

Omarzaman Sayedi, Edward Chappy, Lauren Archer, and Nafiullah Pirzad

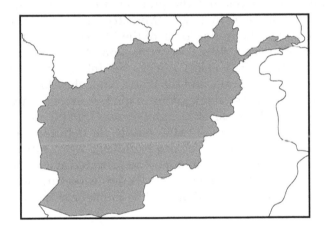

CONTENTS

Background

The Islamic Republic of Afghanistan gained independence from Britain in 1919 and enjoyed relative stability until 1973. Since then, the country has experienced protracted military conflict and civil wars, resulting in the devastation of the health system and its infrastructure. The health workforce is insufficient due to skilled healthcare workers leaving the country, and few have been trained over the last several decades. While improvements have been made, Afghanistan's health indicators remain some of the poorest in the world (see Table 39.1).

In 2011, the Ministry of Public Health (MoPH) declared its mission "to improve the health of the people of Afghanistan through the provision of quality healthcare services and the promotion of healthy lifestyles in an equitable and sustainable manner" (Ministry of Public Health [MoPH] [Afghanistan], 2015). The initial focus of the MoPH was on reconstruction and rapid expansion of services. Also, with support from international partners, including the United States Agency for International Development (USAID), the European Union, and the World Bank, the MoPH implemented several key health sector strategies. One of the key strategies was the development of the Basic Package of Health Services (BPHS) and the Essential Package of Hospital Services (EPHS), which are delivered to population mainly through contracting out to nongovernment organizations. The BPHS delineated the types of services that must be provided at each type of public healthcare facility. The EPHS focused on the infrastructure of hospitals and stated the type of service areas that must be available at all public hospitals (see Table 39.2).

TABLE 39.1

Change in Key Health Indicators

Indicator	Values	Years
Maternal mortality ratio (per 100,000 live births)	1600–327	2002; 2010
Under-five mortality rate (per 1000 live births)	191–97	2006; 2010)
Infant mortality rate (per 1000 live births)	129–77	2006; 2010
Skilled birth attendance (%)	18.9–40	2006; 2011/12
Contraceptive prevalence rate (%)	10–13.8	2006; 2011/12
Total fertility rate	7.2–5.1	2008; 2010

Source: Afghan Public Health Institute, Ministry of Public Health [MoPH], et al. (2011). Afghanistan mortality survey 2010. Calverton, MD; Central Statistics Organization. (2014). National risk and vulnerability assessment, 2011–12. Afghan living conditions survey. Kabul, Afghanistan; Johns Hopkins University. (2008). Afghanistan health survey 2006: Estimates of priority health indicators for rural Afghanistan. Baltimore, MD; UNICEF. (2008). State of the world's children. Retrieved from http://www.unicef.org/sowc08/docs/sowc08_table_8.pdf.

TABLE 39.2

Basic Package of Health Services (BPHS) and Essential Package of Hospital Services (EPHS)

The seven elements of the BPHS	EPHS (provincial hospitals)
1. Maternal	1. Inpatient services
2. Child health and immunization	• General surgical services (operating theater, anesthesia, recovery room services, and sterilization services)
3. Public nutrition	• General obstetrics and gynecology services • General pediatric services
4. Communicable disease treatment and control	2. Emergency department open and staffed 24 hours
5. Mental health	3. Outpatient services (including vaccinations, basic ear-nose-throat, mental health, eye care and dental services)
6. Disability services	4. Hospital pharmacy
7. Regular supply of essential drugs	5. Physiotherapy services
	6. Basic laboratory, blood transfusion services, and blood bank
	7. Basic x-ray and ultrasound services

In 2009, healthcare users in Afghanistan perceived the quality of services as "low." Only 24% and 21% of private and public clients, respectively, rated the quality of private services as "positive," with the remainder rating them as "adequate" or "negative" (Global Health Technical Assistance Project, 2009). Additionally, there is a lack of quality essential secondary and tertiary care, which has led to approximately US$285 million being spent annually by Afghans seeking care abroad (MoPH [Afghanistan], 2013). In light of these challenges, the MoPH has begun to formally address the need for quality secondary and tertiary care services in both the public and private health sectors.

The MoPH undertook several initiatives to reform public and private hospitals with the goal of improving the efficiency and quality of services. These initiatives included implementing standards-based management and recognition systems; establishing patient safety initiatives; and implementing results-based financing schemes. In 2011, the MoPH developed and adopted the National Strategy for Improving Quality in Healthcare to address quality improvement more systematically. An integral part of the strategy was the undertaking of the MoPH-led hospital autonomy plan at 14 national hospitals in Kabul to improve the quality of services. In 2013, the MoPH commenced a harmonization process to align existing quality improvement approaches, which were being implemented by various partners, into a single national healthcare approach. The initiatives laid the groundwork to further expand quality improvement initiatives in the health sector.

Private Health Sector Growth and Government Stewardship

With the adoption of a new constitution in 2004, Afghanistan became a market economy, allowing the private sector to play a greater role in the development of the country, including the health sector. Due to these changes, Afghanistan's health system began to transition from being heavily public sector focused to a mixed health system with more integration of the private sector. Since 2003, the contribution of the private health sector has increased significantly. In 2011/2012, it was estimated that household out-of-pocket health expenditures represented 73% of total health expenditures, of which 62% was spent at private health facilities (Afghan Public Health Institute, MoPH [Afghanistan] et al., 2011). The private health sector also employs thousands of Afghans, which has reduced unemployment and contributed to the economic growth of the country. Figure 39.1 shows the growth of private hospitals since 2003 (Cross et al., 2017).

One of the reasons for the rapid growth of private healthcare facilities was a lack of regulatory policies and procedures, including licensure requirements and quality standards. Due to the rapid expansion of the private health sector after 2002, and the lack of corresponding capacity of the MoPH for effective regulation and monitoring, anecdotal evidence suggested that the private health sector was prioritizing quantity of services at the expense of quality (MoPH [Afghanistan], 2009). In addition, the relationship between the public and private sectors was characterized by a lack of communication and transparency. This resulted in mutual mistrust, which was exacerbated

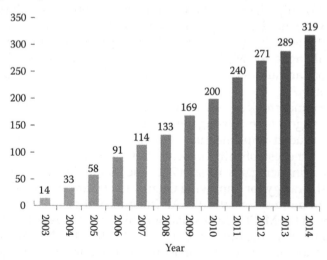

FIGURE 39.1

Number of private hospitals licensed by the Ministry of Public Health, 2003–2014. (From Afghanistan Ministry of Public Health Licensing Department; HPP staff, oral communication, and licensing department files, 2014.)

by the MoPH conducting unilateral inspections with no standardized assessment guidelines.

In 2009, as a response to the rapid growth of the private health sector, the MoPH established the Directorate of Private Sector Coordination (DPSC) and began to identify priorities for improving oversight of the private health sector. Additionally, the MoPH developed the National Policy for the Private Health Sector, along with its strategic plan. The policy outlined the vision, mission, and policy directions for the effective engagement of the private health sector in the delivery of health services. In 2012, the government enacted a regulation that mandated minimum standards of quality for private health centers, paving the way for the development of the minimum required standards (MRS).

Ensuring Patients' Safety at Private Health Facilities: MRS

The growth of the private health sector highlighted the need for assessing and regulating quality in private health facilities. From 2011 to 2013, the MoPH collaborated with the Afghan Private Hospital Association (APHA) to develop the MRS for private hospitals. The intent was to standardize the regulation of quality in private hospitals, improve the culture of quality within the private health sector, and ensure patient safety. The MoPH and the APHA developed and implemented MRS guidelines and an associated MRS checklist to assess quality standards at private hospitals.

The MRS checklist is a user-friendly, Excel-based tool, with five domains, 193 standards, and a total weighted score of 273.5. The objectives of the MRS guidelines and checklist are to: (1) improve the culture of quality and raise standards at private hospitals; (2) increase objectivity in the assessment of private hospitals; and (3) prepare private hospitals for the implementation of national healthcare accreditation. An implementation plan was developed for the MRS, which among other requirements, mandated joint monitoring by the MoPH and the APHA. The joint monitoring made the process more transparent and enhanced open communication between the MoPH and private facilities. The MRS checklist is now a formalized tool used by the MoPH for monitoring private hospitals and is also a self-regulatory tool used by APHA with the goal of improving basic standards of healthcare services.

During 2014 and 2015, APHA conducted baseline assessments of 41 hospitals in Kabul. The MRS baseline scores ranged from 64.3 to 98.3 out of 100 points, with a mean score of 79.1. Facilities with scores greater than 80 met the MoPH's minimum standards. Follow-up assessments of hospitals who had failed to achieve minimum scores were conducted 6 months later and showed an average of an 8 point increase on the MRS checklist. These results demonstrated the heuristic value of the MRS checklist and its effectiveness

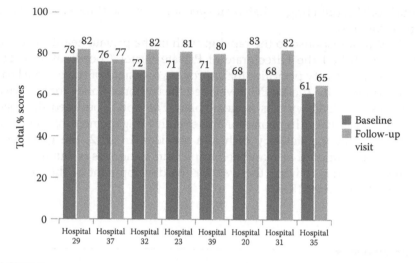

FIGURE 39.2
Distribution of MRS scores among hospitals that conducted baseline and follow-up assessments. (From Sears, K. et al. (2015). *The Impact of Private Health Sector Policy on Health Systems and Outcomes.* Washington, DC, Futures Group, Health Policy Project.)

as a tool for monitoring healthcare services in Afghanistan (see Figure 39.2). The use of the MRS checklist also improved transparency and increased trust between the public and private sectors, which increased the potential for the development of a comprehensive quality improvement system for private hospitals in Afghanistan.

Parameters for the Success of the MRS Experience

The success of the MRS system stems directly from collaboration between the MoPH and APHA. The collaborative approach began with the appointment of a joint taskforce of public and private sector representatives tasked with developing the MRS system and processes. The taskforce met on a regular basis over the course of 2 years to finalize a draft, pilot the system in several hospitals, and sponsor a workshop for all private hospitals to share lessons learned. In 2013, the final MRS guidelines and tools for inspection were mutually agreed upon by the public and private sectors and approved by the MoPH. Subsequent to the approval of the MRS, the APHA conducted orientation sessions for 70 of its member hospitals. These sessions oriented private hospital staff on the contents of the standards and the process for formal inspection by the MoPH and APHA.

Lessons Learned for Other Developing Countries

The private health sector, including private hospitals, plays a major role in the delivery of the health services in many developing countries. Afghanistan's experience with the development of the MRS for private hospitals demonstrates that collaboration between the public and private sectors can lead to constructive outcomes for improving basic standards in private hospitals.

Linking the MRS to other MoPH processes, such as facility inspection licensing and sanctioning procedures, will further institutionalize the approach. Most importantly, systems like the MRS can improve the quality of care, which in turn can drive improved health outcomes and increased efficiency in service delivery (Leatherman et al., 2010).

Potential for Scale-Up and Sustainability

The development of the MRS guidelines and its implementation methodology is one of the first standardized, nationwide approaches taken in Afghanistan to improve quality and safety in private hospitals. A national healthcare accreditation strategy was developed in 2014 that incorporates the MRS and other standards developed by international partners to create a comprehensive quality improvement system for Afghanistan. The MRS and the other standards were separated into categories to develop a system of pre-licensing, licensing, and accreditation standards for all healthcare facilities, both public and private. The same collaborative strategy used to develop the MRS will be used to reach consensus on the development of broader quality improvement initiatives that encompass the whole health system as well as for other health system reform efforts.

Conclusion

Afghanistan's health sector has witnessed considerable growth since 2002. In addition to improved accessibility to primary healthcare services, the MoPH and its partners have made extensive efforts to benchmark and audit the quality of services in the rapidly expanding private health sector. These efforts were solidified when the MoPH and the private health sector collaboratively developed the basic tenets and scope of the MRS. Putting the MRS into practice and tracking key indicators was a major success for improving regulation of the private health sector and ensuring the provision of quality health services for the Afghan population.

40

The Gulf States (Bahrain, Kuwait, Oman, Qatar, Saudi Arabia, and the United Arab Emirates)

Unified Procurement of Pharmaceuticals and Medical Supplies for Gulf Cooperation Council Countries: A Great Success Story

The Gulf Health Council for Cooperation Council States

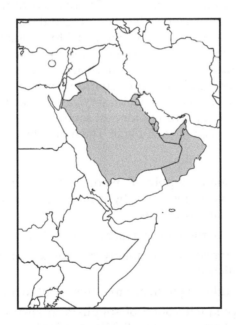

CONTENTS

Background

The group purchasing concept, which involves the ministries of health of the Gulf Cooperation Council (GCC) member countries—namely, the United Arab Emirates, Kingdom of Bahrain, Kingdom of Saudi Arabia, Sultanate of Oman, State of Qatar, and the State of Kuwait—was established in 1976, with the objective of procuring pharmaceuticals and medical supply items that were hard to obtain either because of the small quantity needed or due to their high prices.

The first tender, launched in 1978, covered 32 items awarded to nine companies with the total amount exceeding US$1 million. Prior to the establishment of the Group Purchasing Program (GPP), the GCC purchased drugs and other medical supplies from suppliers by either local and/or international tenders. Drug prices for similar products thus varied widely among the GCC states.

The core function of the GPP is pooled procurement of pharmaceuticals and medical supplies for the ministries of health of the GCC member countries. The continuous annual cost savings obtained over the 3 decades of the joint purchasing arrangement have reinforced the concept that collective procurement is an excellent cost–benefit model for economic and functional cooperation among the member countries. The experience of the GPP during 40 years of centralized tendering for pharmaceuticals and medical supplies has demonstrated that collective procurement can reduce costs and consequently enhance the efficiency of health services. Efficient pool procurement provides the greatest opportunity for cost saving (The Gulf Health Council for Cooperation Council States, 2013a,b). The main objectives and benefits of the GPP are to

- Ensure continuous supply of medicines and medical supplies, through successive deliveries, by minimizing routine administrative and financial procedures
- Ensure the use of the same drugs by all member countries
- Improve the application of quality assurance, control procedures, and bioequivalence
- Support the Gulf drug industry to achieve Gulf drug security
- Require the prequalification of suppliers to ensure compliance to good manufacturing practices (GMP) standards
- Allow other health sectors such as specialized hospitals to procure their needs through GPP (Khoja and Bawazir, 2005)

In addition to the pooled procurement of pharmaceuticals and medical supplies, GPP also provides related services, including

- Conducting training in the requirements of GMP and quality assurance standards
- Periodically updating formularies for the tendered items
- Exchanging information among member states about adverse reactions or side effects of any medication

As well as public health-sector medical centers, a number of university and specialized hospitals in Saudi Arabia also participate in the GPP. These include King Saud University Hospitals; King Abdul Aziz University Hospital; the College of Medicine in Qaseem University; King Selman Kidney Center; King Fahd Medical City; King Faisal Specialist Hospital and Research Centers in Riyadh and Jeddah; King Khalid Specialist Eye Hospital; the Medical Service Ministry of the Interior; the Security Force Hospital; National Guard Hospitals; Prince Sultan Ibn Abdul Aziz Humanitarian City; and the Medical Services, Royal Commission, in Yanbu and Jubail. Hospital and medical centers in the other GCC member countries participate in GPP tenders under the umbrella of the ministry of health in each country (Figure 40.1).

The GPP combines the purchasing power of the six GCC member countries into one regional tender. It operates a centralized restricted tendering system where only preregistered/prequalified vendors are invited to participate in a competitive process. The GPP solicits bids in US dollars to provide one standard monetary unit for easy price comparison, thus allowing GCC states to estimate drug costs without concern about currency fluctuation.

The GPP notifies the successful bidders with the final quantities requested by the participating GCC member states (MOHs) and other health sectors. Strict monitoring of suppliers by participants ensures compliance. The quality of the product is ensured through the monitoring of complaints received

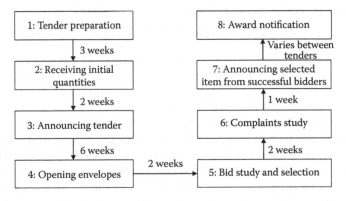

FIGURE 40.1
Mechanism and steps of GPP as outlined by the Gulf Health Council. Note there are 16 weeks from Phase 1 up to Phase 7.

from the ministries of health and other participating entities regarding recalled products or adverse drug reactions. Suppliers deliver the ordered quantity of items directly to GCC member states and other participating health sectors, who in turn reimburse the cost directly to suppliers. Suppliers are expected to execute timely delivery and to comply with the delivery schedule of each participant.

In order to participate in the pharmaceutical tenders (medicines and vaccines), the vendor must either be centrally or duly registered in the GCC member countries with reference laboratories. Participation in the medical supplies' tenders (consumables) is restricted to qualified vendors who have successfully completed prequalification requirements for GPP tenders.

A system for prequalification was developed to ensure eligibility of the new vendors who wish to participate in GPP tenders. In this process, companies that wish to do business are evaluated on the basis of factors such as their competence, discipline, organization, financial strength, and so forth. The prequalification system ensures that only skilled and experienced bidders are allowed to bid for GPP tenders. Tendering companies can therefore be confident that they will not be bidding against inexperienced bidders who may place unrealistically low bids.

To become eligible for GPP tenders, companies must demonstrate that they have the experience, technical capability, available resources, and management systems necessary to competently undertake the work. GPP has rapidly expanded its product portfolio to include the 16 tenders that appear in Table 40.1.

The GPP provides numerous benefits to the GCC member states. These include reducing the cost of procuring drugs and medical supplies through pool procurement; the certification of manufacturers that follow good manufacturing practices; the rapid processing of the tender procedures, which are finalized in 16 weeks; a reduction in labor costs through minimizing administrative and regulatory burdens on the ministries of health in the GCC member states; and ensuring continuous supply of drugs and medical supplies to all participants, all the year round, through regular and successive deliveries. In addition, the GPP helps to support the research fund for the welfare of the GCC member states by deducting 2% of each vendor's awarded quantity.

To ensure credibility, the GPP has developed a transparent tendering system. Gulf and foreign vendors who desire to participate in GPP tenders, and those who have interest, are able to obtain the required information from the official website of the executive, where tender terms and regulations, prequalification requirements, and other information is released and announced. This program utilizes the benefits of the Electronic Connectivity Program, where all aspects of this program can be monitored online. This emphasizes transparency, integrity, and justice.

The GPP enables the exchange and sharing of information among institutions, hospitals, and countries. This information may take the form of

TABLE 40.1

Total Procured Amount in 2015 (US$2,646,312,209)

		US$
1	Medicines	1,372,184,021
2	Vaccine and sera	204,253,223
3	Chemical	1,488,774
4	Insecticides	6,318,344
5	Radio-pharmaceuticals	3,772,359
6	Renal dialysis solutions	22,192,819
7	Hospital sundries	370,038,890
8	Renal dialysis supplies	55,074,761
9	Dental and mouth care supplies	44,731,229
10	Medical laboratory and blood transfusion supplies	294,425,516
11	Orthopedic and spine supplies	151,483,593
12	Rehabilitation supplies	28,807,557
13	Cardiovascular surgery supplies	91,541,124
14	*Linens and medical uniforms	**34,727,851
15	*Ophthalmic supplies	**31,355,396
16	*ENT supplies	**46,175,165

* (launched every 2 years)
** (amount in year 2014)

clinical data, prescribing data, health education programs, and so forth. This sharing of information has contributed to the development of the drug policies in GCC member states, and helped to establish a number of important initiatives, including central drug registration, bioequivalence programs, GCC drug formulary, good manufacturing practice, accreditation of quality central laboratories, along with support to the local pharmaceutical industry.

Over the years, the GPP has had a significant impact on improving the health of the citizens of the Gulf member states. This has been achieved through provision of safe and high-quality drugs. Additionally, this unified action has helped to reduce administration costs and has resulted in a more efficient utilization of the available resources, which is expected to continue to improve performance (The Gulf Health Council for Cooperation Council States, 2009).

The establishment of an electronic common technical document (eCTD), which is due to be finalized by the end of 2017, will ensure that the central drugs registration conforms to international standards (International Council for Harmonization of Technical Requirements for Pharmaceuticals for Human Use [ICH] Guidelines). All cost, insurance, and freight (CIF)-aligned prices of medications in the GCC will be included in the e-connectivity program, which will provide GCC member states and participating drug companies with access to all necessary information.

Sharing Experiences with Other Regional Pool Procurement Systems

The GCC GPP experience has proved valuable in helping to streamline comparable procurement systems in other regional centers. In 2005, a joint World Health Organization (WHO)/GCC delegation was sent to the East Caribbean Island of St. Lucia to review the Organization of Eastern Caribbean States Pharmaceutical Procurement Service (OECS PSS). The OECS PPS combines the purchasing power of nine member states (Anguilla, Antigua and Barbuda, British Virgin Islands, Dominica, Montserrat, St. Kitts and Nevis, St. Lucia, St. Vincent, and the Grenadines) into one regional buyer, and negotiates regional price contracts for pharmaceuticals and medical equipment. Like the GCC member states' GPP, the OECS PSS operates a centralized restricted tendering system and invites only prequalified suppliers to the international competitive process. The main objective of the visit was to review the OECS GPP processes, including the quality assurance system, and to share experiences and expertise regarding best practices. Specific matters under review included

- Procedures and criteria for prequalifying suppliers, including various forms (vendor and product registration documents used by GCC and PPS)
- Procedures and policies on internal and external quality control
- Document management information systems, including computerized functionalities
- Procurement cycles, including tender procedures
- The draft memorandum of understanding (MOU) between PPS and client countries

Conclusion

The GPP, which has been running for more than 4 decades, has proven to be viable and functional. The benefits provided by this program are numerous; not only have GCC member states enjoyed a decrease in the cost of healthcare, but the purchasing process has been made more efficient, drug specifications have been unified, quality assurance has been increased, information exchange has been made easier, and shared pharmaceutical policies have been developed.

41

Iran

Iran's Health Transformation Plan

Ali Mohammad Mosadeghrad

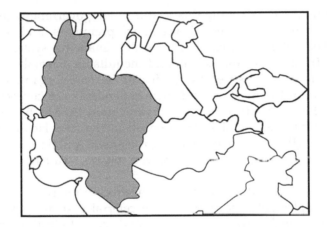

CONTENTS

Introduction

The Islamic Republic of Iran is a middle-income country with a population of about 78 million, with an annual population growth of 1.28%, and a median age of 29 years. The gross national income per capita is (PPP int.) $17,400. Seventy-two percent of the population live in urban areas (World Bank, 2016a; WHO, 2015a). The country's demographic and epidemiological profiles are in transition. Communicable diseases are well controlled;

however, the country now faces a burden of non-communicable diseases in addition to an increase in physical accidents and injuries due to the growth of urbanization and industrialization.

The Iranian healthcare system consists of public, private, and non-government organization (NGO)-funded healthcare. The Ministry of Health and Medical Education (MOHME) is responsible for policy-making, financing, planning, and controlling the health sector at the national level. At the provincial level, medical universities are responsible for providing both medical education and healthcare services. The district health network provides primary healthcare (PHC) services free of charge, and the hospital network delivers secondary and tertiary services (Mosadeghrad, 2014a).

The health system is mainly financed through government general revenues, public and private health insurance premiums, and individuals' out-of-pocket (OOP) payments. The health financing system is highly regressive, fragmented, inefficient, and inequitable. Formal workers and their dependents are insured by the Social Security Organization (SSO), and members of the military and their dependents are covered through the Armed Forces Medical Service Organization (AFMSO). The remainder of the population is eligible to enroll in the Iran Health Insurance Organization (IHIO), which covers government public sector employees, rural households, the self-employed, clerics, students, and so on. (Mosadeghrad, 2014b).

Over the last 3 decades, a number of healthcare reforms and initiatives have been implemented to enhance the referral system, increase capacity for training healthcare personnel, expand access to healthcare services, reduce inequities, and promote quality of healthcare services. Although some improvements have been achieved, the Iranian health system still faces a number of challenges when it comes to access, equity, quality, and efficiency. In order to address these challenges, a series of reforms called the Health Transformation Plan (HTP) have been implemented since May 2014 by the MOHMR, based on the fifth 5-year development plan (2011–2016) to expand access to healthcare services, reduce the catastrophic and impoverishing OOP payments, promote equity, and improve the quality of healthcare services.

Background

The HTP was mainly focused on three departments of the MOHME (curative care, health, and education). The first phase of the HTP began on May 5, 2014 at the Curative Affairs Department of the MOHME, with a view to achieving the following outcomes:

- Reducing inpatients' OOP spending in public hospitals
- Encouraging medical doctors to stay in deprived areas
- Increasing medical specialists' attendance in public hospitals
- Improving the quality of amenities in public hospitals
- Promoting the quality of medical consultations
- Promoting natural delivery
- Financial protection of patients with severe incurable (catastrophic) illnesses
- Improving the air emergency medical services

The second phase of the HTP, which began on May 22, 2014, focused on PHC and public health, and included expanding health services to suburban areas, expanding the Family Physician Program, and enhancing health literacy and self-caring (Moradi-Lakeh and Vosoogh-Moghaddam, 2015). Finally, the third phase of the HTP focused on transforming medical education through 11 service packages. The major source of the HTP funding was a raise in the MOHME budget comprising 1% the value-added tax (VAT) and 10% of freed subsidies (National Institute of Health Research [Iran] [NIHR], 2016).

Accordingly, all uninsured people were encouraged to register and participate in the IHIO. All of the MOHME affiliated hospitals (561 out of the total 878 hospitals) should provide all necessary inpatient services. Patients' OOP payments at these hospitals should be less than 10% of the total medical expenditure. The national tariff for medical services was increased in October 2014 to encourage medical consultants to work full time in public hospitals and provide high-quality services, persuade medical doctors to stay in deprived areas, and reduce informal and illegal payments.

Impact of the HTP

The HTP has had both intended and unintended consequences. The HTP has expanded healthcare coverage horizontally and vertically. Almost 11 million people—primarily informal sector workers, self-employed, unemployed, or those out of the labor force—were insured by the IHIO during the HTP implementation. Most of them were poor and exempt from any contribution. In addition, certain medicines and medical technologies and procedures were included in the insurance package. As shown in Figure 41.1, inpatients' OOP payments in public hospitals decreased significantly (NIHR, 2016; Heidarian and Vahdat, 2015; Piroozi et al., 2016).

The HTP resulted in an increase in the demand for public hospital services, mainly in the form of elective surgeries (Faridfar et al., 2016; Rezaei

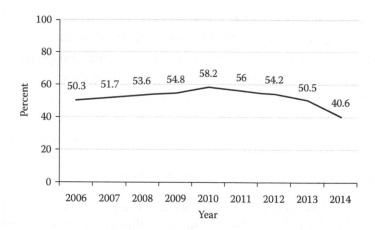

FIGURE 41.1
Patients' OOP payments. (From NIHR. (2016). Health transformation plan factsheets. Retrieved from http://nihr.tums.ac.ir)

et al., 2016). Even patients from private hospitals shifted to the public hospitals. An increase in the medical tariff was an incentive for public hospitals to admit more patients and provide sometimes unnecessary services. Consequently, public hospitals' income has increased (Sajadi and Zaboli, 2016). However, medical insurance companies were unable to reimburse hospitals and subsequently, hospitals faced difficulties in managing their daily activities.

Patient satisfaction in public hospitals has increased (Faridfar et al., 2016; Goudarzian et al., 2016). The number of complaints from public hospitals has decreased; however, complaints about private hospitals and outpatient services and nursing care in public hospitals have increased (NIHR, 2016). A study conducted in a public hospital also reported a lower patient satisfaction due to a rise in patients' numbers without increasing staff and other resources (Hashemi et al., 2015).

About 53% of medical doctors were completely satisfied with the HTP in summer 2014. In August 2014, 813 medical consultants were residents in public hospitals, mainly in deprived areas. Forty-two percent of medical doctors who worked in deprived areas stated that they would stay there if the HTP continues (NIHR, 2016). However, as Figure 41.2 indicates, physicians' satisfaction has decreased mainly because of payment issues.

Only 25% of nurses were satisfied with the HTP in autumn 2014. Dissatisfaction was due to higher workloads and inadequate payment (NIHR, 2016). Many nurses felt that the new medical tariff was in favor of medical doctors as they are paid on a fee-for-service basis.

The utilization of medical services in public hospitals has increased due to a fall in patients' OOP payments (demand side) and a rise in medical tariff (supply side). Expanding insurance coverage, reducing patients' OOP

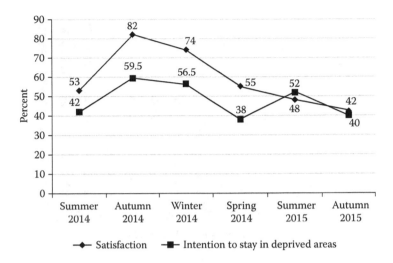

FIGURE 41.2
Physicians' satisfaction with the medical tariff and their intention to stay in deprived areas. (From NIHR. (2016). Health transformation plan factsheets. Retrieved from http://nihr.tums. ac.ir)

payments, and increasing the medical tariff increased the inflation rate in the health sector, which was higher than general inflation (Figure 41.3).

Prospects for Further Success and Next Steps

The HTP increased the demand for expensive hospital services. The utilization of hospital curative services was far higher than expected. Thus, the total healthcare cost as a percentage of GDP in Iran grew from 6.6% in 2013 to 7.5% in 2014 (Figure 41.4).

The average of general government expenditure on health as a percentage of total government expenditure was 9% between 2003 and 2013. It increased to 16.2% in 2014 (Figure 41.5). The GDP growth in Iran is predicted to be 2.5% between 2012 and 2023. The government budget balance is negative (NIHR, 2016). As government debt is increasing, continuing to increase the funding for the HTP reform may be a challenge, and it would be very difficult to lobby for an increase in the MOHME budget.

In retrospect, the HTP was implemented too quickly. For instance, it would have been better to expand insurance coverage over 5 years. An increase in patients' demands due to HTP implementation was beyond the insurance companies' resources, and their debt to the hospitals has increased.

The methods used for revenue collection, funds pooling, and purchasing healthcare services affect the health systems financing, and as a result

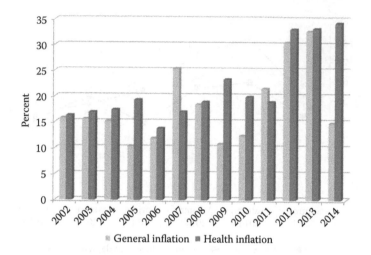

FIGURE 41.3
General and health inflation. (From NIHR. (2016). Health transformation plan factsheets. Retrieved from http://nihr.tums.ac.ir)

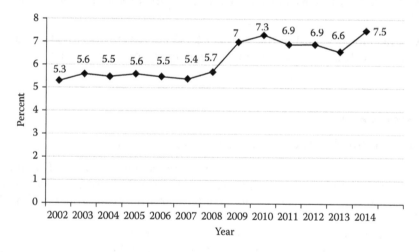

FIGURE 41.4
Health spending as a share of GDP. (From NIHR. (2016). Health transformation plan factsheets. Retrieved from http://nihr.tums.ac.ir)

should be reformed coordinately. A progressive tax should be considered by the government, as should a single-payer, national health insurance scheme. Alternative payment models, such as population-based and bundled payment models should be considered instead of the fee-for-service model.

The governance and stewardship roles of the MOHME including regulating the entire health system, monitoring and evaluating its performance, and enhancing the capacity of citizens to demand accountability should be reinforced for effective HTP implementation. Evidence should be used to guide

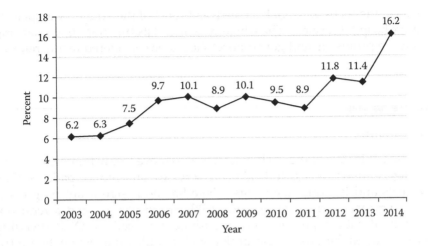

FIGURE 41.5
Government expenditure on health as a percent of total government expenditure. (From NIHR. (2016). Health transformation plan factsheets. Retrieved from http://nihr.tums.ac.ir)

health policies and orient the reform. Therefore, a comprehensive information system should be created to provide information on resource allocation, healthcare service utilization, and the outcomes.

An enhanced access to curative hospital-based services was achieved at the expense of the budget for cost-effective prevention programs. A balanced investment in both medical care and public health is needed to improve population health. The MOHME should focus more on PHC, community health services, health promotion, and disease prevention interventions instead of spending most of its budget on curative actions, such as hospitalization and medication. The HTP should highlight the importance of the establishment of an integrated health system with a comprehensive scope of health-related and clinical services.

Transferability of the HTP

The implementation of Iran's HTP provides other developing countries with some important lessons on how to design and implement a comprehensive health reform to improve the accessibility, affordability, and quality of healthcare services. Merely reforming individual components of the health system is not sufficient: a broad health transformation with balanced goals is needed to strengthen the health system. The HTP in Iran focused simultaneously on the health, curative care, and education pillars of the health system.

However, the focus was not balanced, and most of the budget was spent on curative hospital services. The whole system and its functions (i.e., financing, healthcare provision, and governance) should be considered in any reform.

Conclusion

The main objective of the HTP in Iran was to move toward universal health coverage, enhance access to healthcare services, and reduce patients' OOP payments and informal payments. There has been significant progress in increasing insurance coverage and healthcare utilization and a reduction in financial catastrophe and impoverishment caused by OOP spending. However, an ambitious reform design and its quick implementation introduced some challenges. While significant success has been achieved, there is more to be done.

42

Jordan

Health Care Accreditation Council of Jordan: Driving System Reform, Patient Safety, and Quality

Salma Jaouni Araj and Edward Chappy

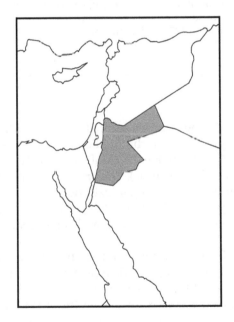

CONTENTS

TABLE 42.1

Comparative Data for 2000 and 2015

	Year	
	2000	**2015**
Population	**5,039,000**	**9,531,712[a]**
Total number of hospitals	86	110
Total number of private hospital beds	3212	4345
Total number of public hospital beds	3229	4783
Total number of RMS hospital beds	1755	2269
Total Number of MoH primary healthcare centers	335	677

Source: Department of Statistics [Jordan]. (2016). Jordan Population and Housing Census report, 2015. Retrieved from http://census.dos.gov.jo/wp-content/uploads/sites/2/2016/02/Census_results_2016.pdf
[a] 6,613,587 Jordanians and 2,918,125 non-Jordanians.

Background

Jordan is a middle-income country located in the Middle East. Health services in Jordan are provided by the public and private sectors. The public sector includes the Ministry of Health (MoH) and the Royal Medical Services (RMS) (military hospitals and clinic). The private sector includes private hospitals and clinics, international organizations, such as the United Nations Relief and Works Agency for Palestine Refugees in the Near East (UNRWA), non-government organizations (NGOs), and other charitable societies (see Table 42.1).

Jordan's health indicators have been internationally lauded. In 2010, Jordan was ranked the leading medical tourism destination in the Arab world and fifth globally by the World Bank (Khammash, 2012; Kronfol, 2012). Average life expectancy at birth increased from 66 in 1980 to 74.4 years in 2013. From 1981 to 2015, infant mortality rates declined from 42 to 15 deaths per 1000 live births (World Bank, 2016b). In 2012, deaths due to communicable diseases were 53 per 100,000 compared with the average international rate of 178 per 100,000 (WHO, 2015f).

In 2013, according to the World Bank, health expenditure in Jordan amounted to 7.2% of the GDP (World Bank, 2016b). This was higher than the average level of expenditure in other countries in the Middle East, which stood at 4.7%. The public sector is funded through the MoH budget, while the private sector is accessed both by fee-paying clients and by those covered by private health insurance.

The 2015 census results revealed that 54.9% of the population is insured, where 68.14% of Jordanians are insured. The MoH, including its Civil

TABLE 42.2

Population Data: National Census 2015

Nationality	Jordan	Syria	Egypt	Palestine	Iraq	Yemen	Libya	Others
Population	6,613,587	1,265,514	636,270	634,182	130,911	31,163	22,700	197,385

Source: HCAC. (2011). Primary Health Care and Family Planning Centers Accreditation Standards , Amman, Jordan; HCAC. (2013) Hospital Accreditation Standards. Amman, Jordan.

Insurance Program (CIP) for civil servants, accounts for 41.7% of the insured, while the RMS accounts for 38%. Only 12.4% of the population is covered by private insurers (Department of Statistics [Jordan], 2016).

Population growth is a major concern in Jordan (High Health Council and WHO, 2016). The country has made some progress in slowing the rate of growth through education, media campaigns to increase awareness of the impact of rapid population growth, and encouraging the use of different family planning methods. Although population growth rate remained at 2.3% in 2014, it rose to 5.3% in 2015 due primarily to the increase in the number of refugees flowing into the kingdom (Ghazal, 2016; World Bank, 2016b) (Table 42.2).

Since 2000, the government of Jordan has introduced several reforms in the health sector, giving priority to the quality and safety of services, and accessibility. There has been an increase in the number of facilities at the primary, secondary, and tertiary levels (High Health Council and WHO, 2016). The MoH has also focused on improvement in the treatment of non-communicable diseases, family planning, maternal and child health, and nutrition. Interventions in these areas are dependent on donors who offer both technical and financial assistance.

With the support of the WHO and the World Bank, Jordan has reviewed its healthcare financing mechanisms and is working on a universal health coverage plan. The improvements needed in the health sector were included in the Ministry of Health Strategic Plan for the years 2013–2017, the High Health Council Health Sector Strategic Directions for the years 2015–2019, and the Government of Jordan's Vision 2025 (High Health Council and WHO, 2016; Ministry of Health [Jordan], 2008; Ministry of Planning and International Cooperation [Jordan], 2015).

The Jordanian health sector continues to face a number of challenges. There is no requirement for re-licensure of healthcare facilities and limited inspection or regulatory enforcement of initial licensure requirements. Additionally, Jordan has no requirement for re-licensing of healthcare professionals or for medical or nursing continuing education. No malpractice legislation or system of redress for patients harmed by providers of services exists in the country. No nationally accepted clinical guidelines or pathways have been adopted. Because of the attraction of higher pay, many doctors and nurses leave Jordan to work in other Gulf countries, which is a drain on the system. Since 2010, the influx of Syrian refugees has increased the burden on the healthcare system.

Details of the Success Story

In 2003, the Minister of Health and other health sector leaders from the RMS, the Private Hospital Association (PHA), the healthcare professional councils, and medical schools met to discuss how to address some of the health system challenges and how they might improve the quality of healthcare services. The Minister of Health requested that the United States Agency for International Development (USAID), a major funder of healthcare projects in Jordan, partner with the MoH to come up with a comprehensive solution to address the many challenges in the system pertaining to quality and patient safety. With financial and technical assistance provided by USAID, all key stakeholders agreed to establish a national healthcare accreditation body to develop standards for healthcare facilities and programs along the continuum of care. From 2004 to 2007, all stakeholders were engaged in deciding what kind of agency should be established, who would be on the board to oversee the process, how it would be funded, and how it would be sustained after donor funding ended (United States Agency for International Development, 2013).

In 2007, the bylaws of the new organization were endorsed by all sectors, and in December of that year, the Health Care Accreditation Council (HCAC)—a private, non-profit, shareholding company—was created to act as the national healthcare accreditation agency of Jordan. The HCAC board was made up of representatives from the MoH, the PHA, the teaching hospitals, the medical and nursing councils, and the insurance commission, along with five members of the public who would provide legal, financial, business, economic, and academic expertise. The mission of the HCAC was to foster the continuous improvement of the quality and safety of healthcare facilities, services, and programs through developing internationally accepted standards, building capacity, and awarding accreditation. The HCAC is recognized by the International Society for Quality in Healthcare (ISQua), and currently holds ISQua accreditations for the organization, its surveyor training program, and standards (Donaldson et al., 2015).

To help the new organization in its initial start-up phase, the USAID funded the Jordan Health Care Accreditation Project to institutionalize accreditation and ensure the sustainability of patient safety efforts in Jordan. The project continued until March 2013. During that time, technical assistance was provided to the HCAC board and staff. Working together, the HCAC developed several sets of standards, trained surveyors, helped healthcare facilities meet the standards, developed several certification courses, and awarded accreditation to private, public, and RMS hospitals, primary healthcare facilities, and programs (see Table 42.3) (HCAC, 2011, 2013).

TABLE 42.3

Health Care Accreditation Council Program Outcomes

HCAC-accredited hospitals	17
HCAC-accredited primary healthcare centers	102
HCAC-certified breast imaging units	10
Certified consultants	11
Certified quality professionals HCQP	135
Certified infection control professionals HCIP	75
Certified risk management HCRM	67
Leadership and management HCEL	54
Surveyors	66

Source: Health Care Accreditation Council, *Primary Health Care and Family Planning Centers Accreditation Standards*, Amman, Jordan, 2011; HCAC, *Hospital Accreditation Standards*, Amman, Jordan, 2013.)

Impact of the Success Story

The HCAC is the driver of healthcare quality improvement and patient safety promotion in Jordan. The HCAC works at the micro level by building the capacity of healthcare professionals to improve quality and patient safety. In addition, through its consultation and education department, hospitals are helped to understand and meet the standards. The training empowers trainees to become the agents of change in their hospitals and primary healthcare (PHC) centers.

At the meso level, the HCAC accreditation, national quality and safety goals, standards, and recognition programs have driven institutions to embrace quality management and patient safety systems. A study, conducted in 2011–2012 by the USAID-funded Health Systems Strengthening Project II (2014), showed that there was increased use of family planning methods by clients in accredited versus non-accredited healthcare centers (United States Agency for International Development, 2014a). Additionally, the study found patients in accredited health centers managed their diabetes and hypertension more effectively than in non-accredited health centers.

A study conducted by El-Tohamy and Al Raoush (2015) showed that the HCAC's accreditation had a significant positive impact on hospital leadership commitment, employee involvement in quality improvement activities, and teamwork between departments, and that it increased the use of continuous quality improvement strategies. The study also showed an increase in customer satisfaction scores. The authors concluded that applying total quality management (TQM) philosophy as a managerial approach and using accreditation as a tool for quality improvement supports sustainable positive change at the health institution level.

At the macro level, the HCAC board has lobbied for mandatory accreditation; the enforcement of present licensure regulations; the passage of malpractice legislation; and the need for better data collection, analysis, and data-based decision-making. The HCAC has also promoted the need for the re-licensure of facilities and professionals, and for linking continuing professional education to re-licensure. The parliament, senate, and government have drafted laws and regulations to make the necessary changes. If passed, the legislated changes will complement the accreditation process and build a stronger healthcare system in Jordan.

Among the many results of the HCAC's lobbying, a clear change in the MoH's approach to quality and patient safety. The MoH has increased the budget and personnel of its Quality Department; and has formed quality monitoring committees chaired by the MoH secretary-general to ensure that accreditation requirements are being addressed and progress is made. In 2014, the MoH had five hospitals and 102 primary healthcare centers accredited. The 2014–2017 MoH strategy aims to achieve HCAC accreditation of an additional 11 hospitals and 27 primary healthcare centers (Ministry of Health [Jordan], 2008). The Government of Jordan's Vision 2025 and the National Healthcare Strategy both state that accreditation is the preferred tool for quality improvement and patient safety. The Private Hospitals Association Law of 2015 states that private hospitals need to be accredited by 2020 (Ministry of Planning and International Cooperation [Jordan], 2015).

Prospects for Further Success and Next Steps

The HCAC started as a healthcare accreditation agency, first working to improve the quality of care in hospitals (HCAC, 2011). The next set of standards developed was for PHC centers (HCAC, 2013). Additional sets of standards were developed based on the need for accreditation of breast imaging units and disease-specific programs like cardiology and diabetes. The HCAC has evolved from an accreditation agency to an organization that partners at the micro, meso, and macro levels to improve quality and safety of healthcare services for all Jordanians and to help other countries in the region create their own healthcare accreditation agencies.

The HCAC has had an impact on the healthcare system and the quality and safety of heath care services in Jordan, but there is more to do. Working with the MoH and other partners, the HCAC will work toward universal accreditation in the country. It will continue to establish increasingly challenging national quality and safety goals and focus on the generation of patient safety data and tools. The HCAC will focus research efforts toward finding best practices in patient safety and quality improvement for Jordan and the region, and supporting research on the value of accreditation. Finally, the HCAC will continue to lead in efforts to improve healthcare quality in the region.

Transferability of the Exemplar

The HCAC has become a model in the region for national healthcare quality improvement. The HCAC has provided technical assistance to help countries in the region embrace quality and patient safety. In addition, the HCAC has consulted with healthcare professionals from five countries in the region, helping them learn how to create or improve their own organizations. The WHO's Eastern Mediterranean Region Office (EMRO) has been showcasing the HCAC success story across the 22 countries in the region and utilizing the HCAC's expertise to support several countries' efforts to establish their national accreditation agencies.

43

Lebanon

"You Don't Have to be Superman to Save Lives. Give Blood": Improving the Health System through Social Innovation—The Case of Donner Sang Compter

Nasser Yassin, Maysa Baroud, Reem Talhouk, Sandra Mesmar, and Sara Kaddoura

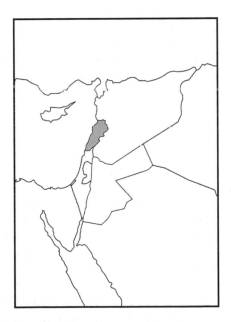

CONTENTS

Background

The health system in Lebanon is pluralistic and fragmented (Chami and Mikhail, 2015). The private sector is greatly involved in healthcare provision, and most healthcare spending involves out-of-pocket expenses (Elgazar et al., 2010). Non-governmental organizations (NGOs) attempt to fill some of the gaps, especially when it comes to the provision of primary healthcare to the poorest elements of society. Although they have received less attention, initiatives led by social innovators have also tackled significant problems in the health system. Social innovation aims at providing novel solutions and adding value to the ways we address social problems (Mulgan et al., 2007).

This chapter highlights the emergence of *Donner Sang Compter* (DSC), an NGO that aimed to create an innovative, efficient, and effective blood donation system in Lebanon, despite the political and economic instability in the country and the Middle East region. Leading this social initiative was Mr. Yorgui Teyrouz, an active Scout member in Lebanon for 15 years and a previous volunteer with the Lebanese Red Cross. Teyrouz was motivated to create a database of blood donors after he was faced with the challenge of finding blood units for a close friend undergoing serious surgery in 2006.

DSC, founded in 2006 (and whose name means "to give blood without expecting anything in return"), has developed innovative ways to recruit volunteers and to raise funds for its activities. It effectively utilized social media to reach out to potential volunteers and blood donors, and in less than 10 years has managed to connect 60,000 blood recipients with donors.

Currently, the wider Middle East region is at a critical juncture in its history, undergoing significant political and social transformation. It is a moment that has shown that both governmental interventions and the private sector have proven to be inadequate when it comes to providing equitable and high-quality healthcare in the region, making it an opportune time for social innovation. Post-Arab Spring transformations have been challenging, but have created new opportunities for change. In many places, citizens, particularly young people, are experiencing the breakdown of barriers to change and are becoming increasingly aware of the need for further transformation. With record levels of unemployment, illiteracy, and indeed the lack of access to healthcare in many countries in the Middle East, which existing institutions do not have the capacity to address, social innovation may provide the answers.

A safe and reliable blood supply is considered an essential requirement of healthcare, as it plays a role in saving lives in both routine and emergency situations. Globally, increases in both life expectancy and surgical interventions have led to an increase in the demand for blood (Custer et al., 2004; Riley et al., 2007). To meet the demand, many systems rely on blood donations from non-remunerated volunteers (NVDs), family or replacement donors, or paid donors (Ala et al., 2012; Al-Drees, 2008; Bates et al., 2007; Marantidou et al., 2007).

Lebanon's health system is ill-equipped to meet the health needs of its population (Ammar, 2003). During the civil war (1975–1992), there was a breakdown in many sectors including the public health sector, and since the end of the war, healthcare has been fragmented and is highly dependent on the private sector (Ammar, 2003). To date, Lebanon still lacks a national blood bank and the necessary infrastructure to support it. While the Lebanese Red Cross has tried to fill this role, the absence of a national blood donation plan means that patients and their families must rely on an informal replacement system, whereby if a patient requires a blood transfusion, the hospital's blood bank requests that the patient's family and friends replace the blood units used. This has resulted in a system that cannot guarantee the safety, quality, availability, and accessibility of blood units. The scarcity of donors with rare blood types, lack of proper care, poor legislation, and insufficient funding, combined with ineffective donor coordination, has hindered the establishment of an effective blood donating system.

Having experienced firsthand the agony and failures of the blood donation replacement system in Lebanon, Teyrouz set out to build a network consisting of strong ties between potential blood donors and health professionals, attempting to bridge the communication gap between donors, patients, and healthcare providers. Today, DSC aims both to improve the blood donation system in Lebanon and to raise awareness about voluntary blood donation. Instead of a fragmented system, where local blood banks control their own unit needs, DSC provides a centralized database of potential donors and runs blood donation drives in partnership with these local blood banks (*Donner Sang Compter*, n.d.). Boasting a community of over 100 volunteer workers, DSC has managed to develop a solid system for running blood drives across the nation—establishing an effective system, which is almost unique in the greater Lebanese healthcare context.

Planting the Seed through Social Media

DSC's social media endeavors began in 2007, when a Facebook page was launched to reach and recruit potential blood donors. DSC knew that targeting Lebanese youth through social networking sites would be an efficient and effective approach—and it was. The DSC database grew from an initial 40 members, all personal acquaintances of Teyrouz, to 3000 members, in less than one year. DSC utilized social media in running blood drives. DSC's campaigns focused on the heroic aspect of the donation process, using slogans, such as "You don't have to be a superman to save lives," "Be my Blood Brother," "The donor saved my life," and "Do we need to beg for blood to save a life? Don't be cold-blooded. Be a donor." The success of these blood drives was contingent on the personal approach; donors were made to feel like heroes whenever they donated blood.

After consents were obtained, pictures of volunteers donating blood were posted on the DSC Facebook page. The donors were tagged, which meant that each individual's donation could be used to encourage their friends and colleagues to do the same. By effectively using the social network of each tagged donor, DSC was able to increase their network exponentially, thus connecting with many more potential donors.

Communication through social media was crucial to the success of DSC. In 2011, DSC participated in TEDxBeirut (Teyrouz, 2011). The presentation highlighted the importance of volunteerism, social solidarity, and the value and simplicity of the blood donation process, further illustrating the magnitude of DSC's outcomes, which in turn motivated donors to return for more voluntary blood donations. DSC was quickly gaining recognition within the community. Patients in need of blood transfusions trusted DSC enough to reach out and ask them for blood donor contacts. DSC established a call center to preserve the anonymity of blood donors and help eliminate repeated donation requests from the same donors. Since its foundation, DSC has helped around 60,000 patients via the call center alone, simply by linking donors to patients in need. Considering Lebanon's population of 4.5 million, and in light of the failures of the current healthcare system, these numbers represent a towering achievement.

Partnering with Hospitals

Fearing that blood units might be unfairly allocated, with some people favored over others, the Lebanese authorities would not allow DSC to run its own blood bank. As a result, each blood drive required the sponsorship of a hospital. While DSC organized the drive, the sponsoring hospital would provide the necessary healthcare professionals to handle the blood donation, screening, and storage.

Initially, because the organization was so new, DSC encountered some resistance from Lebanese hospitals. This led to DSC's collaboration with a consultancy company to assess the opportunities and challenges associated with launching a blood collection bus. The purpose of the venture was to collaborate with hospitals to increase stock for all blood banks by becoming mobile. Again, they succeeded beyond all expectations. In 2014, in one highly successful blood drive via the blood collection bus, school and university students donated nearly 500 blood units to a well-known university hospital in Beirut.

Partnering with the Community

Because of its successful, well-coordinated blood drives and highly effective social media and awareness campaigns, DSC was quickly recognized as a reliable healthcare partner. In numerous instances, members of the community have approached DSC for help, and to form partnerships. Some of DSC's most successful partnerships have involved raising awareness of other local issues during the drives. One such collaborative blood drive, held in 2013, which attracted many donors, simultaneously supported breast cancer patients and promoted the prevention of violence against women. DSC has even formed partnerships with movie theaters, using the theater as a donation center. Allowing donors to watch movies while giving blood minimized donor stress, encouraged volunteer recruitment, and strengthened DSC's ties with the community.

Next Steps and Transferability

DSC is currently working on various projects. Plans are underway to collaborate with other NGOs like the National Organization for Organ and Tissue Donation and Transplantation (NOOTDT). DSC is also working on obtaining a license to run their own blood bank, which would allow them to recruit and train their own phlebotomy staff. This would allow DSC to conduct blood drives independently of hospital staff, with only a single hospital representative required, thus increasing the number of blood drives, while reducing the partner hospital's costs. Another vision for the future is the DSC mobile application. The current donation system involves calling the donor when there is demand. The new system, due to be implemented in the near future, will let the donor schedule their donation. It will also keep track of previous donations, and support the scheduling of subsequent donations.

By gaining the trust and respect of the community, DSC has managed to create a family of volunteers who work together proactively. While DSC's focus has been on recruiting volunteers, it has also tackled the issue head-on by normalizing the relationship with hospitals. DSC's work showcases the ways in which social innovation, propelled by accessible social media, can be used to enhance health systems. DSC has shown that health system issues can be overcome through perseverance, empathy, and innovative thinking.

Conclusion

The incredible success of DSC shows how individuals and communities can work together to overcome health system challenges in developing countries, even in the face of considerable turbulence and uncertainty. Through the innovative use of social media, DSC was able to establish an effective blood donation organization, thus filling a significant gap in the Lebanese health system. Through networks and partnerships with hospitals and communities, one very important component of the Lebanese health system has been significantly improved.

44

Oman

Al-Shifa Electronic Health Record System: From Simple Start to Paradigm Model

Ahmed Al-Mandhari, Abdullah Al-Raqadi, and Badar Awladthani

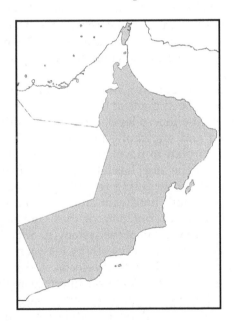

CONTENTS

Background

As part of a national 5-year annual strategic plan that began in 1976, the Ministry of Health (MoH) in Oman has instituted several initiatives to facilitate the delivery of efficient and effective healthcare services on par with international best practice. The introduction of the electronic health record system known as *Al-Shifa* represents a success story for Oman. *Al-Shifa* closely follows healthcare practices in Oman and covers a wide range of hospital administration and management processes. *Al-Shifa* aims to improve the quality of healthcare services and patient safety through the provision of accessible, secure, and accurate records of patient data. Such a system helps in the efficient utilization of available resources through the secure sharing of health information among healthcare providers. This has implications for lowering the cost of delivering healthcare services and creates a database that can be utilized by researchers and administrators in order to chart the pattern and trend of disease in the country (Al-Raqadi, 2013; Ministry of Health [Oman], n.d.).

The *Al-Shifa* system is expanding its capacity at vertical and horizontal levels. Major efforts have been made at the macro, meso, and micro levels to enhance its success. At the macro level, the MoH's Health Vision 2050 has incorporated a unified and interconnected electronic healthcare system as an important part of its plan to develop all components of the healthcare system. At the meso level, the MoH has taken steps to ensure the incremental development of the system, including recruiting skilled staff and upgrading the infrastructure of both hardware and software, in order to cater to national needs. In 2010, as an outcome of these developments, the MoH began installing the fourth version of the system (*Al-Shifa* 3+), which has new functionalities that facilitate interconnectivity between institutions and lay the groundwork for centralized medical records. *Al-Shifa* 3+, a client-server system, is a fully integrated graphical user interface application system for hospital management. It is built around Oracle 9i, using an 11g database, and was developed using Oracle Developer 6i with Java running under the Linux platform.

The MoH has developed several frameworks to ensure that all healthcare transactions, such as clinical appointments, laboratory, and radiological reports, are streamlined via electronic channels, such as e-Referral and e-Notification, thus ensuring that responsible stakeholders are notified of any disease or alerts relating to an individual patient's care.

At the micro level, the MoH has recruited qualified and skillful technicians to supervise the running of the *Al-Shifa* system at an institutional level to ensure that all staff understand the program's capabilities and are able to use it efficiently—thus maximizing trust in and utilization of the system.

After the inception of the National Strategy for Oman (Oman Digital Society—e.Oman) in 2003 and its revision in 2010, Oman has taken concrete steps to fulfill its national and international obligations toward streamlining information and communication technology (ICT), transforming communities, and integrating societies (Information Technology Authority, Sultanate of Oman, c.2013). As healthcare information systems have become increasingly crucial to the development of healthcare operations, Oman has worked toward moving its healthcare system into the digital era. This undertaking has been sanctioned by His Majesty (HM) the Sultan, who has urged the country to be receptive to all scientific knowledge. HM has particularly emphasized the importance of computer science as a developmental tool, with information technology (IT) as the backbone of such endeavors (Information Technology Authority, Sultanate of Oman, 2014).

Oman's growing social and cultural stability have also encouraged the development of IT within the healthcare system. As IT is rapidly evolving worldwide, particularly in the healthcare field, the MoH is recognizing the importance of IT in the healthcare system. According to an ICT survey in Oman, published in December 2012, 61% of government employees now have IT skills (Information Technology Authority, Sultanate of Oman, 2014). Furthermore, around 66% of all PCs in the surveyed government entities are connected to the internet, and over 73% of these entities have fixed broadband (Information Technology Authority, Sultanate of Oman, c.2013). An Information Technology Authority was established in 2006 to oversee the implementation of IT in all government agencies.

Details of the Success Story

While other healthcare initiatives, such as Oman's antenatal and immunization programs, have also enjoyed considerable success, the development of *Al-Shifa* is of particular interest (Al Awaidy et al., 2010; Al-Dhahry et al., 2001; Ministry of Health [Oman], 2014). The program, which was developed in Oman, has transformed the healthcare system from one that was entirely paper-based, into one that uses an integrated, streamlined, and easily accessible electronic database capable of providing a comprehensive view of a patient's clinical history (Al-Raqadi, 2013). The Computerized Physician Order Entry (CPOE) system, for example, helps to minimize the need for paper, pens, and telephones at intra- and inter-institutional levels. The system is currently installed in all public healthcare institutions, including seven healthcare facilities run by the Diwan of Royal Court, Internal Security, and the Ministry of Sport—thus providing support for around 86% of health system users in Oman.

Al-Shifa has successfully transformed healthcare institutions at all levels. Furthermore, the new version of this system has introduced an interconnectivity feature linking these institutions. Over successive years, an exhaustive range of subsystems have also been introduced. These subsystems incorporate clinical system laboratories, blood banks, pharmacy, medical stores, radiology, operating theaters, critical care units, emergency care, quality management, and non-medical software components, such as asset management, inventory, and billing.

The implementation of the *Al-Shifa* health record system has delivered a number of benefits. It is estimated that it has saved 60% of medical personnel time (Information Technology Authority, Sultanate of Oman, c.2013). One of the important components of the system is the e-Referral service, which was launched in 2006. This feature of the system improves communication between healthcare professionals, thus facilitating patients' movement through the primary, secondary, and tertiary levels. It has also helped to improve the quality of referrals through more efficient record keeping, reducing the number of duplicate requests, and ensuring complete and accurate data and correct referrals. Currently, 114 healthcare institutions have been connected via *Al-Shifa*. The system also features integrated SMS notifications that remind patients about their medical appointments.

In addition, the system allows access to patients' medical records through a single page view that includes all major components of the healthcare service provided, such as medical examinations, diagnoses, investigations reports, treatment histories, plans of management, test results, medications, and referral details. The system can detect duplicate registry numbers for each patient and can retrieve an automated data capture from the Omani civil card, including photographs, which helps to accurately identify patients. Furthermore, the system has another essential component called *Nabd-Al-Shifa*, which is the data-warehouse and business intelligence (BI) built on top of *Al-Shifa*. This component allows data analysis and trend identification of a wide range of key performance indicators from over 200 institutions, including offline sites. Sophisticated dashboards and portals with graphs and charts assist healthcare and analysis in decision support. To ensure continuous development and smooth running of healthcare services, the system is continuously upgraded.

Details of the Impact of the Success Story

Several key factors have played a role in the success of the *Al-Shifa* system. Along with a number of other factors it was essential to ensure that

- The vision behind establishing the system was clear and in line with national policies.
- The project leaders made a set of tangible goals and specific strategies for the project.

- There was a strengthening of the ICT infrastructure used by the networked healthcare units adopting the system in order to facilitate and secure their full integration.
- There was an immediate upgrade of the technology to migrate from a client-server based to a web-based system.
- The legal framework and the ethical conditions for preserving the privacy of patients and their medical records were considered at the initial stages of creating the system.
- Efficient utilization of the system was guaranteed through empowering the human resources using and managing the system.
- A high level of collaboration between governmental bodies involved in the implementation of the system was created and maintained.

The system has had a positive impact on the quality of healthcare services and patient safety through a number of essential elements that were considered in its structure. One of these is the fact that the system complies with international interconnectivity standards, such as Health Level 7 (HL 7), Health Level 7-Clinical Document Architecture (HL 7-CDA); Digital Imaging and Communications in Medicine (DICOM); SNOMED; Logical Observation Identifiers Names and Codes (LOINC); the International Classification of Diseases, Ninth Revision, and Clinical Modification (ICD-9-CM). Furthermore, the system is composed of interactive modules serving the various specialties in the healthcare system. It contains modules for records clerks, physicians, nurses, and those who work in pharmacies, laboratories, radiology, blood banks, physiotherapy, nutrition, operating theaters, and medical stores, with all records available electronically. In addition, the system provides healthcare analysts and administrators with instant access to the important indicators and matrices related to processes, along with a quality assurance system for quality control.

Implementation: Transferability of the Exemplar

Given that the processes in Omani healthcare services are standardized, the system is highly transferable. It has been utilized in all publicly funded health institutions, including facilities within a number of government authorities. Other allied healthcare systems are negotiating with the MoH for authority to use it within their institutions. The system is built on international interconnectivity standards and protocols, which means it can adapt to the requirements of healthcare systems in other countries.

Prospects for Further Success and Next Steps

After implementation of e-Referral, e-Notification, wide deployment of *Al-Shifa* 3+, and the first phase of national electronic health records using unique identification (Civil ID), the next step is to establish the second phase of the national e-Health record repository by using unique identification. This aims to connect government and private healthcare institutions so patient records can be accessed by both. This repository will be an interactive database to reduce and avoid duplication, manage drug interaction, and alert healthcare providers to any allergies.

The MoH regards the improvement of the ICT infrastructure as the main requirement for the delivery of an efficient and reliable eHealth services management system, and have therefore established central quality management and national statistical and monitoring dashboards to audit health institutions performance.

Oman's Health Vision 2050 aims to have a connected, consistent, and cohesive national health sector that has improved information flow between providers, and better continuity of care with other providers. Future developmental goals include a single national directory for patients, a single provider registry, a single delivery location registry, and a national service registry.

This vision of the health system can be achieved through enhancing and developing seven key factors that extend across multiple areas. These include facility management, human resources capacity building, development of workflow, development of regulatory rules, adoption of international standards, legislation, and the efficient utilization of resources.

Furthermore, implementation of information technology is required to serve various sectors of healthcare such as tele-health, ambulance management, insurance management, enterprise resource planning, m-health, decision support, and tele-education.

Conclusion

Oman's successful introduction and integration of a comprehensive electronic healthcare record system is a major step in the journey toward improving patient safety and quality of care. Through the *Al-Shifa* system, the MoH has made healthcare information available to providers in a simplified and standardized manner while maintaining confidentiality and security.

The system has received a number of prestigious awards. At a national level, it received an HM Excellence Award for the best electronic system in Oman in the year 2010. The system has also been recognized internationally, receiving first and second place in the United Nations Public Service Award in 2010 and 2012 respectively, and first place for the nursing and midwiferies program in the United Nations Public Service Forum in 2014. The system was also awarded best ICT application in eHealth by International Telecommunication Union (ITU) in 2013.

45

Pakistan

Health Systems, Accreditation, and Databases: Pakistan's Perspective

Syed Shahabuddin and Usman Iqbal

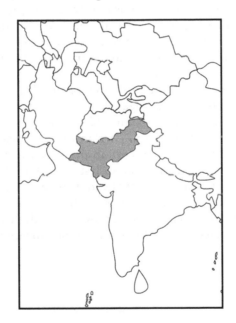

CONTENTS

Overview of Pakistan's Health System

A well-functioning health system requires a trained and motivated work-force, a well-maintained infrastructure, and a reliable supply of medicines and technologies backed by adequate funding, strong health plans, and evidence-based policies (WHO, n.d.a.). This ideal, which exists in most developed nations, is difficult to achieve in developing countries like Pakistan.

Pakistan's health status indicators are poor in comparison with other countries in South Asia. Although Pakistan is a signatory to the Millennium Development Goals set by the United Nations, it has not yet been able to achieve them, and some work is required to strengthen and implement the policies (Afzal and Yusuf, 2013). One of the prerequisite steps toward national health system improvement is to identify the problems that need to be resolved in order to improve the well-being of individuals and communities. If the desired outcomes are to be achieved, problems must be prioritized, timelines set, budgets devised, and human resources allocated.

In developing nations, the process can be extremely complex, and may even falter. This is frequently due to a lack of funding—with allocation of GDP to health being negligible, regardless of whether a project is funded publicly or by the private sector (Islam, 2002). The uncertainty of the political situation can have a negative impact on the progress of such projects: changes in government can mean certain projects are abandoned prior to completion. Poor governance is also an issue (Lashari, 2004). In Pakistan, prior to 2011, the Federal Ministry of Health was responsible for the health-related activity of each province. However, the diverse socioeconomic and cultural constitution of each individual province, with their distinct dynamics and requirements, led to the devolution of healthcare responsibilities to the provinces in 2011.

Role Allocation for Healthcare

Following devolution, healthcare became the responsibility of various divisions, supported by a number of health-related institutions and programs (Ministry of National Health Services, Regulations and Coordination, Government of Pakistan, n.d.). These divisions cover different areas of the Provincial Health System, including the Cabinet Division, the Capital Administration and Development Division, the Planning Division, the Economic Affairs Division, and the Division of Interprovincial Coordination. The Ministry of Health plays an important role in collaborating with international agencies such as the World Health Organization (WHO), which assist with disease eradication programs. The eradication program focuses on two broad categories of disease: communicable and non-communicable. The eradication of communicable diseases, such as polio and tuberculosis, has been the primary focus of both the local and international program.

While non-communicable diseases have been less of a priority, it has become apparent that diseases such as cardiovascular disease, cancer, and diabetes are rapidly increasing (Islam, 2002). Strategies to prevent and combat such diseases are urgently needed. Despite the flaws in Pakistan's health system, the overall infrastructure is excellent—from the basic remote area health units, to the district hospitals. That these resources are sometimes underutilized may be an issue related to poor governance.

Urban and Rural Healthcare

In Pakistan, healthcare facilities are provided by both public and private sector hospitals and sometimes by public–private partnerships. The community healthcare system is divided into urban and rural regions. The urban population, which is relatively affluent, has access to a range of both private and public healthcare facilities. This is not the case for the rural population. Rural populations are disadvantaged in numerous ways—including distance, poverty, and lack of education and awareness. As the World Bank has observed, the effectiveness of private medical facilities may be seriously compromised by a number of factors, including quackery, insufficient preventive care, lack of functioning regulatory mechanisms for consumers, a concentration in urban areas, and their focus on profits (World Bank, 1998). However, private facilities play an important role in improving community health, and their links to both the public system and to non-government organizations (NGOs) helps to facilitate uniform policy development and implementation. In Pakistan's health system, NGOs also provide healthcare to those with limited access and finances.

There are a number of (mostly private) institutes in Pakistan that provide free services to patients with specific medical complaints, such as the Sind Institute of Urology and Transplantation (SIUT), the Shaukat Khanum Memorial Cancer Hospital, the Indus Hospital, and the Aga Khan University Hospital (AKUH). These hospitals have introduced the concept of paperless record keeping, using advanced computer technology to create an electronic medical record system. These hospitals are working hard to provide healthcare for no or low profits, and have adopted quality assurance initiatives to ensure safe practices according to the international standards.

The AKUH, a multidisciplinary tertiary care center, renowned for its research and considered one of the most advanced hospitals in Pakistan, plays a particularly important role. Although it is a private hospital, it provides quality and equitable care to all, regardless of income. For those who are unable to pay, care is subsidized through patient welfare and *Zakat* funds (charity).

International Accreditation of AKUH

One important feature of the AKUH is its prioritization of quality care: from the hiring of staff and faculty and the purchasing of equipment, to the administration of the facility. This effort has been acknowledged internationally, with the granting of ISO 9001 (Quality Management System) certification in 2004. This certification was followed by international recognition in the form of achieving Joint Commission International Accreditation (JCIA) after being found to meet standards set by the Joint Commission International (JCI) in 2009 and again in 2015 (Birkmeyer, 2004: Joint Commission International, 2013; Shahian et al., 2007). The AKUH is the only hospital in Pakistan to have achieved JCIA.

Importance of Healthcare Databases

Healthcare databases are increasingly important to healthcare organizations. Quality of care can be enhanced substantially by the development of comprehensive and accurate databases containing vital information about prevalence, incidence, natural history, treatment, associations of disease, drug exposure, and healthcare utilization patterns. An accurate and up-to-date healthcare database is essential to monitoring the overall state of any healthcare system (Martin, 2008). Some countries, such as Taiwan, who launched a single-payer national health insurance program in 1995, covering 99.9% of the Taiwanese population, have well-established healthcare databases. In the United States, the Department of Veterans Affairs, Medicare, Medicaid, and other health organizations, all maintain large, but discrete, healthcare databases (Hsing and Ioannidis, 2015).

AKUH Cardiac Surgery Database

In developing countries like Pakistan, where the healthcare facilities are provided by both public and private sector hospitals and sometimes public–private partnerships, such databases are still under development. In Pakistan, a small number of private hospitals are in the process of establishing databases, along with additional health information technology. AKUH's cardiac surgery database, which is one of the first of its kind in Pakistan, provides an example of a successfully integrated database.

From the time the field was first established in 1994, cardiothoracic specialists have recognized the importance of creating and maintaining accurate records and databases in order to streamline the treatment of individual cases and facilitate research. Initially, a basic hard copy database was maintained at AKUH; however, the digital revolution has enabled the development of more sophisticated databases. Subsequently, research officers were hired to organize databases, and with the help of IT personnel, computerized databases were created. A dedicated research officer is now responsible for collecting data regarding preoperative details, operative information, and postoperative outcomes.

These include the status of the patient prior to surgery, and whether the surgery was performed electively or on an urgent/emergent basis. Information relating to anesthetic management, details of operative procedure, and perfusionist strategies (related to management of heart lung machines) are also part of the data collecting proforma. Outcomes, including postoperative complications and discharge information, are recorded and follow-up data is acquired from subsequent clinical visits and via telephonic communication. Death within 30 days of procedure, irrespective of whether the patient is in hospital or not, is considered a surgical mortality and recorded with underlying cause.

The development of a national cardiac surgery database was a key step toward comprehensive improvement in quality of care in this specific field. Utilization of the database has already improved many aspects of patient care, ensuring uniformity of care by regularly generating quality indicator reports, and facilitating more accurate risk stratification. Outcomes in terms of major morbidities and death have been improved. The database has also generated original research and was instrumental in formulating a book on risk stratification for the Pakistani population (Qadir et al., 2012; Saifuddin et al., 2015). The AKUH has recently been chosen to participate in JCI's International Cardiac Surgery Benchmarking Project, a pilot program to address international clinical cardiac indicators. The hospital's practice and data collection methodology has been reviewed and validated as part of the program. In this context, external feedback on outcomes not only serves a regulatory function but also directs toward self-assessment and provides further impetus to improve quality.

Challenges

There are a number of significant challenges to establishing well-conceived, comprehensive, and accurate healthcare databases. These include problems surrounding data heterogeneity, veracity, velocity, use, storage, ownership, along with issues of security and confidentiality (Collen, 2012).

These challenges can be overcome by defining the objectives of the specific database, creating a document in which all the steps involved in collecting, entering, cleaning, and analyzing the data are standardized and recorded so that staff can refer to the document when required. This document, which is known as the standard operating procedure (SOP) at AKUH, also functions as a training manual for new participants, and ensures the validity of long-term analyses by defining variables and detailing their changes. The SOP also contains the data collecting tool.

The data is generated and owned by the Aga Khan University. Confidentiality and privacy is ensured by storing hard copies securely. The computerized data is accessible to authorized persons only and provided for research after consultation with the section head. Staff are trained and monitored to ensure accuracy. Collaboration with a larger international database is required in order to provide regular feedback and, if possible, on-site verification and validation, ensuring the accuracy of the database.

Wider Application

The model provided by the AKUH's cardiac surgery database could have applications in related fields. Similar healthcare databases can be used for epidemic prediction, disease prevention, education purposes, research purposes, and to design policies by stakeholders. Additionally, it could facilitate research on healthcare utilization, health economics, and biomedical research—providing information for guiding national health policies. Extensive longitudinal healthcare data provides opportunities for researchers to monitor a wide range of evidence-based medicine. Clinical, personal, and risk factor information can also provide information for research into rare conditions. This is particularly useful when clinical trials are not always practical due to cost and ethical concerns (Wiederhold, 1980).

In summary, despite adequate infrastructure, Pakistan's healthcare system requires significant improvement. Basic healthcare indicators such as infant mortality rate are poor, and the system has failed to achieve its Millennium Development Goals. There is an urgent need for better strategies to utilize funds, human resources, and infrastructure. While the overall situation may appear gloomy, some institutions are attempting to improve the situation by ensuring quality assurance and acquiring international accreditation. Maintaining databases in specific fields will continue to provide performance measurements and help to redefine the benchmarks. The provision and audit of such data can guide resource allocation and help strengthen policies.

46

Qatar

Successful Implementation of a Deteriorating Patient Safety Net System: The Qatar Early Warning System

David Vaughan, Mylai Guerrero, Yousuf Khalid Al Maslamani, and Charles Pain

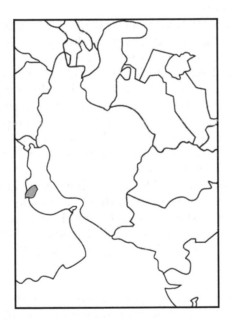

CONTENTS

Background

Qatar has one of the fasting growing populations in the world, largely due to the immigration of workers. Population growth is exceeding the capacity of the hospital system; therefore, despite the country's wealth, there are clear economic imperatives to improve the effectiveness and efficiency of health-care delivery.

Increased wealth has resulted in a marked increase in the diseases of affluence, especially obesity, diabetes, and cardiovascular diseases, instances of which are likely to increase over time. Greater affluence also means that there is a growing demand for quality improvement, along with greater accountability from healthcare providers. A key pillar of Qatar's national development strategy, Qatar National Vision 2030, is to ensure that the population is physically and mentally healthy.

As part of its national development strategy, and in order to meet the Qatar National Vision 2030 goals, the Qatari health system has, in recent years, undertaken a large number of reforms to improve the healthcare system. The Supreme Council of Health (SCH) has introduced a number of initiatives, including the registering and licensing of all healthcare professionals, and ensuring that they undertake an annual program of professional development. The SCH has also mandated that all providers report against a set of internationally validated indicators (for hospital mortality rates, methicillin-resistant *Staphylococcus aureus* [MRSA] infections, and so on), and is introducing a national insurance system.

In addition, the Institute for Healthcare Improvement has entered into a multiyear agreement with Hamad Medical Corporation (HMC). The intent of this strategic partnership is to assist the development of capacity and capability in quality improvement expertise across HMC, and to catalyze the drive to improve quality of care delivered by HMC. The main elements of this partnership are

- A large-scale safety collaborative focusing on hospital-acquired conditions, such as pressure ulcers, central–line associated blood stream infections, and ventilator-associated pneumonia
- The development of internal capacity and capability in quality improvement by training large numbers of staff in the requisite skills and knowledge

HMC provides >90% of hospital care in Qatar. As the largest provider, HMC has a very clear and well-defined strategy for quality, and all activities across HMC align with this strategy. Examples include working on clear organizational priorities (e.g., identification of deteriorating patients and sepsis). These organizational priorities have become a focus of improvement across the system.

Details of the Success Story

Consistent with experience in many other health systems, root-cause analyses of unexpected deaths in HMC showed a consistent pattern of unrecognized deterioration (Chan et al., 2010). In many cases, harm could have been averted if clinical deterioration had been detected earlier. Investigations of these adverse events have shown clear evidence of worsening of vital signs, often hours prior to cardiac arrest, but no action had been taken, in part because the significance of the worsening of vital signs went unrecognized, and in part, when the significance was recognized, nurses did not feel empowered to escalate their concerns to physicians.

In order to reduce such unnecessary deaths, the Qatar Early Warning System (QEWS) was designed. This system was developed by drawing on best practice internationally, and features two key elements: a vital signs chart and a response trigger (Hughes et al., 2014).

The vital signs chart consists of two color-coded zones, a yellow and a red zone. As patients' vital signs worsen, they move from the normal zone, to the yellow, and then the red zone. The charts allow the clinician to track the vital signs over time and trigger a response. Depending on the color zone, one of two responses is triggered: if a patient falls into the yellow zone (a sign that the patient may be "drifting" into trouble), a clinical review by the admitting team is undertaken within 30 minutes. If the vital signs fall into the red zone, the patient must be reviewed within 10 minutes by the rapid response team. In addition, other physiological (e.g., pain) and laboratory (e.g., glucose) values also trigger a yellow or red response.

A number of challenges were encountered during the development and implementation of the program. The diversity of both the healthcare workforce and the served population was sometimes problematic, not only because of the communication difficulties posed by the mix of languages, but also because of variable training and education, and the differing expectations and demands of different groups. There was some initial resistance to making the program a priority, and some clinicians needed to be persuaded of the rationale and evidence base underpinning such a system. There were also certain logistical difficulties to overcome, including the need to develop both paper and electronic versions of vital sign triggering tools. Despite these challenges, however, the system has now been implemented across all facilities and patient groupings.

Factors Contributing to the Early Warning System's Success

A key element of the program was the development of a robust and representative governance structure. This gave the program clinical credibility and allowed clinical peers to address clinical objections. Aligning the regulatory requirements with clinical needs ensured that executive mandate was received. Establishment of a multidisciplinary steering group chaired by a respected senior clinician lent the program a credibility, authority, and expertise that helped to overcome many challenges. Parallel to the establishment of a central governing authority, each facility was required to identify its local governance and implementation group.

The use of previously validated, evidence-based charts helped facilitate acceptance by clinicians and, in addition, reduced the burden of work required to develop local systems. However, the charts did require some modification and adaptation to local circumstances. All charts were tested pre-implementation using a plan-do-study-act (PDSA) approach, a useful tool in quality improvement projects.

All facilities and departments were required to define in advance the composition of their rapid response teams. Some resistance was encountered, as many clinicians reasonably felt that development of such teams without dedicated resources would increase the burden of work on clinicians. Utilizing their existing data for cardiac arrest rates, alongside international data on activation rates for rapid response teams, reassured them that it was unlikely that the quantity of work would increase substantially. In almost all cases, the existing cardiac arrest team was also used as a rapid response team, though some took the opportunity to change the membership of their teams when appropriate. In at least one facility, the medical leadership was changed from a senior resident to a consultant physician or anesthesiologist.

A comprehensive education curriculum and strategy was developed. A major challenge was training more than 5000 nurses in the use of the system over a short period. The curriculum defined four levels of training. Initially, a 40-minute online training module, which all front-line staff were required to complete, introduced the concepts and principles of the program. All nurses then received bedside training in which various scenarios describing deteriorating patients were outlined. More than 5000 nurses and 1500 doctors were trained over a period of 6 weeks prior to implementation, and 3 months after the training module was activated, over 10,000 staff had undertaken online training. All team members of rapid response teams are required to have advanced life support training. All front-line staff will eventually be required to undertake a recognized program that trains them in the initial response and management of deterioration (e.g., ALERT, DETECT Junior). Ongoing training on topics such as crisis resource management, teamwork, communication, and debriefing will also be provided to members of rapid response teams.

An easy-to-use online data system was created that allowed all facilities to input their data and to compare results within and between units and facilities. A large number of secondary measures were defined and developed, which, although not mandatory, were provided to allow facilities to identify and improve areas where their performance might be enhanced.

Taking a systems perspective, along with the alignment of organizational resources, were the final key success factors. These organizational resources included medical and nursing education, information, and communications technologies, and accreditation and quality improvement resources.

What's the Nature of the Success?

Initial data following the implementation of the program suggests a substantial reduction in cardiac arrest rates of around 40%; this compares very favorably with data from other systems (Jones et al., 2011). The data relating to activation rates of the response team is even more encouraging. International literature suggests that most systems will achieve an activation rate of 10/1000 discharges, with mature academic health systems ultimately achieving a rate of 40/1000 discharges (Jones et al., 2011). Given that there appears to be a dose–response relationship (higher activation rates result in better outcomes), higher rates are a surrogate measure of success. Within 3 months of implementation, activation rates across the system range from 25–70/1000 discharges. Interestingly, the single nurse-led response team has the highest activation rates, suggesting that there may be less reluctance on the part of staff nurses to call their nursing colleagues.

Implementation: Transferability of the Exemplar

The QEWS provides an example of successful healthcare development and implementation, and one that will likely result in substantial clinical benefits. The approach taken has lessons for other large-scale improvement initiatives across Qatar and within other systems.

The approach taken is widely applicable and involves taking a systems perspective, ensuring good governance, agreeing on standards used throughout the organization, defining educational, training and other requirements, and ensuring all units use the same key performance indicators (KPIs). Because QEWS is a key foundation of the HMC quality strategy, implementation of further elements of the strategy are more likely to be successful; these include broadening the program to include sepsis pathways and disease-specific pathways, for instance, myocardial infarction and stroke.

The implementation of QEWS was based on the Between the Flags program, which was originally established in New South Wales (NSW), Australia (Hughes et al., 2014). Although there are many differences between the two health systems, our theory of change was that the successful implementation of QEWS could be achieved using the same principles as were used in NSW. This would strongly support the hypothesis that there is a "recipe" that can be used to implement safety programs at scale in diverse health systems.

Prospects for Further Success and Next Steps

The key factor which will ensure ongoing success is to ensure local ownership, oversight, and improvement at a facility and hospital level; this will be strengthened by the development of robust local governance systems, which will both oversee local data and performance and provide assurance to hospital boards that there are systems in place to reduce the risk to patients. In order to minimize the burden on busy staff, we have recommended that the local governance system be integrated into existing committee structures, such as facility level cardiopulmonary resuscitation (CPR) committees or equivalent.

A critical part of the improvement work HMC is undertaking is developing capacity and capability in quality improvement with the U.S.-based Institute for Healthcare Improvement (IHI). Part of HMC's work with IHI includes a harm-reduction collaborative. A number of the elements of the harm-reduction collaborative have been deliberately aligned with the QEWS, both to maximize the impact of such interventions, to reduce time load and confusion among staff, and to ensure that knowledge and skills developed in the collaborative are used to improve elements of the QEWS as required. The common elements include standard handovers using Situation Background Assessment Recommendation (SBAR), reliably measuring vital signs, and escalating care appropriately. We have therefore ensured that definitions and measures are aligned, that a single reporting tool can be used, and that all related work is visible in terms of governance oversight.

Final Messages

Large-scale implementation based on strong evidence and good design that ensures integration with other initiatives (ideally integrated by means of a well-designed and -executed strategy), undoubtedly provides the best opportunity to deliver comprehensive system improvement.

Acknowledgments

We wish to acknowledge the support of the following: Her Excellency, Dr. Hanan Al-Kuwari; Professor Ann Marie Cannaby; Professor Mike Richmond; Mr. Colin Hackwood; Nursing Research and Education, Hamad International Training Center; Hamad Informatics and Communications Technology; and the QEWS team.

47

The United Arab Emirates

Abu Dhabi Healthcare Reform: Improving Quality through a Single Payment System

Subashnie Devkaran

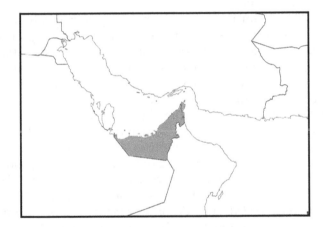

CONTENTS

Background

The United Arab Emirates (UAE) is a federation of seven emirates. The capital and largest emirate is Abu Dhabi, followed by Ajman, Dubai, Fujairah, Ras al-Khaimah, Sharjah, and Umm al-Quwain (Table 47.1). Since independence

TABLE 47.1

UAE Demographics (July 2016)

Indicator	Value
UAE population total	9,267,701
Ratio of Emirati to expatriates	1:9
Deaths per day	47
Births per day	261

Source: United Nations.

in 1971, the UAE has focused on the delivery of high-quality healthcare. The Ministry of Health, established in 1972, is the federal body responsible for healthcare delivery, healthcare policy, healthcare professional practice, and education (Douglas, 2015).

In the early 2000s, reforms to the UAE health system, involving devolution of healthcare regulation, resulted in decentralized funding, decision-making, and independent health authorities for Dubai and Abu Dhabi. The major reforms were predicated on numerous factors. First, there were increases in per capita healthcare spending caused by immigration-driven population growth and the increasing burden of lifestyle diseases and chronic diseases due to sedentary lifestyles and aging. Second, there was diminished trust in local healthcare services and a perception that healthcare in the UAE was inferior to that of many developed countries. Many Emiratis chose to travel to the West for treatment (particularly to Germany, Switzerland, and the United States), even when the procedures were available in the UAE. The costs of sending Emiratis abroad for lengthy treatment regimens created many challenges. In addition, the UAE 2021 Vision set ambitious targets to increase the quality of healthcare to international best practice standards (Table 47.2).

TABLE 47.2

UAE 2021 Vision Indicators

Indicators	2012 Result	2021 Target
Deaths from cardiovascular disease per 100,000 population	211	158.2
Prevalence of diabetes	19.02%	16.28%
Deaths from cancer per 100,000 population	78	64.2
Average healthy life expectancy	67	73
Physicians per 1,000 population	1.5	2.9
Nurses per 1,000 population	3.5	6
Prevalence of smoking	21.6% (men) 1.9% (women)	15.7% (men) 1.66% (women)
Percentage of accredited health facilities	46.8%	100%

Source: UAE Vision 2021.

In 2007, under the new Dubai Health Authority, Dubai advocated the adoption of private health insurance and private providers were promoted. The new Health Authority–Abu Dhabi took a more radical stance by mandating private health insurance for all its residents in 2006 (Vetter and Boecker, 2012). This chapter focuses on the improvement story of the Abu Dhabi health system and its transformation from a fully government-funded sector to a predominantly private sector in just 1 decade (2005–2015).

Details of the Success Story

The Emirate of Abu Dhabi has become one of the most prosperous places on the globe, with more than 10% of the world's oil and 3% of all natural gas reserves (Statistics Centre [Abu Dhabi], 2016). It was expected, therefore, that the government would continue to invest heavily in the health sector to provide free "world-class" healthcare to its residents. However, in 2005 it became clear that the government was not going to make further investments without a clear understanding of the population's health status and medical needs, and without hard data on the current health systems' performance and financial accountability. Consequently, the government demanded a stringent long-term vision for the health system, favoring a predominantly private provision system (Vetter and Boecker, 2012).

Due to the many interdependencies and the scope of the reform, the major challenge was delivering tangible and measurable improvements within a short time frame. Further complexity was added by persistent complaints from users of the existing health system, and vociferous opposition from change-resistant factions within the system (Vetter and Boecker, 2012). These factors resulted in a loss of faith and withdrawal of support by the political decision makers. Thus, the administrators of the reform prioritized a critical path to leverage time. Step one comprised the rapid introduction of a tiered health insurance scheme to pay for access. One framework for evaluating the overall reform process is set out in a number of recent publications dealing with health reform (Doetinchem et al., 2010; WHO, 2001). Following these suggested guidelines, reform involved continuously increasing the trust of all relevant stakeholders in the reform process, as well as trust in the health system itself. The holistic and concerted use of five "control knobs" to achieve desired outcomes advocated "financing, payment, organization, regulation, and behavior." The health reform program in Abu Dhabi made conscious use of all five control knobs in a sequenced and concerted fashion, achieving considerable success. Abu Dhabi is now known in the region not only for its relatively seamless introduction of health insurance (financing), but also for establishing an independent regulatory organization (Vetter and Boecker, 2012).

The Reform Time-Line

The first component of the reform involved the regulatory devolution of the federal Ministry of Health to allow each emirate autonomy over a number of policies. Abu Dhabi and Dubai created their own health authorities. Next, in July 2005, the ruler of Abu Dhabi passed Law No. 23, the Abu Dhabi Health Insurance Regulation Bill. This law obliged all employers/sponsors in Abu Dhabi to provide health insurance for expatriates residing and working in the Emirate of Abu Dhabi. Free insurance coverage was provided by the Abu Dhabi government for all Emiratis. The approval of the new vision for Abu Dhabi by the Executive Council followed in March 2006. Following this, there was a focus on developing the private healthcare sector and increasing public–private partnerships to benefit service quality and shift the cost burden from the government. Management of local public hospitals was contracted to international organizations such as the U.S.-based Cleveland Clinic and Johns Hopkins Medicine International to encourage knowledge transfer of best practices (Douglas, 2015).

In order to increase regulatory and payment transparency, the government entity then legislated a division of responsibilities. The Health Authority—Abu Dhabi (HAAD) was mandated to regulate the healthcare industry and to develop Abu Dhabi's health policy, while Abu Dhabi Health Services Company (SEHA) was made responsible for managing government-owned healthcare facilities (Vetter and Boecker, 2012).

Data standards were released in January 2008 to regulate the automatic data flows from the e-claim submissions (Table 47.3). Once valuable information was received from the e-claims, the regulators turned their immediate attention to quality. The introduction of diagnostic-related groups removed the volume-based, fee-for-service structure. Clinical coding audits improved coding quality and consequently, data integrity. Pharmacy benefits management enabled the use of e-prescriptions and permitted automated monitoring of potential harmful drug interactions and overdosing, while service providers benefited from faster processing of insurance claims.

The Impact of the Abu Dhabi Healthcare Reform Program

When implementing major healthcare reforms, it is often difficult to quantify success in terms of one-to-one outcomes. However, if numerous positive customer satisfaction survey results are any indication, it appears that trust in the system is improving steadily. Perhaps a more tangible result can be seen in the significant increase in private sector investment in the provision sector (Health Authority [Abu Dhabi], 2014).

TABLE 47.3

The Abu Dhabi Reform Time-Line

	Reform Time-Line
July 2005	Health Insurance Law released
March 2006	Vision for the Health System approved by the Executive Council
June 2006	First expatriate insured in health insurance scheme
Quarter 1 2007	Management service agreements signed with Johns Hopkins International, Cleveland Clinic, Bumrungrad International, and VAMed/University of Vienna for the large public hospitals
January 2008	Government entity GAHS splits into a regulator, HAAD, and an owner of the healthcare assets, SEHA
January 2008	Data standards released
April 2008	Health insurance for nationals starts
October 2008	First e-claim submitted
April 2009	Pay for quality scheme introduced
August 2010	DRGs implemented for the basic product
July 2011	Clinical coding audits become reimbursement relevant
April 2012	Pharmacy benefits management becomes mandatory

Source: Adapted from Vetter, P. and Boecker, K. (2012). *Health Policy*, 108 (2–3), 105–114.

As a consequence of the reforms, the insurance claim format was uniquely redesigned, and now contains most of the critical clinical information available in the health record: all diagnoses, procedures, drugs, investigations (including key results, such as cholesterol or HbA1c tests), along with the treating clinicians, are encoded in each claim. By making doctors and hospitals comparable in a standardized and fair manner, the regulator can quickly become the true informed voice of the general public and guardian of patients' interests (Vetter and Boecker, 2012).

In what is a clear validation of the perceived competency of the improved system, the number of patients the HAAD approved for treatment abroad halved between 2010 and 2013, as new international hospitals began offering specialist treatments (Koornneef et al., 2012). The UAE, which had been pushing for the accreditation of providers to global standards for some years, escalated their campaign after the advent of mandatory health insurance in 2006. Since then, some hospitals have completed three accreditation cycles, predominantly by the Joint Commission International (JCI), a U.S.-based non-profit organization. So far, 131 healthcare organizations in the UAE have received a JCI Gold Seal, representing 16% of the JCI's global accreditations across 70 countries; this compares with just one accreditation before 2006 (Joint Commission International [JCI], 2016). The JCI has also assisted the HAAD in developing its standards for licensing hospitals.

In terms of access, virtually all residents are now covered by insurance and can therefore access the basic healthcare that they require with the freedom to choose their provider (Koornneef et al., 2012). According to Vetter and

Boecker (2012), by 2012, 95% of residents had access to healthcare. From 2009 to 2013 there was a 21% (681) increase in the number of hospital beds. The increased market competition promoted the development of new services and increased efficiency of existing services. By 2013, there was a reduction in the service/specialty gaps with a 20% growth in the number of emergency physicians and a 41% growth in neonatologists over one year. Ten new private hospitals have opened in the last 5 years. Over the past 5 years, the number of doctors per 10,000 population has increased by 9% and nurses by 24%, with the private sector responsible for 74% of the increase in the number of physicians (JCI, 2016). Currently, healthcare providers are independent, predominantly private, and internationally accredited.

Transferability of the Exemplar

Within the UAE, the model of the Abu Dhabi reform is considered an exemplar and is gradually being replicated within the other emirates. In Dubai, mandatory insurance is now being rolled out under a February 2014 law requiring the population of the entire emirate to be covered by 2016 (Douglas, 2015). Sharjah is expected to establish a health authority and implement policies in line with Abu Dhabi. As a federal law on mandatory insurance was drafted in 2013, the northern emirates are likely to follow.

Universal coverage remains a challenge internationally, and lessons from the successful implementation of a single payment system in Abu Dhabi may help other countries meet this challenge. WHO (2013) suggests that GCC governments bear 64% of total healthcare costs in the region. Given the decline in oil prices, Gulf countries now face the challenge of continuing to use oil revenues to fund increasing healthcare costs. GCC governments are increasingly making health insurance mandatory in a bid to reduce costs and improve healthcare standards. This is expected to drive demand for medical services as out-of-pocket expenditures decrease, which in turn is expected to draw private investment into the healthcare sector.

Prospects for Further Success

A number of interventions and policies could sustain progress and assist the UAE in achieving its 2021 targets. A transparent public reporting system is currently being developed, with the HAAD working on an Abu Dhabi Healthcare Quality Index, which could guide public decision-making about service providers (Koornneef, 2012). Although regulatory devolution allows each emirate to adapt to changing population needs, this could create federal fragmentation. Emerging variation in the regulatory infrastructure increases the logistical burden as providers must navigate different regulatory systems in what is a relatively small market. Integration and harmonization across emirates could support efficiency and thereby allow providers to leverage the economies of scale. Minimum standards for health professional licensing may address staffing shortages. Alignment of policies on healthcare information will support the vision of a unified patient record.

Conclusion

The Abu Dhabi reform program has progressively attained the triple aims. Not only is healthcare in Abu Dhabi affordable, due to the tiered insurance system, standards of care are high, as demonstrated by the number of accredited organizations, and care is accessible—with 95% of the population covered by the end of 2012 (Berwick, 2003; Vetter and Boecker, 2012).

Ayers and Braithwaite's (1992) model of "responsive regulation" asserts that regulatory interventions are more likely to succeed if they are responsive to the culture, context, and conduct of the regulated organizations. As a responsive regulator, the HAAD's successes include

- Beneficial partnerships with major international healthcare brands diversifying the provider mix
- Increased number of internationally accredited facilities
- Improved access due to compulsory insurance
- Increased bed capacity and healthcare professionals
- Responsive regulation to manage emerging public health challenges
- Meaningful use of data

By 2021, use of administrative data for pay-for-quality initiatives, public reporting on outcomes, and patient engagement initiatives may advance patient-centered care. Furthermore, as trust in local healthcare grows, so too will healthcare investment. Should the 2021 vision become a reality, the UAE will not only be a preferred place to live and work, but a place to receive world-class healthcare as well.

48

Yemen

Improvement of Basic Health Services in Yemen: A Successful Donor-Driven Improvement Initiative

Khaled Al-Surimi

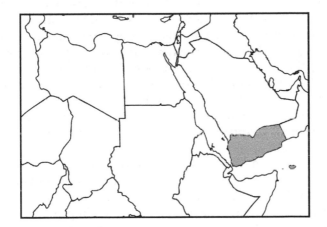

CONTENTS

Background

The Republic of Yemen (c. 25.5 million population) consists of 21 administrative and geographical units called governorates and 334 districts (WHO, 2009, 2016a). While the past few decades have seen significant attempts at comprehensive public sector reform based on principles of decentralization, democratization, civil service modernization, and financial restructuring, Yemen still faces a number of economic and developmental obstacles to sustaining economic development and political reform and achieving its strategic development goals (WHO, 2009). These include a relatively high annual population increase of 3%; a highly dispersed population, with 70% living in isolated rural hamlets; low levels of education; large gender disparities; high unemployment and limited job opportunities; a fragile infrastructure with limited roads and services; water scarcity; and non-functional administrative and financial reforms. Average Yemeni life expectancy at birth is 62.5 years, which is low when compared with the global average of 67.5 years, the Arab states average of 68.5 years, or Japan's average of 82.7 years. This low average life expectancy is one of the factors accounting for Yemen's comparatively low ranking on the Human Development Index (HDI), where Yemen ranks 160th of 182 countries, making it one of the least-developed countries in the world (United Nations Development Programme, 2014a).

The health system in Yemen is made up of three tiers: primary, secondary, and tertiary care (Ministry of Public Health and Population [MoPHP] [Yemen], 2000). While morbidity/mortality rates remain relatively high, health indicators in Yemen have been steadily improving over the last decades, despite a lack of coherent healthcare policies. The health system suffers from multiple shortcomings, including a severe shortage and maldistribution of qualified staff, a lack of essential medicines, and insufficient allocation of funding. Additionally, there is a marked discrepancy between the country's health priorities, available resources, and management (United States Agency for International Development [USAID], 2014b). The healthcare system lacks coordinated monitoring and evaluation systems that could help build an effective referral system or facilitate the integration of basic services at the healthcare delivery point.

Despite these disqualifications, several health system improvement initiatives have been introduced to improve health system performance in Yemen in the last 20 years. The landmark initiative occurred in 1998 after reforms instituted by the MoPHP (2000). One of the main components of the health reform strategy was introducing the concept of a district health system (DHS). The key improvement aim behind establishing the DHS was to provide the foundations to support other reform elements, such as management decentralization, community participation, and inter-sectoral cooperation. Access and availability of care at the community level was improved through the provision of an essential service package targeted at district health system facilities, such as district hospitals, health centers, and health units.

The 1998 health reform strategy also recommended a redefinition of the role of the public sector and encouraged the participation of the private sector. Other significant structural reforms included the development of community co-management, cost-sharing, essential medicines policy, and realignment of the logistics system; introducing outcome-based management systems at central and community levels; establishing hospital autonomy and inter-sectoral cooperation; and encouraging a greater focus on donor coordination and sector-wide approaches to donor funding (MoPHP, 2000; World Bank, 2000).

In 2007, MoPHP and its partners engaged in a comprehensive review of the 1998 health sector reform strategy, assessing the ongoing status quo of the health sector, developing benchmarking, and setting new policies and future directions. This review resulted in the development of a new national health sector strategy with a comprehensive set of targets for 2025. The new national health sector strategy focuses on strengthening system performance, specifically the following strategic areas:

- Leadership and governance
- Planning
- Service delivery processes
- Health workforce development
- Management information systems
- Infrastructure
- Medicines and health technology
- Health economics and financing
- Monitoring and evaluation (World Health Organization Regional Office for the Eastern Mediterranean (EMRO-WHO), n.d.).

Donor-Driven Improvement Initiative

Development assistance to Yemen from other nations and international agencies, including the World Bank and the United Nations, has increased steadily over the years (USAID, 2014b). This development assistance has made a significant contribution to improving health system performance. Improving health system quality performance is an essential element in helping countries to meet health goals and improve health outcomes (Donaldson, 2004). Donors who have supported the Yemeni health and population sectors over the years have largely focused on strengthening management and support services at DHS level. Such support has most often been given through providing training and essential resources. More recent efforts led by the World Bank, the European Commission, and the German Technical Cooperation Agency (GTZ) have focused on developing innovative approaches to improving quality of healthcare provision at the DHS level.

The Yemeni German Reproductive Health Program (YGRHP) Quality Improvement Project (QIP) is an example of a particularly successful donor-driven improvement initiative. The YGRHP, which was implemented in seven governorates from 2004 to 2013, was specifically concerned with improving the health sector, with an emphasis on reproductive health, at both management and service level. The program was actively engaged in reproductive health education and promotion (including family planning), among targeted groups, in particular youth and rural communities (German Technical Cooperation Agency [GTZ], 2012). The QIP, which was implemented during the second phase of the YGRHP (2007–2013), was primarily aimed at strengthening the quality management of DHS at seven governorates and their districts. The YGRHP chose to develop the QIP based on a European Foundation Quality Management (EFQM) framework. The EFQM is a system-based approach for managing and improving quality and striving for excellence. Figure 48.1 displays the main elements of the EFQM Excellence Model (Moeller, 2001; Nabitz, et al. 2000).

While all health facilities (HF) in the seven targeted governorates were invited to apply for inclusion in the QIP each year, participation in the program was voluntary. Key staff from selected HFs were then provided with the friendly guidance and support needed to facilitate quality improvement. This guidance involved training staff members to trust one another and work as teams to identify quality-related problems and opportunities, and to develop and implement necessary action plans. The voluntary nature of the QIP helped to create a cooperative

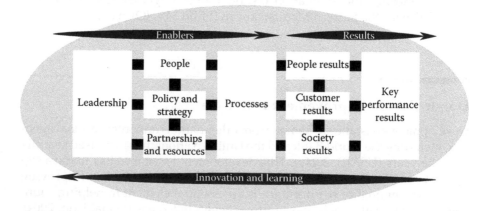

FIGURE 48.1
European foundation quality management (EFQM) excellence model.

atmosphere, and encouraged all HF staff in targeted governorates and districts to work together in order to continuously define and adjust quality standards and objectives, measure results, learn, introduce change, and improve results. The key elements of the QIP initiative (GTZ, 2010) comprised the following:

Field Visits by Quality Assessors or Sadiq ("Friend" in Arabic)

The role of the *Sadiq* in QIP was slightly different to that of the traditional supervisor in the health system hierarchy. During the field visit, the *Sadiq* advised HF staff, explaining the QIP approach, holding friendly meetings with each staff member, listening to them, making observations, and then reporting the findings at a plenary meeting attended by all staff. At the meeting, the quality assessor played the role of facilitator, helping staff to reach agreement on specific problems and opportunities and helping to develop an action plan related to their needs, including assessing individual training requirements along with tailored logistical support.

On-the-Job Training

The QIP team provided experts in three main areas:

1. HF quality management
2. Hygiene and infection control
3. Reproductive health services

Management trainers taught staff how to keep patient records and how to use data to produce charts showing month-by-month changes in patient numbers and progress toward selected improvement targets.

Quality Assessment and Evaluation

After 14–18 months of friendly guidance and support, the QIP team conducted field evaluations. This usually resulted in the selected HFs receiving quality certification valid for 1 year.

Ongoing Support

The QIP also provided ongoing support for those who didn't achieve the required performance key indicators. Ongoing support became the basis for annual re-evaluation and re-certification.

TABLE 48.1

YGRHP QIP Success and Achievements, 2010

Governorate	Estimated Population	Number of Public HFs	Public HFs with RHS	HF/RHS Certified or on Way to Certification through QIP
YGRHP governorates				
Abyan	485,752	125	44	23
Al-Mahweet	555,717	145	103	23
Amran	966,483	132	105	12
Hajjah	1,668,389	190	112	43
Ibb	2,377,501	229	165	35
Mareb	267,291	95	61	26
Sana'a	1,017,256	197	114	23
Subtotal	7,335,379	1,113	704	185 (26%)
Non-YGRHP governorates				24
All 21 governorates	22,198,000	3,073	1,719	209 (12%)

Source: GTZ. (2010). Quality improvement for health care providers: With friendly guidance and support. Ministry of Public Health Population, Republic of Yemen. Retrieved from https://www.giz.de/expertise/downloads/giz2010-en-ygrhp-quality-improvement.pdf

Project Success and Achievements: Quality Certificate

Successfully evaluated HFs received a certificate signed by the MoPHP. This certificate was awarded in a ceremony in the HF's governorate. The ceremony was witnessed by local authorities including the governorate's governor, and received media coverage. Table 48.1 summarizes the number of certified HFs, as well as those that were on their way to certification in the targeted governorates in 2010.

Lessons Learned and Transferability

One valuable lesson the implementation of the YGRHP QIP has provided is to avoid a traditional hierarchical and top-down supervision approach. The problem with a top-down supervision approach is that staff are unlikely to divulge details of problems if they are afraid of being blamed and disciplined. Thus, the idea of the *Sadiq* as a facilitator of the QIP process was welcomed by HF staff. The *Sadiq* was viewed as someone who is an expert but also a good friend to every member of staff; a mentor who will listen, respect opinions, make tactful observations, and offer friendly guidance and support when required. The QIP's *Sadiq* was chosen from among senior managers of hospitals, health centers, and health authorities (i.e., MoPHP and governorate and district health offices). Great care was taken in selecting the *Sadiq*, as personality, attitudes, and communication skills were considered as valuable as expertise. Once selected, *Sadiqs* were given additional training to help establish mutual trust and good rapport with both managers and staff of participating institutions. Because participation was entirely voluntary, many of the HFs who participated in the QIP may have already had a positive view of the benefits of such a program; and if not, there was no penalty for leaving.

Due to the friendly guidance and support provided by the QIP, the initiative has been successfully implemented in a total of 209 (12%) health facilities in Yemen. Anecdotal evidence shows a number of positive outcomes. For example, there have been significant increases in the uptake of basic health services such as family planning, an increased demand for trained birth attendants, and increased utilization of antenatal and other services. As a result, the MoPHP and YGRHP have called for other development partners at all levels, including international donors, to establish QIP as the main mechanism through which Yemen improves and sustains the quality of healthcare ensuring regular certification/re-certification of healthcare facilities that meet minimum quality standards.

The program has also been successfully replicated in Morocco. The Moroccan QIP expanded from 188 health facilities to 665 facilities in 2 years, and has become the country's main mechanism for the continual monitoring, evaluation, and improvement of its healthcare system and institutions (GTZ, 2010, 2012).

Conclusion

The success of the YGRHP QIP demonstrates that QIP is not merely the product of theoretical work done by experts sitting in offices. Rather, it is the product of learning through practice in health facilities and the communities they serve. The YGRHP QIP was not an attempt to re-invent the wheel. Rather, it showed us that learning from each other in a friendly way, and finding solutions that work in specific contexts while avoiding traditional top-down hierarchies, can be an effective way to bring about change and improvement.

Part V

South-East Asia and the Western Pacific

Yukihiro Matsuyama and Jeffrey Braithwaite

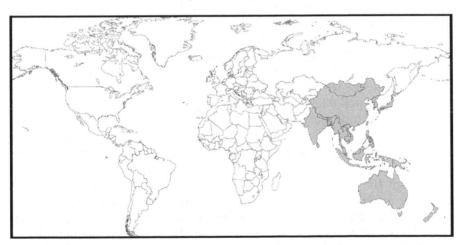

In this final section of the book, we traverse the world once more, this time moving to span two of the World Health Organization's (WHO) regions, South-East Asia and the Western Pacific. This is an extended geographic area, made up of countries that occupy very big and very small landmasses, and with even greater differences between the populations (China and India, with 1.4 billion and 1.3 billion people, respectively, and Fiji and Hong Kong, with 892,100 and 7.2 million people respectively). These countries are defined in large part by their position in two of the biggest bodies of water in the world—the Indian and the Pacific oceans. The nations included in Section V are a diverse group, with vastly different health systems: lower-income Papua New Guinea and Fiji; middle-income China, India, and Malaysia; and high-income Australia, Hong Kong, Japan, New Zealand, and Taiwan. Their success narratives are as diverse as the participating countries' geography.

Hong Fung, Eliza Lai-Yi Wong, Patsy Yuen-Kwan Chau, and Eng-Kiong Yeoh narrate a success story of high-risk in-patients, analyzing the accomplishments of the Hong Kong acute care system in providing more integrated care for elderly patients once they leave hospital. Malaysia too, as Ravindran Jegasothy, Ravichandran Jeganathan, and Safurah Jaafar point out, has had considerable success in reducing the death rates of high-risk patients—with their rates of maternal morbidity in steep decline over the past few decades. Jeffrey Braithwaite and colleagues Clifford Hughes and Charles Pain report on Australia's involvement with hospital-based rapid response systems (also known as medical emergency teams), led for over 2 decades by co-author Professor Ken Hillman, a Sydney-based intensivist with a long-standing interest in the safety of patients. These systems are now widely embraced in many acute settings across the world.

The case studies from China and Taiwan take a different tack. Hao Zheng discusses the way in which the implementation of new information technology (IT) systems in tertiary hospitals in the largest Chinese cities, Beijing and Shanghai, have resulted in technological advancements as well as more efficient treatment of patients. Yu-Chuan (Jack) Li, Wui-Chiang Lee, Min-Huei Hsu, and Usman Iqbal are also interested in technology as an enabler of improved care, in their case, the development of Taiwanese electronic health records, the use of smart cards, the application of a cloud system for storing confidential data, and the MyHealth Bank for accessing health information. This is four stories in one, and, allied to Zheng's Chinese success story, shows how something every health system struggles with—making good use of emerging digital capabilities and health information technology capacities—can become a success story worthy of emulation.

Although the cases presented by Fiji, India, Japan, Papua New Guinea, and New Zealand contrast markedly in their specifics, they are all about strengthening capacities to provide better care across entire health systems. There are multiple ways to do this; in Paulinus Sikosana and Pieter van Maaren's story, despite Papua New Guinea's struggles with poverty, crime, and falling national income, a home-grown policy reform, restructuring health services around a provincial health authority, is noteworthy. In Fiji's case, decentralizing the health services' responsibilities and decision-making capabilities proved to be a worthwhile initiative, and one that was achieved despite earlier setbacks; it's a useful lesson for other developing countries. The lesson of persistence is a crucial one—ably communicated by Jalal Mohammed, Nicola North, and Toni Ashton in this case, along with many others in this volume. In Japan, a relatively rich country, the narrative selected by Yukihiro Matsuyama centers on universal insurance and creating sustainable financial arrangements. For India, as told by Girdhar Gyani, strengthening the coverage of basic, affordable care to a huge population is a prime consideration.

Finally, we can point to a story by Jacqueline Cumming, Jonathon Gray, Lesley Middleton, Haidee Davis, Geraint Martin, and Patricia Hayward from New Zealand, which has parallels with those of Fiji and Papua New Guinea, but in a high-income country. The success of strengthening quality improvement expertise in the health system through the establishment of Ko Awatea, an agency intent on promoting improvement through innovative means, is of value to developed and developing countries alike. This New Zealand chapter, in concert with those of Fiji, India, Japan, and Papua New Guinea, provides lessons in how to take a systems approach, emphasizing collaboration, training and empowering staff, and capacity building.

49

Australia

Two Decades of Evolving a Patient Safety System: An Australian Story of Reducing Harm to Deteriorating Patients

Jeffrey Braithwaite, Ken Hillman, Charles Pain, and Clifford F. Hughes

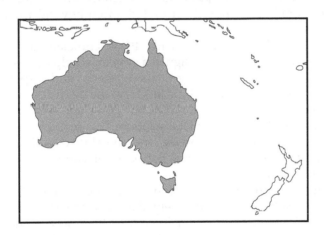

CONTENTS

Background

This is a story about an innovative Australian patient safety system, designed by clinicians and refined through 2 decades of endeavor and experimentation. Its latest evolution into a state-wide system was stimulated by top-down endorsement after a major enquiry and was delivered through middle-out expertise sponsored by the Clinical Excellence Commission in New South Wales: the Between the Flags (BtF) system (Coiera, 2009). The precursor to BtF was the medical emergency team (MET) concept, one of the most successful improvement initiatives in the last 20 years.

A Historical Perspective on Managing Patients' Deterioration

Over 30 years ago, many inpatient deaths and cardiac arrests were recognized by clinicians as being potentially preventable. It may seem amazing, therefore, that hospital patients who deteriorated were only visited by a "crash team" after they deteriorated, often beyond the point of no return.

This was so for decades. In the early 1990s, clinicians at the Liverpool Hospital, in Sydney, Australia, designed a system to help colleagues identify deteriorating patients earlier using defined criteria, and responded with a MET comprised of experienced clinicians from the intensive care unit (ICU). The MET system was designed by front-line clinicians who recognized the problem and were able to construct a solution. This required content knowledge, a collective front-line response, and the ability to design new care models on the ground. Management, policymakers, and regulators were not involved at this point.

At that time, this kind of organization-wide, patient-centered system could not have been developed and implemented in many major teaching hospitals: they were too big; there was too much red tape; there were competing medical egos and too many warring clinical tribes. Having ICU staff responding to ward-based patients in decline wasn't the way things were done and changing a system could threaten medical autonomy. Indeed, patients in virtually all health systems were "owned" by the admitting doctor, not the intensive care physicians, who were not authorized to attend to patients if they deteriorated. There was also a diffusion of responsibility, and patients fell through the cracks in the clinical accountability system (Hillman et al., 2011).

One of the authors of this chapter, Ken Hillman, had tried unsuccessfully to implement an early warning response system at a large London teaching hospital in the mid-eighties, but inertia and overt obstruction made it impossible. At the time of the implementation of the MET system, the administrative and medical hierarchies were less entrenched at Liverpool, which was then a fledgling teaching hospital, and so less likely to inhibit innovation and impede adoption of new ideas. Liverpool at the time was an institutional version of the Galapagos Islands: an evolutionary incubator, ready for change, with an experimental culture.

Impact and Spread

Ken Hillman's test-bed activities at Liverpool inspired some early adopters in the United States and the United Kingdom in the early 1990s. In fits and starts, initially low-level publications and conference presentations encouraged other clinicians around the world to slowly examine, and then eventually embrace, the MET concept (Winters and DeVita, 2011). Dissemination was by subtle clinical networks and informal discussions, with advocates latching on to the idea and visiting one another. Change remained incremental, and wholly bottom-up. Small numbers of hospitals participated, but increasing curiosity and adaptation occurred over the next 10 years, with small-scale conferences and localized publications in modest journals. Evidently, clinicians must feel it is their system, and their local initiative.

A large demonstration study was eventually funded by Australia's National Health and Medical Research Council (NHMRC), enrolling 23 hospitals (the Medical Emergency Response and Intervention Trial [MERIT]). The results, published in 2005 in *The Lancet*, were inconclusive in some ways but demonstrated a significant reduction in mortality in the intervention hospitals (Chen et al., 2009a; Hillman et al., 2005).

By the mid-2000s, the concept had reached policymakers in many countries. Often, there were triggering events such as the severe acute respiratory syndrome (SARS) epidemic in Ontario, Canada, leading to physician-initiated and government-funded implementation of systems in every hospital. An outreach medical response program emerged in the United Kingdom, with doctors and nurses working together with policymakers to develop recommendations for adoption. Standardized implementation occurred in every hospital in the Copenhagen district of Denmark. In the United States, Ken Hillman had discussions with the doyen of systems redesign, Dr. Don Berwick, with the Institute of Healthcare Improvement then taking a lead advocacy role for MET implementation.

Australia had signaled a significant change to the silos of clinical team practice. It was clear that ICU expertise could be delivered quickly and effectively across unit boundaries, but there were still obstacles to implementing the MET concept across the whole health system. The Clinical Excellence Commission (CEC) had embarked upon a clinical (bottom-up) review of success factors of early recognition, and appropriate escalation to a MET call. This informed the development of the BtF system, which was based on color-coded, standardized observational charts with clinician-derived prompts for escalation, which were able to be customized to the local context (Hughes et al., 2014).

Then in 2005 in New South Wales (NSW), 16-year-old Vanessa Anderson was struck on the head by a golf ball. After admission to Royal North Shore Hospital in Sydney, she died in her bed without anyone recognizing that she was deteriorating. The resulting Garling Inquiry recommended that a system be introduced in all NSW hospitals, using a five-element design proposed by the Clinical Excellence Commission, based on Ken Hillman's original MET ideas (Garling, 2008). This subsequently became a mandatory feature of NSW hospitals. A major top-down mechanism had now been invoked. The initiative was now sanctioned at all levels: the ward, the clinician-management team, and executives and policy directors in hospitals.

Implementation: Transferability of the Exemplar

To give effect to Garling, two of the authors, Cliff Hughes, CEO of the CEC, and Charles Pain, the CEC's director of health systems improvement, forged a partnership, bridging the interests of clinicians and policymakers. Physicians were again key to the acceptance of the policy by other clinicians. By 2012, every state hospital in NSW had adopted the BtF system (Hughes et al., 2014).

Elsewhere, from the late 2000s to the early 2010s, the MET concept was spreading internationally, like a Mexican wave. METs increasingly became known as rapid response systems (RRSs). The success of MET adoption was demonstrated not only by the widespread uptake of the system, but by the enthusiastic response of staff, especially bedside nursing staff and junior doctors who no longer felt abandoned and could be genuine advocates for their patients by calling for expert help (Santiano, 2009). Nursing staff would even move from hospitals that didn't have an RRS.

As is often the case with real-world change, the evidence followed adoption success, rather than leading the way. Over time, well after the initial bottom-up experimentation era, there were before-and-after studies, then RCTs such as MERIT, and then meta analyses (Aneman et al., 2015; Chen et al., 2009b, 2014; Cretikos et al., 2007; Jones et al., 2012; Maharaj et al., 2015). Another dimension to transferability, finally, was the engagement of government or a key sponsor in the upper echelons of health systems to mandate the RRS (Hughes et al., 2014).

The Recipe for Success, and Prospects for Building Further Success

The MET-RRS-BtF success was created around a real patient safety problem. For entrenched organizational and historical reasons, patients were managed in organizational silos, within clinical disciplines—medicine and surgery, cardiology and orthopedics. Movement between these silos was, and remains, uncommon. Thus, clinical culture can trump patient safety: better to ignore patient deterioration, arrest or death than upset the time-honored way of doing things. The MET changed that.

The ingredients for success can be readily categorized. The problem had to be recognized. Patients at risk had to be identified. Then a system of responding had to be developed around patients' needs. Staff with appropriate training, skills, and experience had to be organized and dispatched to patients, based on their immediate clinical condition. There are many situations where a similar approach can be adopted. The required ingredients are easy to specify, but, as with any recipe, the process is more complex.

Begin with clinicians and a real-world clinical problem. Have them redesign the system around the patient. Define and identify the patient population and then construct a response, experimenting with options to meet patients' needs. Acknowledge that ultimately, universal take-up will best succeed with effective governance. This is where, later, middle-out approaches and top-down support come in. Appreciate that leading with top-down and middle-out approaches at the start of a program rarely achieves these results.

Hospitals that have implemented an RRS have reduced serious adverse events, such as cardiac arrests and mortality by about one-third (Chan et al., 2010; Chen et al., 2009a). There are very few interventions that have had such an impact on patient safety in acute hospitals, and no top-down or middle-out initiatives that we can point to, nationally or internationally (Benning et al., 2011; Landrigan et al., 2010).

Next Steps: New Applications of the MET Experience

One, perhaps counter-intuitive application, generalizable from the MET-RRS-BtF experience, lies with today's over-treatment of the frail elderly in acute hospitals. The present system does not necessarily work in their interests and, additionally, contributes greatly to the unsustainable costs of healthcare (Hillman et al., 2015).

To apply the MET-RRS-BtF experience to this problem, first find motivated clinicians who already recognize the challenges, and want to work to address them. Define the problem from the patient's perspective, and identify the patient population: in this instance, frail elderly patients who are often subject to futile treatment (Cardona-Morrell and Hillman, 2015). Then, develop an appropriate response. This will be more complicated than implementing METs and RRSs. Again, it involves a multidisciplinary approach, with staff working together to improve outcomes and, in this case, to significantly reduce the unsustainable costs of unnecessary care and financial and clinical burdens on elderly patients.

The MET movement took decades to arrive at BtF. Perhaps we can shorten the timescale for reshaping the system of dealing with the frail elderly. That could become another legacy of the MET-RRS-BtF model.

50

China

Self-Service Encounter System in Tertiary Hospitals

Hao Zheng

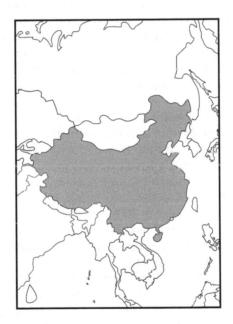

CONTENTS

Background

Health reform has been a fundamental part of each of the Chinese central government's National Five-Year Plans (the 13th such plan runs from 2015 to 2020). In 2009, a new round of health reforms was initiated, with more ambitious goals to provide equitable, affordable, high-quality, and cost-effective health services for all citizens (Li, 2016; *The Lancet*, 2008; 2015).

According to statistics published by the National Health and Family Planning Commission [China] (NHFPC) in September 2015, there are 989,844 health institutions in China. Although hospitals account for only 2.7% of all health facilities, they provide 39% of health services to the population; and while only 7.5% of hospitals are accredited as tertiary hospitals, they provide 48% of hospital services (National Health and Family Planning Commission, 2015a,b). People tend to choose to receive care in hospitals, especially tertiary hospitals, due to the nationwide lack of local, community-based primary healthcare facilities and the huge gap in quality between hospital-based and community-based services.

The lack of an effective health workforce provides another challenge. The unequal distribution of doctors and nurses further affects the efficiency of health delivery. In 2014, more than 85% of doctors reported that they work more than 40 hours per week, with workloads increasing relative to the level of hospital—for instance, nearly 92% of doctors in tertiary hospitals work overtime (Chinese Medical Doctor Association, 2015).

The health reforms launched in 2009 aimed at realizing two major goals: to achieve and sustain universal health coverage, and to enhance the quality of care (*The Lancet*, 2008; 2015). Subsequently, the Ministry of Health (MoH) has initiated a series of annual national campaigns, called "China Medical Quality Champions" (Ministry of Health [China], 2009) to ensure continuous quality improvement and safety in healthcare with a different focus each year. In 2009, the MoH also launched the China Healthcare Quality Indicators System (CHQIS) to assess the quality of health services in hospitals (Zhao, 2009). With growing awareness and recognition of patient safety and quality improvement in healthcare, China's health system is undergoing a significant shift, committing resources to provide safe, high-quality care, initially in tertiary hospitals in major cities.

Self-Service Encounter System in Tertiary Hospitals

Visiting any outpatient department in a tertiary hospital in a major city in China involves long lines and overcrowded waiting rooms; indeed, from published data on hospitals' websites, 70% of tertiary hospitals in Beijing and Shanghai average more than 8000 outpatient visits per day. In order to cope with such large numbers of patients, hospitals have had to find innovative ways to improve management and to increase efficiency of care delivery. One recent innovation that has contributed to improving hospitals' efficiency and patients' experience in outpatient departments in tertiary hospitals is the development and introduction of an integrated health information system (IHIS).

The IHIS contains the many components needed to manage every aspect of a hospital's operation, including a laboratory information system (LIS), policy and procedure management system, picture archiving and communication system (PACS), medication management system (MMS), and electronic health record (EHR) (Chen et al., 2010; Yuan, 2013; Zhang, 2012). This complex system now includes a self-service encounter system (SSES) composed of a self-service registration machine (SSRM), a self-service payment machine (SSPaM), and a self-service printing machine (SSPrM) so that patients are able to manage various administrative aspects of their care themselves (Chen et al., 2010, 2013; Gao, 2011; Guo et al., 2012; Liu, 2012; Lu, 2014; Wang et al., 2008; Wang et al., 2013; Xiao et al., 2012). Patients can choose to use the self-service registration machine to register with preferred doctors, pay through the self-service payment machine, and use the self-service printing machine to check the status of treatments shown clearly on the screen of the machine, and to print out results.

Every patient is assigned a different barcode each time they register at the hospital. This assigned barcode serves as his or her identity in the system. This barcode can only be used for a specific hospital visit and can't be transferred between hospitals. For patients with a medicare number, the assigned barcode will be logged chronologically under that number, representing one specific hospital visit. Patients can choose to use the medicare number or the assigned barcode as their identity for the hospital visit. The doctors' prescriptions will be recorded under the patient's name/medicare number/barcode. After confirmation by the patient/payee, the system will prioritize the treatments, and automatically schedule the patient for laboratory tests or radiology examinations depending on their medical condition—those in more urgent medical situations will be given higher priority. The system estimates the waiting time, and patients are able to undertake required pathology tests or radiology checks. Patients need not wait for their pathology or radiology reports, as these are usually released within 24–48 hours, and can be printed out once the patient scans his/her medicare card or the barcode at any SSPrM in the hospital in the next 30–60 days. Details of prescribed drugs are also registered and are packed ready for patients to pick up at a designated window in the pharmacy.

Impact of the Self-Service Encounter System

While there is not yet evidence-based research evaluating the overall effect or impact of IHIS and SSES, the immediate benefits to patients, as well as medical and administrative staff were reported to be positive (Chen et al., 2010, 2013; Gao, 2011; Guo et al., 2012; Liu, 2012; Lu, 2014; Wang et al., 2008; Wang et al., 2013; Xiao et al., 2012; Yuan, 2013; Zhang, 2012). Benefits to patients include

- A significant reduction in waiting time. Rather than waiting in long lines, patients follow the system's instructions for treatments. For example, in a regular busy tertiary hospital in Shanghai, the waiting time for patients to undertake prescribed laboratory tests has been shortened to about 20 minutes at peak times and about 5 minutes at other times between 7:00 am and 5:00 pm weekdays.
- Ease of use: while hospital volunteers can help patients, especially the elderly, to use the machine, the majority of patients feel comfortable using it themselves.
- The generation of computerized medical records: patients can easily check on SSPrM to follow tests and treatments prescribed.
- Patient privacy is safeguarded. The provision of unique identity codes means that only patients have access to their reports.

Benefits to healthcare professionals include

- Improved work efficiency: repeated or duplicate tests/procedures are reduced through automating manual processes.
- More effective communication is achieved through rapid dissemination across units.
- The use of guidelines and protocols is supported. The system facilitates the standardization of clinical procedures, which may contribute to a reduction of errors and improved quality of care.

Benefits to hospital managers and administrators include

- The system automatically collects real-time data following every administrative, medical, and operational procedure in the hospital, thus providing evidence for workload management, process management, and performance-based assessments, as well as recommending policy direction and changes to improve safety and quality.

- Hospital operations and workflows are monitored in order to coordinate the use of resources, especially in busy hours. For instance, more staff and facilities are assigned to provide necessary services during peak periods.

Dependency on the system has proved to be a major challenge. While a malfunction in one component of IHIS usually won't disrupt the other components or the system as a whole, server or network problems can lead to a total system breakdown. A backup and recovery system must be installed to ensure data security and to restore the system in about 10 minutes (Chen et al., 2010; Yuan, 2013; Zhang, 2012). Information technical support has to be on standby 24 hours, 7 days a week, in case of system breakdown to avoid immediate overcrowding in the waiting room.

Transferability

The success of the IHIS in China's hospitals sets a strong example to encourage further integration of information technology across healthcare in other countries. It has simplified medical processes for patients and reduced workloads for health professionals. More importantly, the system has proved that health information technology (HIT) encourages patients to actively partner in their own healthcare and facilitates interdepartmental communication between health professionals, leading to a better quality of patient care.

Next Steps

Currently, each hospital has a different IHIS and SSES. Each was developed and installed by different suppliers and are not comparable or interoperable. With more hospitals introducing IHIS in China, the more ambitious goal is to link individual hospitals' systems to support more straightforward information sharing, thus reducing waste and driving savings of health resources.

Another potential opportunity is to make full use of the big data gathered by IHIS. At the moment, IHIS is mainly used to track patient flows, to simplify clinical processes, to reduce workloads of health professionals, or to respond to inquiries for information. The huge volume of data stored in each hospital's information system has been largely wasted, and should be more effectively mined and analyzed to further support evidence-based care delivery. In addition, more significant real-time data analysis functions are expected to be integrated into IHIS to provide further insight in medical practices.

The HIT annual investment has increased by more than 20% for 5 constitutive years since 2009, reaching 27.52 billion RMB in 2014, which accounted for 0.3–0.5% hospital revenues (China Industry Research, 2015). The Healthy China 2020 strategy research report (Chen, 2012) pointed out that 61.1 billion RMB would be designated to build the National Electronic Health System. This was further emphasized in the 13th National Five-Year Plan, with the goal clearly set to establish three digital national databases by 2020. These databases will comprise health profiles, health information, and medical records, along with a national online platform that integrates information at the national, provincial, municipal, and county levels to allow real-time information update and sharing (Norton Rose Fulbright, 2015).

Conclusion

The use of the IHIS and its associated SSES is still in its early stages in China, nevertheless it already successfully coordinates patients, clinical practice, and management to facilitate information flow and to improve the efficiency and effectiveness of care delivery. It will be further integrated into the health system to eventually change the way in which medicine is practiced.

51

Fiji

A Context-Specific Approach to Primary Care Strengthening in Fiji

Jalal Mohammed, Nicola North, and Toni Ashton

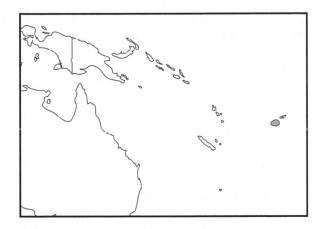

CONTENTS

Background

Two major healthcare reforms have been attempted in Fiji. The reforms differed significantly in both approach and outcome. The first was radical and ambitious, but failed to be supported by Ministry of Health (MoH) personnel and was eventually abandoned. The second, more successful, reform, was tailored to local context (i.e., context specific). It adopted a more gradual and circumscribed approach involving incremental strengthening of community-based health centers and refocusing of ambulatory hospital services.

Universal healthcare in Fiji is mainly provided by the MoH through four divisions (Central, Eastern, Northern, Western) and their subdivisions that deliver healthcare to nearly 1 million people across 332 islands (Ministry of Health and Medical Services [Fiji], 2015a). Each division delivers healthcare through nursing stations (basic care only), health centers (comprehensive primary care), and subdivisional and divisional hospitals (ambulatory and inpatient care at all levels).

Starting in 1979, a series of critical government and external reports highlighted community dissatisfaction with healthcare and declining health outcomes. Criticisms that the MoH did not effectively delegate responsibility, authority, and planning to regional divisions, were related to poor staff morale, high turnover, shortages of staff and drugs, and a mismatch between population changes and staffing levels (Coombe, 1982; Dunn, 1997; Government of Fiji, 1979, 1996, 1997; Ministry of National Planning [Fiji], 2009). Recommendations were for a more responsive healthcare system with improved accessibility (Mohammed et al., 2016a,b; Australian Agency for International Development [AUSAid], 2008). In response, the MoH initiated two periods of reform through decentralization: the first from 1999 to 2004, and the second from 2009, with a brief period of recentralization between.

The first far-reaching reform involved a collaboration between the Fiji government and the Australian Agency for International Development (AUSAid). The reforms involved strengthening healthcare delivery in the four geographic divisions and developing management capacity, reflective of the approaches used in other Pacific countries. However, political instability, coupled with a lack of support from MoH personnel (who viewed the reform as being driven externally by AUSAid), hindered the establishment of the devolved structure (Mohammed et al., 2016a). By the end of the 5-year implementation period, only limited delegation, along with some restructuring of the delivery and organization of services, had been achieved. These changes, however, fell far short of the reform goals (Mohammed et al., 2016a,b).

In 2009, a less ambitious decentralization program was initiated, aiming to improve access to primary care through the strengthening of health centers in the Suva subdivision (one of five in the central division), accounting for approximately one-quarter (217,597 persons) of Fiji's population. This initiative addressed reports that lower-level services were often bypassed by users who self-referred to divisional hospitals, which they perceived as providing better care, indicating that health center resources were underutilized, while divisional hospitals were being used inappropriately (AUSAid, 2008; Ministry of Health [Fiji], 2010; Roberts et al., 2011; WHO, 2000). Over a period of 2 years, services at the six health centers in the Suva subdivision were expanded, enabling the divisional hospital outpatient service to be closed to self-referrals, and designated a tertiary hospital, by February 2011.

This reform initiative followed a *coup d'état* in 2006. A priority of the new government was to improve physical and financial access to healthcare (Ministry of National Planning [Fiji], 2009). With the goals of decentralization widely perceived as benefiting the population, the reform was given some support by both MoH personnel and the general public.

Globally in resource-constrained health systems, there is strong support for expanding primary healthcare to encourage the utilization of lower-level health services and reduce inappropriate utilization of expensive hospital services (Feeney et al., 2005; Kruk et al., 2010; WHO, 2000). The failure of the first healthcare reforms strongly influenced the approach to the second initiative, recognizing the importance of incremental reform in a politically unstable and fragmented society. In light of the documented failure of the first prescriptive approach to radical healthcare reform, this exemplar has been chosen to examine a contrasting approach, whereby health reforms were undertaken using an incremental, context-specific approach.

Details of the Success Story

Fiji's constitution guarantees a right to health, which is reflected in universal health coverage with an emphasis on primary healthcare (see Figure 51.1). Primary healthcare strengthening is thus central to Fiji's health reforms and to the aims of achieving accessible, responsive, and quality outcomes, as well

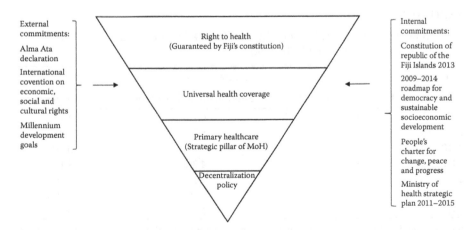

FIGURE 51.1
Framework for primary healthcare in Fiji.

as universal health coverage (Government of Fiji, 2013; Ministry of National Planning [Fiji], 2009).

Starting in 2009, first-contact care was decentralized from hospital outpatient services to the six health centers in the Suva subdivision in order to enhance both access to health services and the responsiveness of primary healthcare, and to encourage the use of outpatient services (Ministry of Health and Medical Services [Fiji], 2016).

Implementation was deliberately incremental, involving the closure of ambulatory hospital services as health centers were expanded. The first three health centers were strengthened in early 2009, then the remaining three in early 2011, after which the divisional hospital ceased accepting self-referrals (Ministry of Health [Fiji], 2011a). Health center strengthening involved upgrading infrastructure and equipment, increasing pharmaceutical and consumable supply, and introducing limited diagnostic services. This was made possible through an increased allocation of government health expenditure to central division health centers following decentralization (from 4.7% in 2008 to 9.2% in 2014; see Table 51.1) (Ministry of Health and Medical Services [Fiji], 2015b). While a centrally defined basic package of health services ensured the delivery of essential health services in all health centers, larger health centers with space were upgraded to provide basic diagnostic services including blood tests, x-rays, and basic scans (Ministry of Health [Fiji], 2010). Access to first-contact healthcare was enhanced by extending hours of operation from 8 to 16 hours per weekday and 8 hours per weekend day (Mohammed et al., 2016b) Health centers underwent structural improvements to cater for increased numbers of users and staff.

During implementation, continuous monitoring allowed for feedback from health centers to MoH planners, and for problems and deficiencies—such as the inadequate supply of pharmaceuticals—to be

TABLE 51.1

Government Current Health Expenditure Allocated to the Central Division, Including Suva Subdivision (2008–2014)

Year	Central division		
	Divisional hospital	Subdivisional hospitals	Health centers
2008	29.4%	6.1%	4.7%
2009	29.6%	5.5%	5.0%
2010	29.2%	5.7%	5.3%
2011	33.5%	4.2%	6.1%
2012	30.1%	4.2%	7.9%
2013	26.9%	4.8%	10.3%
2014	24.4%	5.5%	9.2%

Source: Fiji Health Accounts National Health Expenditure (2011–2014). Note: These figures reflect both decentralized and non-decentralized health centers. Of the total divisional population, 58% live in the Suva subdivision.

identified and remedied. Incremental upgrades to equipment at all health centers—none of which met even the minimum standard equipment requirements prior to decentralization—were made before and after decentralization. Human resources needs, deemed key to the success of the decentralization policy, were continually revised throughout the decentralization process. The number of medical officers and nurses employed in the six health centers increased by 44% and 30%, respectively, following decentralization. New posts for laboratory assistants and radiographers were created at larger health centers to introduce diagnostic services (Ministry of Health [Fiji], 2010, 2011b).

Details of the Impact of the Success Story

In the Suva subdivision, decentralization has resulted in increased utilization of health centers, reflecting the increased availability of community-based services and removal of divisional hospital self-referrals (except after-hours). Comparisons of utilization rates prior to decentralization in March 2008, and following the closure of hospital outpatient services in March 2011, reveal an average increase in utilization of 150% at the six health centers (range 98–225%) and a decrease in utilization of hospital outpatient services by 21% (Ministry of Health [Fiji], 2008, 2011c, 2011d). A close inspection of the first three decentralized health centers shows that the most significant increases in utilization occurred following the closure of hospital outpatient services (see Table 51.2).

TABLE 51.2

Utilization Rates at the First Three Health Centers to be Strengthened

	Health Center A		Health Center B		Health Center C	
	Outpatients seen	Percentage change	Outpatients seen	Percentage change	Outpatients seen	Percentage change
Baseline month	3525	—	4061	—	2429	—
One month post-decentralization	4124	16	6239	54	2568	6
Six months post-decentralization	6703	90	5275	30	3196	32
One month post-closure of divisional hospital to self-referrals	7116	102	7658	89	6135	153

Implementation: Transferability of the Exemplar

Internationally, there has been a marked shift in approaches to reform, involving a move away from a prescribed set of common elements to taking a more context-specific approach (Green et al., 2007; Healy et al., 2006). An incremental approach to health reform is not unique; however, primary care reforms in the Suva subdivision show that reforms need to be context specific. In Fiji's case, changes were gradual and progress was monitored carefully, thus ensuring greater responsiveness to any problems encountered. In addition to MoH support, the harnessing of local "ownership" and engagement from health professionals at lower levels was essential to the reform's success. The approach is transferable not only to other divisions within Fiji, but also to neighboring Pacific island countries that have experimented with prescribed approaches to health reforms but have failed to achieve intended outcomes. Like Fiji, many of these countries are remote and sparsely populated, have centralized administrative systems, and have limited funding and skilled personnel.

Prospects for Further Success and Next Steps

Utilization rates—which provide the MoH's only measure of success—have limitations, in that they do not provide insights into whether visits are first, repeat, or follow-up. Users have no choice but to utilize health centers; further studies are needed to examine whether primary healthcare is acceptable to users. Such studies could examine issues such as waiting time, other barriers to access, whether the type or scope of primary health services are appropriate for users, and why some people opt out of the public health system (Goddard and Smith, 1998). Penchansky and Thomas (1981) offer a possible framework for such an evaluation, which considers personal, financial, and organizational factors in the utilization of healthcare.

Conclusion

Two separate attempts at decentralizing Fiji's health services, each employing a different strategy, indicate that a context-specific, incremental approach has been more successful than a prescribed approach to reform. The first, a major prescriptive reform approach, failed to be supported by MoH personnel and was abandoned. The second more gradual and circumscribed approach, has allowed the MoH to respond to feedback and apply lessons learned as decentralization has been implemented. Wider acceptance and support for the reforms, ensuring local ownership and drive, has, in Fiji's case, accompanied context-specific approaches.

52

Hong Kong

Integrating Care for High-Risk Elderly Patients after Discharge from Hospitals in Hong Kong

Hong Fung, Eliza Lai-Yi Wong, Patsy Yuen-Kwan Chau, and Eng-Kiong Yeoh

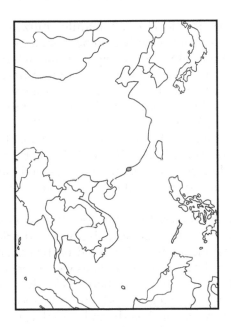

CONTENTS

Background

Hong Kong has a pluralistic healthcare system comprising a highly subsidized public sector funded by general government revenues, along with a private sector that is predominately accessed by fee-paying patients and those who are covered by employment-related benefits. In 2012–2013, private health insurance accounted for only 7% of total health expenditure, and public health expenditure accounted for 2.6% of gross domestic product (Food and Health Bureau [Hong Kong], n.d.). This supported 80.6% of inpatients admitted to 42 public hospitals with 27,440 beds, and 28.9% of outpatients treated in 73 clinics in the whole territory (Census and Statistics Department [Hong Kong], 2015a; Hospital Authority [HA] [Hong Kong], 2015). All these public facilities are operated by a statutory public corporation, the Hospital Authority (HA).

Healthcare services in the HA are mainly utilized by the elderly. In 2013–2014, the total number of elderly patients discharged from Hong Kong's public hospitals totaled 644,836 (41%), representing 51% of total patient days (HA [Hong Kong], 2015). The ratio of utilization of hospital beds between persons aged less than 65 and elderly aged 65 or above was 1:9 (Lo, 2013). By 2034, persons aged 65 or over will make up 30% of the whole population (Census and Statistics Department [Hong Kong], 2015b). Currently, 74.6% of the elderly in the community have at least one chronic disease (Census and Statistics Department [Hong Kong], 2015a). This combination of greater longevity and chronic disease has substantially increased the demand and burden placed on the health system, and the provision of integrated elderly care has become a high priority.

In 2012, the HA developed the Strategic Service Framework (SSF) for elderly patients—incorporating goals, objectives, and priorities for the next 5 years. The SSF was formulated with broad participation from physicians, nurses, and other healthcare professionals, as well as patient representatives. To meet the objectives for the integration of elderly services, the HA has implemented programs to integrate primary and secondary care through chronic disease management; health and social care through high-risk elderly management; and public and private healthcare through programs for public–private partnership.

Among these programs, an integrated program for discharged elderly patients has evolved, which has proved to be an effective intervention for reducing hospital readmissions. The following section will discuss the design of the program and how it has improved care.

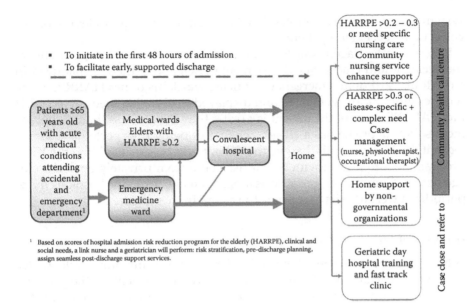

FIGURE 52.1
Components of the integrated care and discharge support (ICDS) for elderly patients in hospital and after discharge.

Integrated Care and Discharge Support for Elderly Patients

The key components of the Integrated Care and Discharge Support for Elderly Patients (ICDS) program appear in Figure 52.1.

Risk Assessment System

The Hospital Admission Risk Reduction Program for the Elderly Living in the Community (HARRPE) utilizes routine data from electronic patient records to develop a validated score to predict the risk of elderly patients aged over 60 experiencing unplanned readmissions within 28 days of discharge.

The risk assessment is composed of 14 variables taken from patient sociodemographics, prior service utilization in the past year, presence and number of comorbidities, and current hospital discharge. The HARRPE score ranges from zero to one. The higher the patients' scores, the higher the probability of their readmission. The scoring system to successfully identify high-risk elderly patients aged over 65 years old was validated by a receiver-operating characteristic curve analysis of a complete cohort in 2006 (Tsui et al., 2015). The HARRPE model is computerized and built into the clinical information system, so that healthcare professionals can plan discharge strategies for targeted high-risk elderly patients.

When a patient aged over 65, with acute medical conditions, presents at the accident and emergency department (AED) and is then hospitalized in a medical ward or an emergency medicine ward, his or her HARRPE score will be automatically generated and displayed in his or her medical record. If the HARRPE score of the patient is greater than 0.2 and less than 0.4 (which means that he or she has a 20–40% chance of being unexpectedly readmitted within 28 days of discharge), the patient will be recruited into the ICDS program. Most patients with >40% risk come from privately operated old-age homes. Community geriatric assessment teams from the hospitals make periodic outreach visits to support the carers in these homes.

Integrated Discharge Support Service

When a patient is registered in the ICDS program, a link nurse collaborates with a geriatrician to perform a comprehensive assessment for the patient's pre- and post-discharge plan. The role of the link nurse is to connect the health and social care organizations that can best provide the care needed by the elderly patients on discharge to their home in the community.

For those patients with a HARRPE score between 0.2 and 0.3, or those requiring specific nursing support at home, an Enhanced Community Nurse Service—which provides follow-up home visits by community nurses—will be provided. For those with HARRPE scores greater than 0.3, or those requiring complex care, case managers, along with a multidisciplinary team of nurses, physiotherapists, and occupational therapists, will take care of the patient. The patient may be referred to fast track clinics or geriatric day hospitals for continuing treatment and rehabilitation. Such intensive follow-up under ICDS typically lasts for 4 weeks.

The home support team (HST) under the ICDS is usually provided by a non-government organization (NGO). After the patient is discharged, the HST is responsible for providing caregiver training and transitional home-care support. The home support service is provided for an average of 9 weeks (Labour and Welfare Bureau and HA [Hong Kong], 2011). Standardized information is used by case managers and NGOs for assessment and discharge planning, home visits, telephone consultations, case conferences, and closing case summaries (Yiu et al., 2013).

Community Health Call Centre

The Community Health Call Centre (CHCC) is a nurse-led program that was established to proactively integrate information sharing, medical informatics, and tele-nursing practice. A telephone nursing consultation service was first set up in the eastern region of Hong Kong in January 2003, and became fully functioning by June 2004 (Ho, 2006). In 2009, a patient support call center (PSCS) was set up to centralize all services (HA [Hong Kong], 2014). By 2011, the service covered all of the Hong Kong Special Administration Region. The following year, another team, mental health direct (MHD), was established to provide a coordinated 24-hour mental health service. Both PSCS and MHD are located in the CHCC.

Nurses in the CHCC contact the patients as soon as they are discharged from the ICDS. A total of 92 clinical protocols for complaints, such as abdominal pain, symptoms of diabetes mellitus, and shortness of breath have been developed to help the CHCC nurses provide timely advice to the patients. Patients can also call the PSCS themselves, during daily office hours. Their calls will be answered within 20 seconds.

Overall Results

The integrated discharge support service demonstrated positive outcomes for its elderly patients, improving both functional outcomes and quality of life. This significantly reduced carers' stress and increased the satisfaction of both carers and patients (Labour and Welfare Bureau and HA [Hong Kong], 2011; Ng et al., 2011). Furthermore, implementation of the program has led to significantly reduced emergency admissions to medical wards, decreased acute patient days in medical wards, and less frequent AED presentation.

Two studies have been conducted to evaluate the ICDS (Hui et al., 2014; Lin et al., 2015). In 2012–2013, the average length of hospital stays in the eastern region of the New Territories went from 5.16 to 4.79 days within 90 days of exiting the ICDS program. Both patients and carers showed significant improvement in their quality of life (Hui et al., 2014). Another study carried out in the western region of Hong Kong Island demonstrated a 40% reduction in AED attendance, a 47% reduction in acute hospital admissions, and a 31% reduction in hospital bed days, just 6 months after implementation of the ICDS. Patients' functional ability was also found to have significantly improved. Unnecessary and frequent readmissions to hospital were therefore 25–50% less likely, representing savings of up to HK$200 million (US$30 million) annually in the HA (Lin et al., 2015).

Evaluation of the telephone nurse consultation service, via a randomized control study from September 2005 to January 2006, showed a decrease in total AED attendance by 36.5% and emergency admission by 35.8%, just 2 months after the introduction of the service (Ho, 2006). Patients and caregivers also rated the program highly (HA [Hong Kong], 2014).

Studies have shown that the relative risk reduction of patients who had received the CHCC service were 27% and 26%, respectively, in the 90-day utilization rate of AED attendance and AED medical admission (Ng, 2014).

The success of the CHCC has also been recognized beyond the medical world—in 2012 it was named Best Innovation and Research in the Hong Kong Information and Communication Technology Awards (Ng, 2011).

Summary

The ICDS has successfully integrated health and social care. It has combined components of well-evaluated programs, which have been connected and extended into an integrated program serving the whole territory. All programs incorporate communication and data interchange, protocols and guidelines, evaluation, and staff straining. A well-established infrastructure provides the cornerstone of the program's success.

Information technology (IT) is essential in the integrated program. The HA has created highly accessible electronic patient records (EPR) for all patients, which are shared by all public hospitals. IT provides platforms for the ICDS to make use of EPR for information sharing, build up unifying protocols, standardize care plans and procedures, and monitor performance. IT facilitates collaboration between all of the services: enabling clinicians, care managers, link nurses, and social workers to effectively join forces for the benefit of the patient.

Risk stratification and assessment in the ICDS provides evidence about the use of data analytics to drive change. It applies not only to risk stratification but also case management as well as specialist disease managements to prioritize intervention strategies. Outcome evaluation is highly dependent of data analytics.

Acknowledgment

We would like to thank to Dr. Elsie Hui, Shatin Hospital, New Territories East Cluster who provided us with Figure 52.1.

53

India

India's Road Map to "Affordable and Safe Health for All" through Public–Private Partnership

Girdhar Gyani

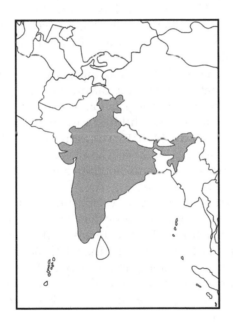

CONTENTS

Background

Health for all, or universal health coverage (UHC), aims to provide accessible, affordable, and appropriate health services for all citizens in any part of the country, regardless of their socioeconomic status, or the class to which they belong. It offers financial protection to an individual during illness, thereby reducing out-of-pocket expenditure while ensuring accessible, affordable, and quality full-spectrum healthcare.

Most nations with UHC spend between 5% and 12% of GDP on health. In India, the government provides about 1%, while the private sector contributes 4%, bringing it up to a healthy 5%. This suggests that if public and private sectors were to join forces, UHC should be possible in India. As per the 12th Five-Year Plan (2012–2017), India is committed to UHC by the year 2022. This is based on the assessment by the High-Level Expert Group (HLEG) on Universal Health Coverage, constituted by the Planning Commission of India in October, 2010.

India, like many other nations, is moving toward becoming a developed nation. No longer a nation where the majority of the population is mired in acute poverty, India now has legislation in place to guarantee a number of human rights, including the Children's Right to Free and Compulsory Education Act of 2009 and the Mahatma Gandhi National Rural Employment Guarantee ACT (MNREGA) of 2005. The majority of the population now receives minimum wage, food, and clothing, and slowly but surely, healthcare is becoming an election issue.

The Indian government, intent on establishing UHC, is working to get the support of private healthcare providers and insurance companies. In the Indian federal structure, where there are 29 states, healthcare is a state responsibility. While each state is pursuing UHC individually, in a manner that best suits their unique demographics, they all have much to learn from one another. Seven states have successfully implemented UHC for the vast majority of their population, and a number of other states are close to experiencing the same success.

The story of how these seven states have implemented UHC by way of government-sponsored health insurance schemes (GSHISs) provides an interesting case study of successful healthcare development. Some of the innovative features common to all these schemes, which use a public–private partnership (PPP) model, include giving patients the choice to visit any public or private provider empaneled by the government. In most schemes, hospitals provide free treatment. These schemes target low-income groups, make impressive use of information and communication technology, and use pre-agreed package rates for payment. The package rates are fixed by the government and are accepted by the private hospitals through a formal agreement. The payment is released by the government to the hospital post-treatment.

This is a win-win formula for the government, for the private health sector, and above all—the population.

Details of the Success Story

The Indian government has a huge healthcare infrastructure by way of primary health centers (PHCs) and community health centers (CHCs) in rural regions. The PHCs and CHCs are supported by district hospitals and teaching hospitals, who deal with secondary and tertiary care services respectively. There is also a wide network of private healthcare providers. About 70% of outpatient department (OPD) and 60% of inpatient department (IPD) services are being catered for by the private sector, which is mainly present in urban areas.

Until recently, it was widely recognized that in most instances, the Indian population was bearing the cost of out-of-pocket healthcare expenses. It is also believed that the payment of unexpected healthcare expenses pushed many families below the poverty line. This scenario, however, is beginning to change for the better. A recent World Bank report, "Government-Sponsored Health Insurance in India: Are You Covered" stated that these schemes were introducing explicit entitlements, improving accountability, and leveraging private capacity, particularly with the aim of reaching the poor (La Forgia and Nagpal, 2012). The report stated that 300 million were covered under government-run schemes by the end of 2010 and estimated that by 2015, this figure will come close to 630 million—around 50% of India's population.

The first state-run scheme was Aarogyasri, which was established in 2007 in the southeastern state of Andhra Pradesh and also covers the population of the newly created state of Telangana, which separated from Andhra Pradesh in 2014. This scheme provides financial protection to families living below the poverty line (BPL), for the treatment of serious ailments requiring hospitalization and surgery through an identified network of healthcare providers. BPL beneficiaries can visit any hospital, either public or private, and are not required to make any sort of payment to the hospital for procedures that are covered under the scheme.

Andhra Pradesh and Telangana have managed to cover as much as 70% of their population under this health insurance umbrella, which provides cover of up to 200,000 Indian rupees (US$3000) per year for individuals requiring serious medical treatment or surgery. Other states such as Tamil Nadu, Karnataka, Gujarat, Maharashtra, and Rajasthan have similar health insurance schemes covering between 30% and 50% of their populations. With the exception of Rajasthan, the schemes are run directly by their respective state governments through trusts. In Rajasthan, the scheme has been recently rolled out through a private insurer, the New India Assurance Company. With a government allocation of 3750 million Indian rupees (US$56.4 million), the scheme is expected to benefit 65% of the state's population.

The seven states, which operate government insurance schemes for the BPL population, have a moderate to high per capita allocation on health: between 700 and 1300 rupees (US$10–19). States like Andhra Pradesh and Telangana contribute a little over 13% of their health budget on insurance schemes—7960 million rupees (US$119 million) and 6500 million rupees (US$97 million) respectively—while Tamil Nadu allocates a little over 9% of their health budget (7810 million rupees or US$117 million) to the insurance schemes (Table 53.1). These states demonstrate that it is possible to achieve UHC for their most vulnerable citizens. In contrast, some large states like Uttar Pradesh, Bihar, Madhya Pradesh, and West Bengal allocate only a small proportion of their budget to health cover—between 300 and 600 rupees per capita (US$4–9)—which is not enough to operate health insurance schemes (Table 53.2).

There are also pan-India insurance schemes run by the central government. One such scheme, Rashtriya Swasthya Bima Yojana (RSBY), launched in 2008, covers BPL households across India, providing a maximum (and very modest) 30,000 rupees (US$450) per annum for most diseases that require hospitalization, and allowing beneficiaries to choose between public or private hospitals. The scheme is information technology (IT)-enabled, with beneficiaries given a biometric-enabled smart card, with portability

TABLE 53.1

Indian States Operating Government Insurance Schemes

State No.	State	Health budget (in millions of Indian rupees)	Health budget (in millions of US dollars)	Per capita spend of health budget (in Indian rupees)	Per capita spend of health budget (in US dollars)	Amount of health budget spend on insurance schemes (in millions of Indian rupees)	Amount of health budget spend on insurance schemes (in millions of US dollars)
1	Andhra Pradesh	57,280	855	700	10	7,960	119
2	Telangana	49,320	735			6,500	97
3	Tamil Nadu	82,540	1,230	1,200	18	7,810	116
4	Karnataka	61,070	910	1,000	15	2,500	37
5	Gujarat	77,760	1,160	1,300	19	3,000	44
6	Maharashtra	89,600	1,340	700	10	3,000	44
7	Rajasthan	60,630	900	800	12	3,750	56

TABLE 53.2

States Not Operating Any Government Insurance for Health

State No.	State	Health budget (in millions of Indian rupees)	Health budget (in millions of US dollars)	Amount of health budget spend per person (in Indian rupees)	Amount of health budget spend per person (in US dollars)	Amount of health budget spend on insurance schemes
1	Uttar Pradesh	73,500	1,100	300	4.50	NA
2	Bihar	49,710	740	500	7.50	NA
3	Madhya Pradesh	47,400	700	600	9.0	NA
4	West Bengal	25,880	385	300	4.50	NA

across India. The scheme has already issued 40 million smart cards with an estimated coverage of 200 million.

In addition, the central government of India runs a number of insurance schemes for specific categories of government employment. These include the Central Government Health Scheme (CGHS), which caters to central government employees, pensioners, and their dependents. The Ex-Servicemen Contributory Health Scheme (ECHS) covers retired defense personnel and their families. Other noteworthy central schemes include the Employee State Insurance Scheme (ESIS), which is tailored to provide health protection to workers in the organized sector, along with their dependents. ESIS is self-financing scheme with funds contributed by employee, employer, and state government. The three schemes together, that is, CGHS, ECHS, and ESIS, cover around 100 million people.

Impact

In all, more than 50% of the Indian population is covered by some sort of health insurance. This includes the BPL population of the seven states that provide government insurance schemes—and which represents 40% of the national population. Another 200 million, around 15% of the population, are covered by RSBY. A further 100 million are covered by various central government health schemes. A small percentage of the population is covered by miscellaneous private insurance and employer insurance schemes.

Implementation: Transferability of Exemplar

While the Indian government still cannot afford to allocate a greater proportion GDP to healthcare, existing models of PPP, where the government procures healthcare from private providers, are a viable option for a successful UHC program.

The extent of coverage may depend on individual circumstances: for instance, healthcare may be provided free to BPL populations, and those with a higher income might receive a 50% subsidy, while those who are more affluent may receive a 20% subsidy.

Those states that have not yet implemented insurance schemes are studying the successful models of those seven states that have. With rising awareness among the population, state governments are being pushed to find innovative ways to provide affordable healthcare.

Prospects for Further Success

In order to launch state schemes for BPL/APL populations in line with those described previously, most states will require a substantial increase in their health spending. In order to establish government insurance schemes for BPL/APL populations, each state requires a health allocation of about 1000 rupees (US$15) per capita. Central government can simultaneously strengthen RSBY low-premium schemes by increasing its cover from the present limits. Indeed, in its budget announcement on 29th February 2016, the central government revealed plans to provide the BPL population with annual cover of 100,000 rupees (US$1,500) per family, and an additional 30,000 rupees (US$450) for senior citizens. The government expects to cover about one-third of the population under this new scheme.

Benefits from GSHISs are largely confined to urban populations for the simple reason that the majority of tertiary care private hospitals are confined to tier-I and tier-II towns. For rural populations, while primary healthcare is available, tertiary and emergency care is less common. CHCs—30 bed, secondary care government hospitals located at sub-district level—are frequently ill-equipped. In order to overcome some of these problems, the private sector is set to take over the operation of some of the CHCs in some states, providing manpower and management, while the infrastructure is retained by the government.

Micro-financing schemes may provide further opportunities. In 2002, the southern Indian state of Karnataka launched the first state health scheme, Yeshawini. With 3.4 million members, and with 823 defined procedures performed in 476 network hospitals across the state, over a million farmers have already benefited from the scheme. Yeshaswini, which is the most long-lived of all state health insurance schemes, is currently the only self-funding scheme in India: members are charged a premium of about 200 rupees (US$3) per annum, and the government is only a reinsurer. Yeshawini could provide a low-cost, micro-financing model for other states to follow.

Conclusion

Despite having only a small proportion of government spending devoted to health, half of the Indian population receives some sort of healthcare cover. This has largely come from the private sector's contribution to healthcare infrastructure. Some of the state governments have successfully utilized the PPP model, with health services procured and delivered to the population at predetermined rates. Governments of developing nations like India will always be short of financial resources, and it would be worth considering incentivizing the private sector to invest in healthcare. Ultimately, the models used by various Indian states should be consolidated to achieve national uniformity.

54

Japan

Universal Insurance

Yukihiro Matsuyama

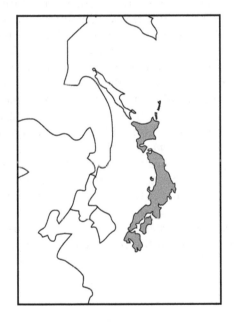

CONTENTS

Background

As the World Health Organization (WHO) indicates in its report, "Health in 2015," universal health coverage, by which a government provides all its people with health insurance, has become an important policy goal in all countries (WHO, 2015c). Possible ways of developing such schemes are many and varied, and depend on the social context and economic development of each country. There is, however, one common principle in the design of universal health coverage: its economic implementation relies on a three-way split between taxes, insurance premiums, and patient contributions. In almost all cases the distribution of the financial burden is as follows: the working generations bear all the cost of their own healthcare, along with that of the elderly, and the wealthy elderly also bear a fair share of their healthcare cost.

Japan guarantees equitable access to healthcare to all citizens via public health insurance and long-term care insurance. There is no doubt that the current system contributes significantly to the fact that, in Japan, both average life expectancy and healthy life expectancy are among the best in the world. A 2011 issue of *The Lancet*, "Japan: Universal Health Care at 50 Years," which investigated the reasons behind Japan's overall health improvement, rated the system highly (*The Lancet*, 2011).

As with all such systems, however, success can also generate its own problems. In recent years, it has become increasingly difficult for Japan to maintain the healthcare system under the current scheme due to a rapidly aging population. While the continuation of health coverage remains a priority, the challenge is to find a way to create a sustainable system—one that will continue to be effective even when the percentage of the population aged over 65 years of age reaches 40%.

Details of the Success Story

Between 1960 and 2014, the average Japanese life expectancy rose considerably—going from 65.3 to 80.5 years for men, and from 70.2 to 86.8 years for women—and is currently the highest in the world. According to an estimation by the National Institute of Population and Social Security Research [Japan] (2012), it will continue to increase, reaching 83.6 years for males and 90.3 years for females in 2050. Moreover, according to World Health Statistics 2015 from the WHO, the healthy life expectancy of Japanese men and women was 75 years in 2013, which also ranks as the worlds' best (WHO, 2015f). Both the infant mortality rate (2.5/1000 in 1990→1.0/1000 in 2013) and under-five mortality rate (similarly 4.6→2.1) are among the lowest in the world, and continue to improve. One of the major reasons for this success lies in the equitable system of healthcare insurance that is available to all Japanese citizens.

Japan introduced universal health insurance in 1961. In 1973, patients over the age of 70 were given preferential treatment with no co-payment requirement. The implementation of such generous benefits was due to the strong economic growth—more than 10%—that Japan experienced between 1954 and 1973. The growth rate plunged, however, after the first oil shock in 1973, averaging only 3.5% between 1974 and 1983. As a response to this, elderly patients were required to contribute a small amount to the cost of their healthcare. At the same time, the government enacted a new scheme in which all the health insurance programs for those generations still at work would subsidize the financial resources of healthcare for the elderly on behalf of the government.

In order to support the increasing demand for nursing care within a rapidly aging population, a revolutionary system of public long-term care insurance was introduced in 2000, along with a late-stage medical care system for those aged 75 years and older in 2008. While some problems with long-term care insurance have emerged, such as low wages and elder abuse, many elderly patients have benefited from the introduction of the new system (see Table 54.1). The late-stage medical care system was able to publicly clarify the infrastructure of the healthcare available to those aged 75 years and over.

According to the Organization for Economic Cooperation and Development (OECD) Health Statistics published in July 2015 (OECD, 2015c), health

TABLE 54.1

Long-Term Care Services User Ratio by Age Group (October 2014)

Male	65–69	1.9%
	70–74	3.8%
	75–79	7.3%
	80–84	14.1%
	85–89	25.3%
	90–94	41.8%
	Over 95	60.0%
Female	65–69	1.4%
	70–74	3.2%
	75–79	8.1%
	80–84	19.1%
	85–89	36.9%
	90–94	58.3%
	Over 95	76.0%

Source: Ministry of Health, Labor, and Welfare [Japan]. (2014). Long-Term Care Insurance Statistics. Retrieved from http://www.mhlw.go.jp/toukei/list/45-1b.html

spending in Japan as a share of GDP was lower than the OECD average before 2005. Japan's population is aging more rapidly than any other in the world. Despite this, it is predicted that it will be able to maintain its universal health coverage system, which is less expensive than those of other advanced nations, despite providing generous health insurance benefits. One factor in the scheme's continued success is its utilization of an official price scheme, in which the government decides the level of medical fees after taking several factors, including the country's fiscal situation, medical technology progress, and so forth, into account. Medical fees and long-term care fees are revised every 2 and 3 years respectively.

Social factors, including sanitation improvement, equal educational opportunities, greater economic equality, the stable, peaceful nature of Japanese society, along with the healthy lifestyle, have also contributed to the world-class stature of Japan's health indicators. Japanese fat and carbohydrate intake, for instance, are within healthy limits: according to the OECD Obesity Update published in June 2014 (OECD, 2014b), the obesity rate of the population aged 15 years and over in Japan is very low at 3.6%, following India (2.1%), Indonesia (2.4%), and China (2.9%). These rates are far lower than those of the United States, which, at 35.3%, has the highest obesity rate of the 40 countries surveyed. However, the high levels of salt in Japanese staples such as soy sauce and miso, mean that many Japanese consume excessive salt, and are at risk of high blood pressure and stroke. In order to solve this problem, Japan has been working for many years on a salt-reduction education campaign. As a result, the average salt dose per day decreased from 13.5 grams in 1975 to 10.2 grams in 2013. However, this is still twice as much as the 5 grams a day recommended by the WHO.

Details of the Impact of the Success Story

There are 47 prefectures in Japan. In 2013, Nagano prefecture (with a population of over two million) achieved No. 1 overall life expectancy, despite per capita medical expenses that were 10% less than the national average (Nagano Prefecture Healthy Longevity Project Study Team, 2015). In 2013, Nagano prefecture (with a population of over two million) achieved No. 1 overall life expectancy, despite per capita medical expenses that were less than 10% of the national average (Nagano Prefecture Healthy Longevity Project Study Team, 2015). The success of the "Nagano Model," as it is known, is due to a variety of health improvement activities, such as medical check-ups and home nursing care, which Nagano prefecture has been developing for nearly 70 years. One important component of the model's success is the ongoing education program devoted to improving lifestyle and eating habits. This well-organized program is carried out by 11,000 volunteer health counselors and 4500 healthy eating advisors. While other prefectures have established similar programs, the Nagano prefecture continues to lead the way.

Nagano Koseiren, a successful example of integrated healthcare networks in Japan, has played a leadership role in the success of the model. The data health project of the Abe administration is aiming to replicate the success of the Nagano Model across the country by leveraging medical-related national databases.

As mentioned previously, success can generate its own problems. In the case of healthcare systems, the increased average life expectancy combined with the declining birth rate has increased the age dependency ratio, which is the ratio of dependents (people younger than 15 years, or older than 64 years) to the working age population (those aged 15–64 years). As of 1990, just before the collapse of the economic bubble, the age dependency ratio of Japan was 43, the lowest among advanced nations, and its social system was highly flexible. However, by 2013 the ratio reached 60, and is expected to reach 94 in 2050. This means that it will become increasingly difficult to reform the current health insurance system in which the balance between benefits and cost burden favors the elderly.

Implementation: Transferability of the Exemplar

Although the Japanese health insurance system can be given a high rating if we consider it on the basis of its world-class health indicators, there are two defects in the institutional design. As described previously, the first defect is that the balance between benefits and cost burden is so favorable to the elderly that it has become difficult to correct it politically. However, as over 60% of household financial assets (1684 trillion Japanese yen [US$14.93 trillion] as of September 2015) belong to those aged 60 years and over, the government should carry out reforms to transfer the cost burden to the elderly.

The second defect is that the healthcare system, which secures financial resources and delivers healthcare services, lacks localized governance schemes (by prefecture), mainly because there are so many small- and medium-sized insurers and healthcare institutions. While the medical fees are a uniform price directly controlled by the government, there are more than 3000 insurers. The healthcare delivery system depends on private institutions that compete fiercely against each other. Moreover, national hospitals, national university hospitals, and public hospitals also replicate services and compete for investment with subsidies. Even if they are located in the same healthcare district, they do not share patient information to improve the quality of medical care. This results in excess hospital beds and wide regional disparities in healthcare expenses per capita. For example, in

2013, Fukuoka prefecture's medical expenses were 38% more than Niigata prefecture's.

Prospects for Further Success and Next Steps

The government has revised healthcare related laws to establish prefectural governance of the healthcare system; 1717 national health insurers are scheduled to be consolidated into 47 insurers in 2018. By 2025, each prefecture will have formulated a regional healthcare vision and taken control of local healthcare finances. The government has begun utilizing a public healthcare fund as an incentive.

The establishment of a universal social security numbering system is underway, with many people having already been assigned a number, and this will improve the efficiency of government administrative procedures. Beyond this, such a system will also help the government achieve a fairer balance of benefits and contributions in the social security system by enabling a more accurate picture of the income and financial assets of each citizen. In addition, discussions are underway regarding the introduction of a health-specific numbering system as part of the government's health infrastructure reform.

Conclusion

When people live longer, healthier lives, it can be difficult for a nation to avoid a rise in the ratio of health spending to GDP. In every country, disease prevention and management is an important area of health reform. However, while costs may be postponed, improved health does not guarantee that the lifetime healthcare expense per capita is reduced. When a country introduces universal health insurance, the benefits should not be too generous, especially for the elderly, because it makes future reforms very difficult. Moreover, the choices of medical care utilization in the late elderly have increased along with advances in medical technology. The kind of terminal care an elderly person chooses, whether life-prolonging medical care or natural death, depends on the individual's values. Therefore, to incorporate an option relating to the balance between benefits and cost burden into universal health insurance would be an effective way to simultaneously increase patient satisfaction and control healthcare costs.

55

Malaysia

From Maternal Mortality to Maternal Health: The Malaysian Experience

Ravindran Jegasothy, Ravichandran Jeganathan, and Safurah Jaafar

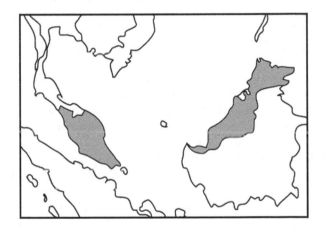

CONTENTS

Background

This chapter outlines the results of a recent Malaysian investigation into maternal mortality through a system of clinical audits that were anonymous and non-punitive. The system classifies every maternal death using the ICD Classification of Deaths (WHO, 2010a).

Malaysia has successfully reduced maternal mortality using a comprehensive approach that involved

- The overall socioeconomic development of the country
- The provision of health services specifically focusing on the issue of access
- The specific efforts and initiatives for the reduction of maternal mortality, one of which was the audit of maternal deaths by the Confidential Enquiry into Maternal Deaths (CEMD)

The reduction of maternal mortality can be divided into three distinct phases. The first phase was from 1933—when what was then Malaya was under British rule—to 1957, when the nation gained independence. During this period, maternal mortality was high and was identified as a high-priority health problem. This led to a strong political commitment to reducing maternal mortality from the founding fathers and the government of Malaya, and the foundations were laid for the development of maternal and child health services. The passing of the Midwives Ordinance in 1954, laid the foundations for the professionalization of midwifery. Midwives in Malaya were henceforth regarded as professionals, in contrast to many other developing countries, where such staff frequently went missing from their posts (Pathmanathan et al., 2003).

The second phase was from 1958 to 1975. During this period, the maternal mortality rate (MMR) was still moderately high, but was rapidly declining. The health system was strengthened by making healthcare more accessible to the disadvantaged. Partnerships with traditional birth attendants (TBAs) were also strengthened as an interim short-term measure while adequate numbers of skilled birth attendants (community nurses and midwives) were being trained (Government of Malaysia, 1990; Pathmanathan and Dhairiam, 1990). TBAs, who were trained and integrated into mainstream services, now provided their services under supervision, ensuring that they did not conduct deliveries, which had in the past sometimes proved harmful. This was a particularly important innovation, and one that helped further reduce the mortality rate.

During the third phase, from 1976 to the present, the relatively low MMR underwent further decline but then plateaued. It was decided during a national meeting in 1987 that the existing system of maternal mortality audit held at the local and state levels should be escalated to a formal national audit that could be utilized by policymakers who were in the position to make system changes whenever required. This phase saw the consolidation of past gains through the introduction of several specific initiatives to further lower MMR, such as the meticulous auditing of maternal deaths via the CEMD, which began in 1991.

The System

The CEMD evaluates all maternal deaths including those that occur in the private sector and at home. All deaths, including fortuitous deaths of non-citizens, are studied. This is important as there can be important lessons to learn in every death.

The secretariat is based in the Family Health Division of the Ministry of Health. The national-level team is headed by a senior obstetrician and gynecologist and includes other obstetric and gynecological specialists, physicians, anesthetists, forensic medicine specialists, nursing personnel, and family physicians. It is co-chaired by the director of the Family Health Division. All cases evaluated by the panel are anonymous. If details are insufficient, clarification is sought from the state-level secretariat. Finance is provided under the operational budget of the Ministry of Health (Suleiman et al., 1999).

The initial use of the term *substandard care* in the CEMD was changed to *remediable factors* to ensure a more positive attitude toward the caregivers. This is in line with the patient safety movement, which emphasizes that many remediable factors are systemic in nature rather than the fault of particular individuals.

Triennial to biennial reports are distributed to health personnel and obstetric and gynecological specialists in both public and private sectors. Bulletins, case summaries, and technical reports are produced to educate and inform all categories of personnel (Suleiman et al., 1999).

The Benefits

There has been improvement in the reporting systems of maternal deaths. This contrasts positively with figures reported in 1991, when the CEMD data showed a doubling of the MMR as compared with that reported by the Department of Statistics, Malaysia (Ravindran and Mathews, 1996).

To overcome the disparity in reported rates, efforts were made to improve reporting by encouraging the active capture of maternal deaths. Soon after the introduction of the CEMD, the Department of Registration was requested to include on the death certificate of every woman who had died, information as to whether she was pregnant or had delivered in the past 42 days.

The CEMD reports provided evidence-based information to support budget requests in the Ministry of Health. This resulted in budget allocations for alternative birthing centers in rural and urban settings, provision of communications systems for remote areas, as well as equipment for hemoglobin estimation to provide for effective management of anemia in pregnancy.

Funds were also provided for patient-kept maternal records to ensure a better continuity of care by the health and hospital sectors (both public and private). These record cards encouraged mothers' "ownership" of their health, and in addition, carried important educational messages regarding nutrition, frequency of antenatal visits, and warning signs of obstetric emergencies.

In addition, funds were allocated to human resource skill improvement through training. Training modules were developed for the most important causes of maternal mortality—postpartum hemorrhage, hypertensive disease of pregnancy, heart disease in pregnancy, and the management of venous thromboembolism. Obstetric lifesaving skills courses were introduced to improve the competency of caregivers.

The CEMD allowed for improvement in work processes based on the remedial factors in care identified in the audit. Examples of these included the use of the partogram in the hospital setting and at home, protocol development (such as for anemia), conduct of combined inter-disciplinary clinics for medical disorders in pregnancy, and the creation of the red alert system in hospitals, which allowed for rapid mobilization of multidisciplinary specialists for obstetric emergencies.

There is now a changing trend in maternal deaths from direct obstetric causes to indirect maternal deaths and fortuitous deaths. This change indicates that efforts in training as well as improvements in the quality of obstetric care have had an impact (Karim and Ali, 2013).

The empowerment of midwives has been a key component of the CEMD activities. This includes the color coding system used in Malaysian antenatal care, designed to streamline referrals by midwifes to the hospitals. A woman given a red code by a midwife could be admitted to a specialist hospital immediately (Ravindran et al., 2003).

Midwives are now allowed to continue heparin for thromboprophylaxis, give antenatal steroids to mothers with preterm labor, and provide intramuscular magnesium sulfate under guidance from Ministry of Health protocols.

A curriculum for an advanced diploma in midwifery was developed, incorporating the lessons learned from maternal deaths. There was increased emphasis on practical skills in the management of the major causes of deaths, emergency care, and the referral system. Some labor wards in the public hospitals allow midwifery-led care for selected patients in specialist hospitals.

In 2009, following a number of high-profile cases of infant abandonment, there were discussions regarding the provision of services for the termination of pregnancy, and in 2012 the Ministry of Health issued termination of pregnancy guidelines. These guidelines utilized the provisions of existing laws, which had previously been amended in 1989 following representation by women's groups.

What Would Be Needed to Replicate the System?

The attitude of leadership toward its female population is critical to the reduction of maternal mortality: women must be regarded as an integral part of society, and their right to better care during the most vulnerable period in their lives—their reproductive years—must be considered a priority.

To be sustainable, it is vital that the system is nonpunitive, and that anonymity is guaranteed. It is tempting to mete out administrative admonishment in various forms, but the fear of punishment may compromise honest reporting of medical incidents. A comprehensive root-cause analysis should be performed to enable systemic deficiencies to be remedied. A problem with the system demands that the system be corrected rather than individuals.

The enquiry should be chaired by someone with the authority to implement system-wide remedial changes. Having only a clinician as chair would not be wise, as clinicians may not have administrative authority. A system of co-chairmanship has worked well for Malaysia and has many benefits to commend it.

The system should blend well with the health administrative system in any country. The CEMD system is found at the health district, state, and national levels in Malaysia; the health district, which is the basic administrative unit of the health services in the country, is the key to implementation of any health-related recommendations and remedial measures.

The CEMD system is not anonymized at the health district or state level. However, the report is anonymized when it is sent to the national level. This important distinction ensures that remedial actions are taken speedily at the ground level but system-wide improvement occurs after national-level investigations. This ensures prioritizing scant health resources according to areas of need. For example, postpartum hemorrhage as the leading cause of maternal deaths was the focus of efforts such as the red alert system, establishment of blood storage facilities at various public and private sector delivery centers, improvement in obstetric retrieval systems, improvement in the provision of emergency care during transit, and the upgrading of skills (Ravichandran and Ravindran, 2014).

As in Malaysia, maternal deaths will reduce over time. Remedial measures will be taken to correct any identified weaknesses in the system. Success will be the tonic that will sustain the system, and more importantly, ensure the patients benefit from the audit system (Ravindran, 1998).

Conclusion

The CEMD has now been incorporated into hospital accreditation systems. The sole accreditation agency for hospitals has developed quality indicators that monitor major causes of maternal death. The CEMD system has thus been incorporated into another systemic improvement process. The CEMD system that has evolved has led to a dramatic fall in maternal deaths over the last decades (Figure 55.1).

There is no shortcut to success. There must be system changes for sustainable progress. The CEMD system was benchmarked against an established system in England and Wales. Competency was emphasized to ensure skilled care at delivery. There was documentation of every instance of progress. All interventions were evidence-based. Frank explanations were provided to top management when things did not go well. Widely disseminated guidelines served to spread the message. There is an A–G for converting maternal deaths into maternal health and this is sustainable and replicable! (Box 55.1).

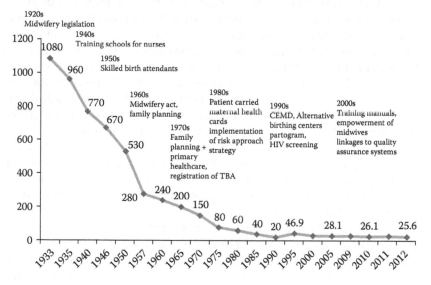

FIGURE 55.1
Maternal mortality rates and key strategies.

**BOX 55.1   KEY LEARNING POINTS
FOR SUCCESS OF THE CEMD**

A   Avoid shortcuts
B   Benchmark
C   Competency
D   Documentation
E   Evidence-based practice
F   Frank explanation
G   Guidelines

56

New Zealand

Ko Awatea: Improving Quality, Promoting Innovation

Jacqueline Cumming, Jonathon Gray, Lesley Middleton, Haidee Davis, Geraint Martin, and Patricia Hayward

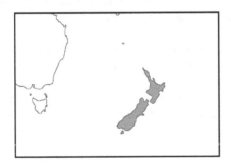

CONTENTS

Background

Over recent years, there has been a growing focus in New Zealand on improving the quality and safety of healthcare and on transforming services to improve health, reduce inequalities, and ensure value for money from the health system (Ministry of Health [New Zealand], 2016). In one New Zealand district health board (DHB)—Counties Manukau Health (CM Health)—a proactive approach to health quality and safety recently led to the establishment of Ko Awatea, an organization that aims to lead the transformation of health services in the twenty-first century.

CM Health faces critical challenges in delivering services to meet the needs of its population (510,000 people), which includes a high proportion of both younger and older residents; high numbers of Māori*, Pacific, and Asian peoples; significant proportions of the population living in deprived areas; and a high level of inequality in health. Key health concerns include high rates of smoking, and growing rates of diabetes and obesity, which will require significant resources to treat in future years (Counties Manukau Health, 2013).

Ko Awatea's mandate is to lead an innovative approach to achieving sustainable, high-quality healthcare services. It aims to bring "positive health outcomes for patients and communities" (Ko Awatea and Counties Manukau Health, 2015), through being "a hub of education, improvement and innovation to support health systems and public services" (Ko Awatea and Counties Manukau Health, 2015).

In relation to quality improvement and innovation, Ko Awatea is involved in a number of high-profile projects, emphasizing quality improvement and integrated care, enhancing skills not only in the health sector (including in hospitals and in primary healthcare), but also in the education and social development sectors, and in the wider community (Ko Awatea and Counties Manukau Health, 2015). Here, the focus is on two recent key initiatives.

The 20,000 Days and Beyond 20,000 Days Campaigns: Improving Community Health

The 20,000 Days and Beyond 20,000 Days campaigns were developed to reduce severe pressure on hospital beds at CM Health's main hospital (Middlemore). The first campaign, 20,000 Days, commenced in October 2011. The aim was to avoid the projected growth in demand for beds, and return 20,000 healthy days to the community before the end of July 2013. The second campaign, Beyond 20,000 Days, ran until July 2014 and aimed to continue giving back healthy days and to further reduce the number of occupied bed-days at CM Health.

The campaigns were designed around collaborative teams with ideas to prevent hospital admissions, reduce length of stay, and improve access to community services. They used design elements from the Institute for Healthcare Improvement (IHI) Breakthrough Series (BTS) collaborative methodology (Institute for Healthcare Improvement, 2003), albeit extending the concept from spreading a shared and well-defined best practice to a much broader topic of reducing demand for hospital care across a range of services. Ideas

---

* Māori are the indigenous population of New Zealand.

were developed by front-line staff, and decision-making processes at CM Health balanced the desire to harness the energy of those with ideas for change with the need to back ideas most likely to succeed. The resources available for approved projects included assistance from a campaign team, which provided project managers, improvement advisers, and training in the theory and practice of the Model for Improvement (Langley et al., 2009). The campaigns were well resourced: NZ$2.7 million (US$1.9 million) for the 20,000 Days Campaign and NZ$2.5 million (US$1.8 million) for the Beyond 20,000 Days Campaign. One-third of the funding went on improvement support, while the other two-thirds went towards new activity in the collaborative teams.

The number of teams varied through the life of the campaigns, with an initial 29 teams participating, 24 maintaining momentum right up until the end, and 19 going on to implement their changes permanently. Teams that implemented permanent changes included those aiming to

- Reduce length of stay for hip and knee patients
- Reduce length of stay for those aged over 64, with hip fractures
- Increase the number of low acuity patients managed in the primary care setting rather than transported to hospital
- Identify high-risk primary care patients and reduce unplanned hospital admissions
- Reduce length of stay and readmission for people with diabetes by changing the model of inpatient diabetes care from reactive review to virtual review
- Facilitate early supportive discharge for stroke
- Reduce overall hospital and GP use for individuals with long-term medical conditions and co-existing severe mental health/addiction issues (Middleton et al., 2014, 2015)

The campaigns applied the model for improvement, which uses Plan-Do-Study-Act (PDSA) cycles—a four-step problem-solving process—to develop and test change ideas (Langley et al., 2009). Teams learned from each other, resulting in a heightened awareness of the conditions that would support the application of the Model for Improvement. These conditions included the benefits of releasing team members to attend learning sessions and learn about PDSAs, and the development of sufficient infrastructure to start regular cycles of PDSAs early. The first campaign ran for a year and 8 months, and the second for a year, to give teams enough time to develop and test change initiatives.

The first campaign saved an estimated 23,060 days, and by 2015, it was estimated the combined campaigns had saved 34,800 days (Middleton et al., 2014, 2015). The evaluations of the campaigns identified five key mechanisms that supported their success:

1. Organizational preparedness to change: participants were aware of local evidence of the need to manage hospital demand, were part of the same organizational culture at CM Health, and there was clear senior management support for the campaigns.

2. Enlisting the early adopter: campaign participants came up with their own ideas for change, providing a strong base on which to build positive momentum.

3. Strong team dynamics: the campaigns enabled teams to develop skills in applying the model for improvement, and the teams described how small-scale measurable cycles were a great way to test whether their idea for improvement actually delivered what was expected.

4. Learning from measurement: key aspects of the PDSA cycles, including agreeing on goals and learning from tests that failed, worked well, but teams were more tentative when assessing how well they measured progress.

5. Sustaining improvement: an adaptive climate was promoted throughout, including the campaign sponsors being prepared to adapt and learn as one campaign transitioned into another. The campaigns' communications—with the tagline, "Wouldn't you rather be at home?"—sought to make the campaigns relevant to what patients valued, emphasizing (particularly in the Beyond 20,000 Days Campaign) the giving back of "well days" to the community (Middleton et al., 2014, 2015).

One of the key challenges for the campaigns was having the successful changes adopted as standard practice. Engaging the support of organizational leaders at all levels early on was important to secure the resources to enable sustained change and ensure that key people took responsibility for leading it.

Target CLAB Zero: Reducing Central Line Infections in Intensive Care Units

Central line–associated bacteraemia (CLAB) prevention is a major challenge, particularly in intensive care units (ICUs). In New Zealand, it was estimated that of 19,000 admissions to ICUs, around half have a central line inserted (Ko Awatea and Health Quality and Safety Commission [New Zealand], n.d.), bringing a risk of infection, complications and increased length of hospital stay, and excess costs of around NZ$20,000 (US$14,000) per CLAB (Burns et al., 2010; Proudfoot, 2013).

Following a successful initiative at CM Health in 2008 (Seddon et al., 2011), Ko Awatea led Target CLAB Zero, a national CLAB prevention collaborative funded by New Zealand's Health Quality and Safety Commission (HQSC). Ko Awatea provided leadership, coordination, and data management across all 25 ICUs in New Zealand's 20 DHBs. The collaborative commenced in October 2011, and aimed to

- Reduce the rate of CLAB in New Zealand ICUs toward zero (<1 per 1000 line days), from an estimated national pre-collaborative rate of 3.32 per 1000 line days
- Share best practice and provide leadership, build capability, coordination, and data management to create sustainable improvement and better patient safety outcomes
- Establish a robust national measurement approach to CLAB to inform the establishment of a national web-based data repository for collection, analysis, and reporting of outcomes (Ko Awatea, 2011)

Key challenges in Target CLAB Zero included the geographic isolation of some ICUs and the variation in the experience of CLAB among ICUs. CLAB rates were higher in some ICUs because the patient mix in larger units is broader, and acuity higher, than in smaller ICUs. In addition, definitions of CLAB infection and the data collected were inconsistent across ICUs, and there was no established national surveillance system for CLAB. Finally, there was no mechanism for shared learning and improvement (Gray et al., 2015).

An IHI bundle of care (Institute for Healthcare Improvement, 2006) was adopted for Target CLAB Zero, which set out best practice requirements for preventing central line infections.

The collaborative involved many activities, including improving the quality of the measurement of CLAB rates; IHI training; team coaching; and national and regional face-to-face and "virtual" learning sessions and meetings. A web-based database was also developed, enabling the display and analysis of data at team and aggregate levels. Teams reported monthly on progress (Proudfoot, 2013).

CLAB rates fell quickly following the collaborative. During the implementation period, from January to March 2012, the rate was 2.17 per 1000 line days. In the post-implementation quarter, April–July 2012, the national CLAB rate was 0.37 per 1000 line days. An estimated four to six cases per month were prevented, saving NZ$80,000–$120,000 (US$54,000–$82,000) per month (Proudfoot, 2013). By March 2015, the HQSC reported that around 260 infections had been prevented, with a saving of around NZ$5.2 million (US$3.5 million). The CLAB rate continued to be below 1 per 1000 line days (Health Quality and Safety Commission New Zealand, 2015).

Six key factors have been identified as supporting the success of the collaboration:

1. The existence of strong international evidence for the effectiveness of the intervention
2. The existence of a proven example of international evidence being successfully applied in the New Zealand context
3. The flexibility of Breakthrough Series methodology
4. The peer-led nature of the campaign: the ability to attract influential clinicians to leading roles was important; clinical respect was leveraged within and across DHBs
5. The involvement of HQSC: HQSC sponsored attendance at learning sessions and leaned weight to the campaign as a national initiative
6. An effective communication plan: targeted messages secured engagement from key stakeholders, and the use of regional and virtual meetings enabled participants to connect despite the geographical isolation of some units (Gray et al., 2015)

Discussion and Conclusions

In a short period of time, Ko Awatea has built a solid reputation for successfully driving innovation and quality improvement. The two examples discussed here show that Ko Awatea's strong collaborative approach, emphasis on building capability, and use of organizing frameworks to guide its work, have successfully led to significant improvements in the quality of care provided not only to its own community, but also across New Zealand as a whole. An emphasis on measurement and evaluation provides the evidence needed to identify how well initiatives are being implemented, whether or not key goals and objectives are being achieved, and lessons for future initiatives.

Gaining strong evidence remains a challenge, however, given the real-world and complex nature of such initiatives (Parry, et al. 2013; Parry and Power, 2016) and, in the case of recent Ko Awatea initiatives, their breadth. Extensions to our understanding of the key initiatives discussed here might have included a greater understanding of the effects of the campaigns on those using services, and the overall economic impact of the 20,000 Days and Beyond 20,000 Days Campaigns, along with an understanding of the costs compared with the benefits of the Target CLAB Zero initiative.

57

Papua New Guinea

Establishment of the Provincial Health Authority in Papua New Guinea

Paulinus Lingani Ncube Sikosana and Pieter Johannes van Maaren

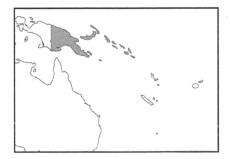

CONTENTS

Background

In 1973, Papua New Guinea's central government faced a political uprising from a number of provinces pushing for self-governance (Reilly et al., 2014). These demands influenced the direction of Papua New Guinea's decentralization policy. The Organic Law on Provincial Governments and Local-Level Governments, enacted in 1977 and revised in 1995, formed the initial legal basis for decentralized governance in the country.

The Organic Law on Provincial Governments and Local-Level Governments was by no means a purposeful legislation designed specifically to improve the health system. The National Health Administration Act (1997) and the Public Hospitals Act (1994) were passed to align health service delivery to the Organic Law. Implementation of these acts, however, resulted in a fragmented health service delivery model.

The Medium-Term Development Strategy 2003–2010 stated that "the reforms embodied in the 1995 Organic Law on Provincial Governments and Local-Level Governments (OLPGLLG) have not solved the problems of the decentralized system" (National Department of Planning and Monitoring [Papua New Guinea], 2004). Health services continued to deteriorate, with dysfunctional service delivery and widespread confusion over functional responsibilities across the three levels of government (National Department of Planning and Monitoring [Papua New Guinea], 2004). The parallel service delivery architecture created bottlenecks that impeded the smooth flow of operational funding to front-line service delivery. There were also concerns that provincial governments tended to prioritize administrative costs over costs for actual delivery of health services.

The Functional and Expenditure Review of Health Services (Public Sector Reform Management Unit, 2001) noted that the health system in PNG "had deteriorated to such an extent that it was almost collapsing" (May 2007). The Organic Law was blamed for the "disconnect" between health officials and provincial governments.

A number of policy options to restructure provincial health services were outlined in the expenditure review of health services in PNG. These included the need to

- Eliminate the requirement in the Organic Law for health staff to report to the district administrator
- Reflect the importance of health by establishing a separate division of health within provincial administrations
- Reintegrate hospitals into the provincial health system (World Bank, 2003, p. 24)

To put into effect these policy recommendations, the government enacted the Provincial Health Authority Act (Government of Papua New Guinea, 2007). The main objective of this legislation was to reorganize the health system architecture into an efficient, effective, and integrated organization within the decentralized system of government.

In addition to Provincial Health Authority (PHA) reform, there are a number of complementary initiatives aimed at improving the quality of healthcare. These include the National Health Service Standards, the Health Workforce Enhancement Plan (2013–2016), and the pharmaceutical reform agenda, in place since 2008. As a prerequisite to adopting the PHA, the

National Health Service Standards guide provinces to conduct health facility audits and develop health service plans. The Community Health Post was introduced in 2013 as part of a revised health referral model to improve access to quality primary health services in rural areas.

Details of the Identified Success Story

The PHA reform can be considered the boldest strategic policy decision that the leadership of the National Health Department has undertaken to improve health service delivery since the enactment of the Organic Law in 1995. The PHA integrates the management of hospital services with that of rural primary health services (public health services) under a single health authority. The reform abolishes provincial health boards and public hospital boards established under the Hospital Administration Act. The legal framework for the PHA literally "challenges" the status quo in the distribution and sharing of power or political control of (health) service delivery within provincial governments. It shifts internal decision-making on health matters from general administrators to health professionals. The chief executive officer of the PHA takes charge of both curative and public health services, all health staff, and health funding within the province. The PHA is an accountability mechanism through which the National Department of Health can monitor health sector performance and ensure adherence to national health standards.

Details of the Impact of the Success Story

The PHA has proved to be a sound model that has established a single authority that manages an integrated health delivery system in the three first-phase provinces. Results from these three provinces demonstrate that the reform is both implementable and politically feasible. The PHA initiative has

- Addressed deficiencies in the definition of roles
- Resolved coordination issues between the central steering role of the National Department of Health and the provincial level
- Streamlined funding modalities that characterized the segmented subsystems of the health delivery system
- Integrated public health services (primary health services) with the provision of curative care

This integration of service delivery has demonstrated a potential to improve the continuity of care and facilitated increased access to other levels of healthcare, both of which are associated with improvements in clinical effectiveness, responsiveness of health services, and health system efficiency.

The combination of a PHA, an experienced, skilled, and motivated health workforce, and political commitment at the local level have resulted in improved health outputs. For example, Es'la district, in one of the pilot PHAs, increased the proportion of women delivering at health facilities from 43% to 73% within 2 years (National Department of Health [Papua New Guinea], 2015). The 2013 and 2014 Annual Performance Reports show that all the three pilot PHA provinces, Milne Bay, Western Highlands, and Eastern Highlands, were among the top six best-performing provinces in the country (National Department of Health [Papua New Guinea], 2014).

Compared with previous provincial health boards, PHA management boards meet regularly and now hold health managers accountable. Direct allocation of health funds from the Treasury to PHAs, revised charts of accounts, and the adoption of facility-based budgeting by PHAs have helped to determine the true cost of providing health services at facility level and have improved accountability and the flow of funds to district and health facility levels. In implementing the National Health Service Standards, PHA executives visit rural health facilities and conduct staff audits, determine available skills mixes, and assess the state of health infrastructure and other physical assets. All this information provides evidence for the development of PHA health service delivery plans. Western Highlands PHA have established a website through which they showcase their success stories (see www.whhs.gov.pg).

Milne Bay, Western Highlands, and Eastern Highlands PHAs started receiving budget allocations directly from the Department of Treasury in 2011. The combined total of K3,035,700 (US$954,720) they received in 2011 was mainly to establish the PHAs and not to support recurrent costs. The additional four PHAs (West New Britain, Manus, Enga, and Sandaun) received their first appropriation directly from the Treasury in 2016. Since 2012, the three phase-one PHAs have been receiving increasing health budgets to deliver both hospital and rural health services (health function grants). The allocation to the three PHAs increased from a combined total of K48 million (US$15 million) in 2012 to K79 million (US$24.8 million) in 2013; K82 million (US$25.7 million) in 2014; K93 million (US$29 million) in 2015 and K127 million (US$29.9 million) in 2016 (Department of Treasury [Papua New Guinea], 2015; N. Mulou, National Department of Health, Health Economics Unit, personal communication, February 2, 2016). This trend in appropriations to the PHAs is incontrovertible evidence of government's political commitment to the PHA reform.

Success Factors

The success of this initiative can be attributed to a number of factors. First and foremost, the establishment of a PHA derives its legitimacy and political support from an Act of Parliament. Secondly, the objectives of the reform respond directly to the conviction that by fragmenting health service delivery, the Organic Law is responsible for the deterioration of the health delivery system in Papua New Guinea. Thirdly, the establishment of a PHA is a voluntary and self-motivated policy initiative agreed to by a provincial governor and the minister of health. The whole of government approach adopted by the National Department of Health galvanized support from other central agencies of government, such as the Department of Personnel Management, the Department of Provincial and Local-Level Government Affairs, and the Department of the Treasury. This intragovernmental approach to reform contributed to the government's decision to fund the PHA reform.

The establishment of a Provincial Health Authority Reform Unit within the National Department of Health and an inter-sectoral National Provincial Health Authority Steering Committee provided the necessary guidance and oversight for the implementation process. The publication of a Provincial Health Authority User Handbook in 2009, detailing change management processes and procedures, was a timely asset to guide the process. An effective Provincial Health Authority Board and strong leadership by the chief executive officer have proven to be essential ingredients for success.

Transferability of the Provincial Health Authority Model

The PHA is a locally context-specific reform that addresses the unintended effects of the Organic Law on health service delivery across the country's 22 provinces. It is firmly grounded in an Act of Parliament and has been successfully piloted in three provinces. According to the independent review, the reform has the potential to achieve its intended objectives and should be maintained (Government of Papua New Guinea, 2015). Four additional provinces are currently rolling out the reform and progressing faster than the first-phase provinces. Given the deplorable state of the existing health services, the PHA model is a welcome opportunity to improve the country's health service delivery.

Transferability to Other Countries

Although the PHA reform is specific to Papua New Guinea, and may not necessarily be transferable to other countries, it is possible to share experiences on the reform process itself. A major success factor of this reform is that it is entirely home grown. Without guaranteed and sustained political support, the reformers adopted an incremental approach rather than "big bang" or "radical" reforms.

Prospects for Further Success

The PHA is only one lever among many strategies necessary to address the ills of the country's health system and promote health system efficiency. Additional and complementary system inputs include variables to improve efficiencies in the utilization of existing health resources, increasing the health workforce, improving procurement and rational use of essential medicines, increased utilization of health information in decision-making, and strengthening health leadership and good governance. An effective and fully functional PHA requires the strengthening of internal organizational structures, processes, and procedures. The oversight role of the National Provincial Health Authority reform unit and the National Provincial Health Authority Steering Committee needs further strengthening. Efforts to institutionalize the Provincial Health Authority Act through the review of the Organic Law require more urgent attention.

Conclusion

The PHA is a home-grown policy reform that has demonstrated the potential to resolve some of the structural issues affecting health service delivery in Papua New Guinea. It establishes an integrated system of delivering health services in which the chief executive officer is in charge of both curative and public health services. All provincial health staffs and health funding fall under the management of a single health authority. Considering that the decentralized governance system in Papua New Guinea is unlikely to change any time soon, the PHA may well be the only opportunity to ensure a better functioning health sector with improved health outcomes. Current challenges affecting implementation of this reform are largely systemic, and will require a more coordinated whole of government approach to improving service delivery.

58

Taiwan

Taiwan's Health Information Technology Journey: From Flash Drive to Health Cloud

Yu-Chuan (Jack) Li, Wui-Chiang Lee, Min-Huei Hsu, and Usman Iqbal

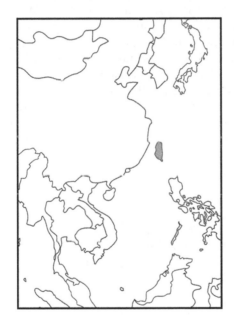

CONTENTS

Introduction

Taiwan is an island nation in East Asia with a population of 23 million, of which 11.5% are aged over 65 years. Taiwan provides universal healthcare coverage, with guaranteed equal access to healthcare services. The National Health Insurance system, first established in 1995 and operated by the National Health Insurance Administration, uses a single-payer system and covers 99.9% of the Taiwanese population.

Taiwan's single-payer system has helped facilitate the nationwide adoption of health information technology (HIT). Taiwan has made great progress in utilizing HIT through the use of flash drive and smart card systems, and is currently working toward implementing a cloud-based system (Li et al., 2009, 2015; Syed-Abdul et al., 2015). Effective use of such technology has allowed the system to be more cost-effective by reducing administrative costs, and by generally improving the quality of the utilized information. This has enhanced collaboration between different providers, and helped unify public health and clinical medicine information systems, which provide health data for research purposes (Yen et al., 2016). This provides solid evidence that the long-held vision of using HIT to transform healthcare systems, and make them operate more effectively, is achievable, and that even greater benefits can be expected in the future (see Figure 58.1).

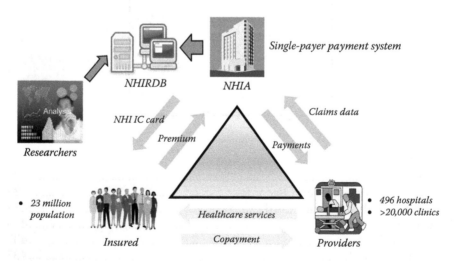

FIGURE 58.1
Taiwan's National Health Insurance administration structure.

Taiwan's USB-Based Health Records

In 2000, Taiwan's Department of Health (DoH) initiated the National Healthcare Information Project to promote adoption of a personal health record (PHR) system and to enhance health information exchange. The first PHR system was a USB-PHR—a portable personal health summary covering all aspects of healthcare. The DoH also created the Taiwan Electronic Medical Record Template (TMT), a local electronic record template that was developed by adopting international standards such as HL7 Clinical Document Architecture, which provides interoperability within healthcare systems. This was developed primarily to achieve functional and semantic interoperability of health information across the country.

The USB flash drive contains software to collect and view patients' personal medical information, such as medications and laboratory results, and may include multimedia files containing endoscopy recordings or ultrasound scans, for example. Information is updated at the reception desk when patients are discharged or following outpatient visits at participating hospitals (Jian et al., 2012).

One of the aims of developing the USB-PHR is to engage consumers in their own care management by empowering them with tools and knowledge that will streamline access to and interaction with a wide variety of health providers, including hospitals. In order to encourage such engagement, patients are able to view their own information. There are no security and privacy concerns, as the USB-PHR provides encrypted flash memory for secure storage and access to health records. The USB-PHR is particularly convenient for older patients, and for those with complex medical histories or who require multiple medications (see Figure 58.2).

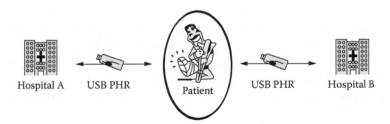

Hospital A　　USB PHR　　Patient　　USB PHR　　Hospital B

FIGURE 58.2
Information collection process from different hospitals. (From Jian, W.S., Syed-Abdul, S., Sood, S.P., et al. (2012). *BMC Health Services Research*, 12(1), 277–284.)

Taiwan's Healthcare Smart Card

In 2001, the Taiwan Ministry of Health and Welfare's National Health Insurance Administration (NHI), began the process of replacing paper-based patient identification (ID) cards with smart cards in order to increase efficiency, reduce fraud and decrease health system costs. Currently, 23 million people are using smart cards in Taiwan (Li, n.d.). The smart cards include the following patient information:

- Personal information, including the card's serial number, issue date, cardholder's name, gender, date of birth, ID number, and picture
- NHI-related information, including cardholder status, information on catastrophic diseases, number of visits and admissions, use of NHI health prevention programs, cardholder's premium records, accumulated medical expenditure records, and amount of cost-sharing
- Medical service information, including drug allergy history, long-term prescriptions, ambulatory care requirements, and certain medical treatments. This information will be added gradually, depending on how healthcare providers adapt to the system
- Public health administration information, including personal immunization chart and instructions for organ donation

Adoption of the smart card system resulted in a faster and more efficient reimbursement process, with hospitals and clinics able to upload electronic health records to NHI. After every six patient visits, card information is uploaded online for data analysis, audit, and authentication.

The Health Smart Cards have replaced the regular paper ID card, the Children's Health Handbook, the Prenatal Exam Handbook, and the Catastrophic Illness Certificate, and as such is very convenient for both card holders and healthcare professionals. The benefits for card holders are numerous—they provide a summary of personal medical information and do not need to be renewed. The cards also offer many benefits to healthcare providers and medical institutions—streamlining previously time-consuming and costly processes and transactions, and drastically reducing fraud (Smart Card Alliance, 2005).

In terms of the card's privacy and security, NHI developed multiple security mechanisms to prevent counterfeiting and safeguard cardholder information, to protect the security of information during transmission, and to block the transmission of computer viruses. A crisis management and response plan has also been implemented (see Figure 58.3).

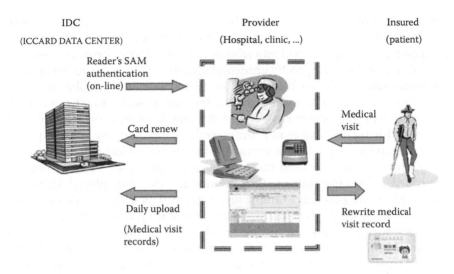

FIGURE 58.3
Health Smart Card and process.

Taiwan's Cloud Era

In order to provide an even more informative and transparent platform for healthcare service providers, and patients, Taiwan's DoH launched NHI PharmaCloud and My Health Bank in 2013 and 2014, respectively (National Health Insurance Administration [Taiwan], 2016).

PharmaCloud

Over the past 20 years, Taiwan's government has successfully provided a wide-coverage/low cost-sharing NHI program. However, increased medical expenditure, along with patient safety issues resulting from misuse of prescription drugs, poses serious challenges to the program. Taiwan's PharmaCloud System was developed to help reduce over-medication and improve medication safety (Huang et al., 2015).

PharmaCloud, which was introduced by NHI in 2013, provides NHI-contracted hospitals or clinics with confidential access to NHI's central database. Practitioners are able to use their personal integrated circuit (IC) card as well as the patient's NHI IC card to monitor a patient's drug use over the past 3 months. Patient privacy is protected through the use of a virtual private network (VPN) system: all enquiries are real-time, and no information can be downloaded onto the hospital system. All providers (496 hospitals and 20,000 clinics) have access to the PharmaCloud.

The PharmaCloud application facilitates the sharing of information within and between specific hospital divisions, and between the hospitals and local clinics. Information is also shared between hospital pharmacies and community drugstores, helping to minimize drug interactions and providing health education information to patients who have two or more chronic diseases.

The PharmaCloud has greatly improved primary care, giving doctors a more prominent role in primary healthcare. While the Taiwanese public can freely select their primary healthcare provider, the system lacks an effective referral mechanism. Physicians have found that many patients overuse medical resources during the treatment process, and doctor-shopping is widespread. In contrast to the health insurance card, which was previously used as a data carrier and is now only used for authentication purposes, PharmaCloud is web-based, able to integrate medical information that is displayed separately along with a computerized order entry system (CPOE) for healthcare professionals. Patients' medication histories along with previous diagnoses and past laboratory examination results are all available on PharmaCloud, thus ensuring healthcare professionals are able to make better informed and more effective treatment decisions. PharmaCloud also improves medication safety, protecting patients from drug interactions and dosage errors. Additionally, PharmaCloud prevents accidental drug duplication and deters prescription fraud—thereby decreasing expenditure (see Figure 58.4).

However, PharmaCloud usage is still relatively low. This could be because many physicians find the sometimes extensive list of data difficult to sift through. Prioritization of information and automatic summarization of data would allow health professionals to find information easily and efficiently.

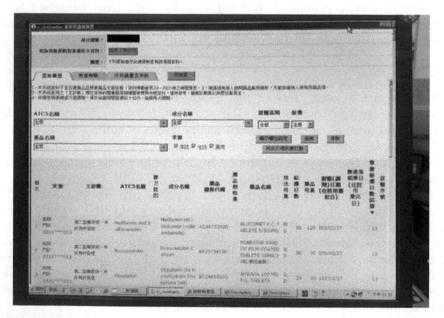

FIGURE 58.4
PharmaCloud physician's screen snapshot.

MyHealth Bank

In 2014, NHI established the official website for the MyHealth Bank system (http://www.nhi.gov.tw/). This site gives users instant access to all information relating to their visits to NHI-affiliated medical institutions (National Health Insurance Administration [Taiwan], 2016; San-Kuei, 2014). The site also contains details of an individual's inpatient and outpatient care; all prescribed, and certain over-the-counter drugs; dental services (excluding orthodontics, and prosthodontics); traditional Chinese medicine; day care for people with mental health conditions; home nursing care; allergies; and vaccination records. There are currently 330,000 MyHealth Bank accounts.

Such access helps individuals better understand and manage their own health. A citizen's medical history can be provided to doctors, facilitating fast and accurate diagnoses and prescriptions, reducing inconsistencies between patient histories, and improving doctor–patient communication as well as medical safety and efficiency.

MyHealth Bank also allows users to download payment and billing information. Since the individual's medical history is private, citizens must apply for this service themselves using their Citizen Digital Certificate (see Figure 58.5). The Citizen Digital Certificate ensures security for all downloaded files.

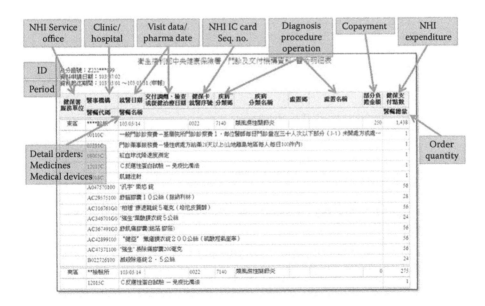

FIGURE 58.5
MyHealth Bank snapshot.

Conclusion

The introduction of HIT by the Taiwanese DoH has been a success. Recent initiatives, such as the USB-PHR, the Taiwanese Healthcare Smart Card, PharmaCloud, and My HealthBank have multiple benefits, empowering patients and sustaining the continuity of care by providing access to patient information at the point of care, in addition to improving quality of care. Plans for future improvements include NHI's development of applications to ensure that My HealthBank data is available for analysis and to make it more accessible to patients.

Discussion and Conclusion

Jeffrey Braithwaite, Russell Mannion, Yukihiro Matsuyama, Paul Shekelle, Stuart Whittaker, Samir Al-Adawi, Kristiana Ludlow, and Wendy James

CONTENTS

Across the pages of the book, we have presented success stories emanating from a third of the world's countries, harnessing local knowledge from well-informed and respected authors who have adduced the elements of success embedded in their well-chosen exemplar. The most telling point we would make at the outset is how much variety is exhibited in the choices of topic and the narratives of the stories. By way of summarizing the wide range of countries, stories, and themes, Table D.1 synthesizes for each country the topic they chose, the broader theme to which this topic belongs, and whether the primary attention of the chapter was in macro-, micro-, or meso-level considerations.

There are patterns that emerge from this rendering. We can see at a glance from the table that the topics range from Ebola in West Africa (Guinea, Liberia, Sierra Leone), through other public health issues such as trying to cope with the brain drain in Ghana, creating stronger primary care services in Fiji, Venezuela, and Estonia, and child abuse and neglect in Serbia. They also focus inside hospitals, as in the acute care topics dealt with by Ecuador, Portugal, Australia, Qatar, and South Africa.

Outside of hospitals, at the policy level, we see authors grappling with topics ranging from the discharge of elderly patients in Hong Kong, national systems of reform such as those offered by Turkey, Iran, and Mexico, making legislative improvements in Russia, grappling with medical training and regulation in Malta, the idea of capital in Chile, the Categorizing Authorization Program in Argentina, the single payment system in the United Arab Emirates, affordability of care in India, and health insurance

439

TABLE D.1

Synthesizing Regions, Countries, Topics, Themes, and Foci

Region	Countries	Topic	Primary Theme	Key focus
The Americas	Argentina	Government legislation and non-government initiatives	Policy, coverage, and governance	Macro
	Brazil	Quality improvement	Quality	Macro
	Canada	Improving stroke outcomes through accreditation	Standards accreditation and regulation	Meso
	Chile	Creating symbolic capital and institutional motivation for success	Policy, coverage, and governance	Macro
	Ecuador	Improving hospital management	Organizing care at the macro level	Macro
	Guyana	Elderly patient care	Organizing care at the meso level	Meso
	Mexico	Monitoring and evaluation system for health reform	Policy, coverage, and governance	Meso
	The United States of America	Improving safety in surgical care	Safety	Meso
	Venezuela	*Misión Barrio Adentro* ("Inside the Ghetto Mission") national primary care program	Policy, coverage, and governance	Meso
Africa	Ghana	Arresting the medical brain drain	Workforce and resources	Meso
	Namibia	Quality management model	Quality	Macro
	Nigeria	The responsive health delivery system	Organizing care at the macro level	Macro
	Rwanda	Community-based health insurance	Policy, coverage, and governance	Macro
	South Africa	Regulation of healthcare establishments via a juristic body	Standards accreditation and regulation	Macro

(Continued)

TABLE D.1 (CONTINUED)

Synthesizing Regions, Countries, Topics, Themes, and Foci

Region	Countries	Topic	Primary Theme	Key focus
	West Africa (Guinea, Liberia, Sierra Leone)	Ebola-affected countries	Organizing care at the macro level	Macro
Europe	Austria	Stroke units	Organizing care at the meso level	Meso
	Denmark	Pathways for cancer patients	Organizing care at the meso level	Meso
	England	The role of the National Institute for Health and Care Excellence (NICE)	Workforce and resources	Macro
	Estonia	Reform in primary healthcare	Organizing care at the meso level	Meso
	Finland	eHealth in clinical practice	Technology and IT	Macro
	France	Care-centered approach: increasing patients' feelings of safety	Safety	Macro
	Germany	"Healthy Kinzigtal" population-based healthcare system	Organizing care at the meso level	Meso
	Ireland	Innovative treatment of hemophilia	Technology and IT	Micro
	Israel	Electronic health records and the health information exchange program	Technology and IT	Macro
	Italy	Management of pharmaceutical innovation	Workforce and resources	Macro
	Malta	Medical training and regulation	Workforce and resources	Macro
	The Netherlands	"Prevent harm, work safely" program	Safety	Macro
	Northern Ireland	Improving maternal and pediatric care	Organizing care at the macro level	Macro
	Norway	Standardization of measuring and monitoring adverse events	Safety	Macro

(Continued)

TABLE D.1 (CONTINUED)

Synthesizing Regions, Countries, Topics, Themes, and Foci

Region	Countries	Topic	Primary Theme	Key focus
	Portugal	Hospital-acquired infection	Collaboratives and partnerships	Meso
	Russia	Legislative improvements to improve healthcare quality	Quality	Macro
	Scotland	Partnership and collaboration prompting collaboration	Collaboratives and partnerships	Macro
	Serbia	Child abuse and neglect	Policy, coverage, and governance	Macro
	Spain	Organ donation and transplantation	Organizing care at the macro level	Macro
	Sweden	Researching and learning from clinical data	Technology and IT	Macro
	Switzerland	Collaborations to improve patient safety	Collaboratives and partnerships	Macro
	Turkey	National healthcare accreditation system	Standards accreditation and regulation	Macro
	Wales	Shared decision-making in practice and strategic improvements	Organizing care at the meso level	Meso
Eastern Mediterranean	Afghanistan	Minimum required standards (MRS)	Standards accreditation and regulation	Macro
	The Gulf States (Bahrain, Kuwait, Oman, Qatar, Saudi Arabia, and the United Arab Emirates)	Procuring pharmaceuticals and medical supplies from Gulf Cooperation Council countries	Organizing care at the macro level	Macro
	Iran	The wide-ranging reforms of the Health Transformation plan	Policy, coverage, and governance	Macro

(Continued)

TABLE D.1 (CONTINUED)

Synthesizing Regions, Countries, Topics, Themes, and Foci

Region	Countries	Topic	Primary Theme	Key focus
	Jordan	Healthcare accreditation council	Standards accreditation and regulation	Meso
	Lebanon	Social innovation and blood donations	Collaboratives and partnerships	Meso
	Oman	*Al-Shifa* electronic health record system	Technology and IT	Macro
	Pakistan	Role allocation, accreditation, and databases, for example, cardiac surgery database	Technology and IT	Meso
	Qatar	Qatar early warning system (QEWS) for deteriorating patients	Organizing care at the meso level	Meso
	The United Arab Emirates	Single-payment system	Policy, coverage, and governance	Macro
	Yemen	Improvement of basic health services in Yemen: a successful donor-driven improvement initiative	Quality	Meso
South-East Asia and the Western Pacific	Australia	Between the Flags rapid response system in emergency departments	Organizing care at the micro level	Micro
	China	Self-service in tertiary hospitals	Technology and IT	Meso
	Fiji	Strengthening primary care	Organizing care at the meso level	Meso
	Hong Kong	Care for elderly patients after hospital discharge	Organizing care at the macro level	Macro
	India	Public–private partnership to increase safety and affordability of care	Policy, coverage, and governance	Meso

(*Continued*)

TABLE D.1 (CONTINUED)

Synthesizing Regions, Countries, Topics, Themes, and Foci

Region	Countries	Topic	Primary Theme	Key focus
	Japan	Health insurance	Policy, coverage, and governance	Meso
	Malaysia	Maternal health	Organizing care at the meso level	Meso
	New Zealand	Ko Awatea Organization for innovation and quality improvement	Quality	Meso
	Papua New Guinea	Provincial health authorities	Organizing care at the meso level	Meso
	Taiwan	Improvements in information technology	Technology and IT	Meso

in Japan and Rwanda. There is a strong emphasis on technology too, with chapters from Finland, Ireland, Israel, Oman, Pakistan, Sweden, China, and Taiwan, as examples of countries that are exploiting the benefits, but also paying the costs and making the investments needed, of IT and communication technology to serve patients better and create better data sources for decision-making among providers.

Mirroring the first book in the series, *Health Reform, Quality, and Safety: Perspectives, Participants, Partnerships, and Prospects in 30 Countries* (Braithwaite et al., 2015), there is a strong theme about quality of care and the safety of patients from Brazil, the United States of America, New Zealand, France, Yemen, the Netherlands, Namibia, Russia, and Norway. Closely associated with quality and safety is the topic of accreditation and its counterpart, standards; chapters dealing with this issue include Jordan, Turkey, Afghanistan, South Africa, Canada, and Norway.

Another theme is the way care is organized, whether that is at macro, meso, or micro levels. Countries or authors grappling with this perennial challenge include Ecuador, Guyana, Nigeria, Austria, Denmark, Estonia, Germany, Northern Ireland, Spain, Wales, Qatar, the Gulf States, Australia, Fiji, Hong Kong, Malaysia, and Papua New Guinea. Rubbing shoulders with the idea of organizing care are a series of other themes including workforce (e.g., chapters from Ghana, England, Italy, and Malta), and collaboration (e.g., chapters from Scotland, Switzerland, and Lebanon).

The following sections employ word clouds to emphasize the important concepts through the book. Word clouds are images that give prominence to the most frequently occurring words across text and were generated using

Tagul (https://tagul.com/). To see the frequently occurring concepts, we made some adjustments to the word clouds by taking out the commonly occurring words. We deleted functors, such as "and," "but," "if," and "the," and frequently occurring concepts that occur in all word clouds in the sections of the book, for example, "health," "healthcare," "system," "patient," "care," "hospital," and "improve."

Current Improvement Initiatives and Enhancement Projects In-Country

In this section, we examine, by drawing on the background part of the chapters, the within-country setting and situation that authors presented as a way of providing background for the exemplar they chose. It attempts to answer the question, "What is the context for fertile projects?" Word Cloud 1 provides a diagram to illuminate the key constructs.

As we can see, the context allows authors to provide an option, in this case presented centered on "service," "quality," "improve," and "nation." Many authors chose hospitals and other providers as the focus of their chapters. Reforms at the national level and population-wide implementations, affecting specific circumstances or settings, were popular.

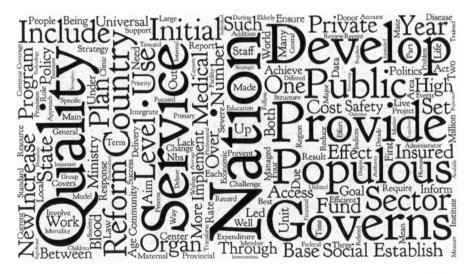

WORD CLOUD 1
Key words relating to the context and setting of chapters.

Criteria for Choosing the Success Stories and a Synthesis of Their Core

Chapter writers were asked to explicate the criteria for success they used to select their chosen case study. Taken together, these stories tell a tale of what success can look like, project by project. Regardless of income disparities across the sample of countries, the differing nature of the health systems, and distinguishing regional features, commonalities emerge. Word Cloud 2 summarizes what the authors had to say about their choice of success story, along with the central features of their narratives.

The criteria for choosing a candidate story were multifaceted including "program," "provide," "develop," "improve," "service," "team," and "quality," for instance. Centrally, authors wanted to show improvement: how this is managed, what services are affected by improvement efforts, how patients benefit or are involved in the improvement strategy, and how quality of care results or patients are made more safe. These considerations were generally the kinds of foci that were judged to be important in selecting a success story.

What Constitutes Success?

Developing the chapter authors' ideas further, we extracted from what the authors presented, and what they said about the impact of their success

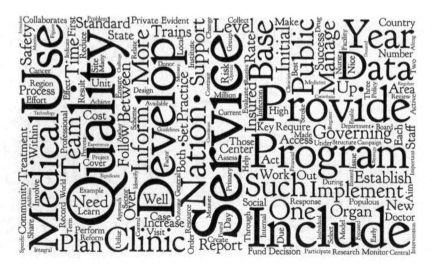

WORD CLOUD 2
Key words concerning the criteria for selecting success stories.

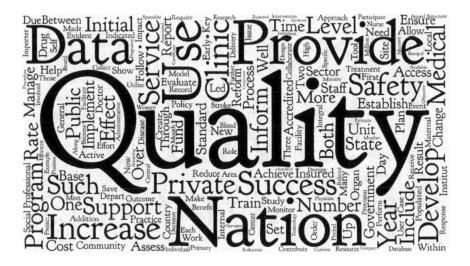

WORD CLOUD 3
Key words regarding the impact of the success stories.

story, in the next word cloud. Word Cloud 3 provides the synthesis of the key factors constituting the criteria for choosing the narrated tale; "quality," "provide," "data," "program," "nation," "implement," and "use" commonly recur.

As the word cloud shows, success comes in many forms. The most important aspects were whether groups' or populations' health was improved, or whether care, and how it is organized, was enhanced. Success was measured in terms of new programs, better provision of services, the development of infrastructure to improve things, and better policy, services, or implementations of new initiatives.

Diffusion of Good Ideas and Their Implementation: Transferability of the Success Narrative within the Originating Country and Elsewhere

We turn to the author's contributions to diffusion and implementation. One current trend in improvement research circles is the idea of "implementation science." This involves the investigation of methods designed to promote the adoption of research results into routine healthcare delivery. It encompasses clinical, organizational, or policy considerations.

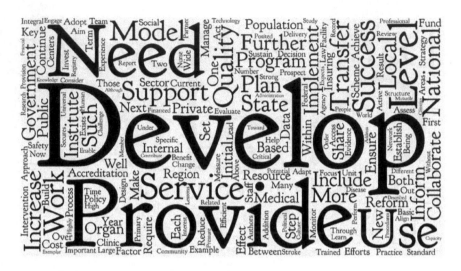

WORD CLOUD 4
Key words relating to the transferability of the success stories.

Our authors provided information about implementation in two modes: first, they discussed transferability of their exemplar elsewhere in their own health system. Secondly, they looked at whether they saw their success story as unique and not likely to be diffusible within other countries, or whether they believed there were lessons to be learned from their chosen example, and the extent to which take-up could be advantageous to other international health systems. Word Cloud 4 provides a synthesis.

As the word cloud highlights, there are wide-ranging ideas on transferability. No one failed to answer the question, although some provided more specific information than others. This shows how rich are the case examples, and how they exhibit considerable propensity for take-up and spread elsewhere. Key issues about implementation and take-up include leverage words, such as "develop," "support," "government," "the State," "provide," "use," "need," "model," and "include."

Prospects for Further Success and Next-Step Change Strategies: Next Generation Improvement

A final word cloud (Word Cloud 5) summarizes what the authors had to say at the end of their chapter. Here, they wrote about what needs to be done further to build on the success they had articulated, and, on the basis of this

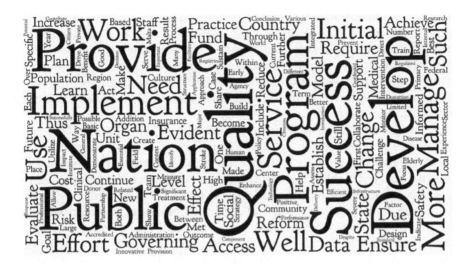

WORD CLOUD 5
Key words regarding the future direction of health system improvement.

knowledge, how else things could be improved across their health system and in other countries.

Again, there was little reluctance from authors about the extent to which they could see how their success story could be of benefit in other countries, health systems, or cultures. Of course, as is well known, it is not advisable to simply drop in an initiative from another country without considering the context and applicability for that new setting. That being said, the sheer groundswell of success across the 60 countries shows commonalities for successful adoption. These include persistence across time, getting the governance and leadership arrangements sorted out for successful implementation, and providing resources, even modest amounts, to fund take-up and adoption. Other success factors include ensuring stakeholders are on board, overcoming political, logistical, and other barriers, and having accountability for implementation assigned appropriately, with individuals and teams committed to the improvement initiative. The key words that summarize the prospects for future success in the word cloud include "quality," "develop," "change," "public," "manage," "work," and other concepts, such as "learn," "implement," "evaluate," "access," "reform," and "data."

Conclusion

A major message from this book is that both developing and developed nations are feeling the effects of changing or aging populations and shrinking health budgets, but nevertheless are creating successful initiatives, programs, and projects despite very challenging environments. Another compelling theme and lesson from countries where the socioeconomic situation is challenging is that improvements can come about relatively inexpensively, and that deceptively simple changes in systems and procedures can be achieved without the need for large allocations of expenditure.

Are there enduring lessons from the book? One is that it may be a good idea in many cases to start with a targeted project. Small-scale, localized improvements can lead to system-wide improvements—from enhancing maternal mortality rates, to extending widespread health improvement or coverage, to looking after the aged poor. Another is that there is a growing realization that the effective use of digital technology, in record keeping, integrated databases, and decision support, are all topics both for the present, and also for the future. More focused lessons include those regarding control of pharmaceuticals, patient education, and "ownership" of the initiatives across a wide range of stakeholders. We discovered that new forms of technology, such as the use of smartphone apps, have their uses. We also found that meta-themes are often part of the aim of smaller-scale projects. Universal health coverage, better policy, or more effectively organized care delivery, for example, are big goals of many health systems. While many are making progress in achieving these aims by running projects at a much smaller scale, they end up being in support of these broader goals.

That is perhaps the key message: one successful case study, if done well, can provide motivation for other successes, and these can eventually build much better health systems for the future. And, if we can aggregate and apply the learnings of this book across the international community, all of us can benefit. This also leads to our next book in this series. We propose to develop a book with our authors on where health system reform is heading over the next 5–15 years. In this compendium, we will tell some new stories extrapolated into the future.

References

Accreditation Canada. (2015). Qmentum accreditation program. Retrieved from https://accreditation.ca/qmentum

Adamski, J., Godman, B., Ofierska-Sujkowska, G., et al. (2010). Risk sharing arrangements for pharmaceuticals: Potential considerations and recommendations for European payers. *BMC Health Services Research*, 10(153).

Adler-Milstein, J., Ronchi, E., Cohen, G. R., et al. (2014). Benchmarking health IT among OECD countries: Better data for better policy. *Journal of the American Medical Informatics Society*, 21(1), 111–116.

Afghan Public Health Institute, Ministry of Public Health, et al. (2011). Afghanistan mortality survey 2010. Calverton, MD: APHI/MoPH.

African National Congress. (1994). A national health plan for South Africa. Retrieved from http://www.sahistory.org.za/archive/national-health-plan-south-africa

African Renaissance Ambassador Corporation. (n.d.). Brain drain in Africa: facts and Figures. Retrieved from http://www.aracorporation.org/files/factsandfigures.pdf

Afzal, U. and Yusuf, A. (2013). The state of health in Pakistan: An overview. *The Lahore Journal of Economics*, 18(special edition), 233–247.

Ahmed, N., Ahmed, F., Anis, H., et al. (2015). An NHS leadership team for the future. London: Reform Research Trust. Retrieved from http://www.reform.uk/wp-content/uploads/2015/11/NHS-Leadership-team-A5-report_WEB.pdf

AIID (Amsterdam Institute for International Development). (2015). The impact of access to quality healthcare in Africa: Research findings on health insurance funds supported programs. Retrieved from http://aiid.org/website/wp-content/uploads/2015/12/The-Impact-of-Access-to-Quality-Healthcare-in-Africa-Research-findings-on-Health-Insurance-Fund-supported-programs.pdf

Al Awaidy, S., Bawikar, S., Prakash, K. R., et al. (2010). Surveillance of adverse events following immunization: 10 years' experience in Oman. *East Mediterranean Health Journal*, 16(5), 474–480.

Ala, F., Allain, J.-P., Bates, I., et al. (2012). External financial aid to blood transfusion services in sub-Saharan Africa: A need for reflection. *PLoS Medicine*, 9(9).

Al-Dhahry, S. H., Al-Awaidy, S. T., Al-Busaidy, S. M., et al. (2001). Poliomyelitis in Oman. II. Toward eradication. *Acta Tropica*, 80(2), 131–138.

Al-Drees, A. M. (2008). Attitude, belief and knowledge about blood donation and transfusion in Saudi population. *Pakistan Journal of Medical Sciences*, 24(1), 74–79.

Alhassan, R. K., Spieker, N., van Ostenberg, P., et al. (2013). Association between health worker motivation and healthcare quality efforts in Ghana. *Human Resources for Health*, 11(37).

Al-Raqadi, A. (2013). National e-health record in Oman. e-Health in Oman. Unpublished document.

Amelung, V., Wolf, S., and Hildebrandt, H. (2012). Integrated care in Germany: A stony but necessary road! *International Journal of Integrated Care*, 12(1). Retrieved from http://doi.org/10.5334/ijic.853

American College of Surgeons. (2011). Business case for ACS NSQIP. Retrieved from http://site.acsnsqip.org/about/business-case/

American Geriatrics Society. (2005). Geriatric medicine: A clinical imperative for ageing population, Part IA policy statement from the American Geriatrics Society. *Annals of Long-Term Care*, 13(3). Retrieved from http://www.managedhealthcareconnect.com/article/geriatric-medicine-clinical-imperative-aging-population-part-ia-policy-statement-american

American Psychological Association (1996). Training guidelines for practice in clinical geropsychology (Draft No. 8). Washington, DC: American Psychological Association.

Ammar, W. (2003). *Health System and Reform in Lebanon*. Beirut, Lebanon: Entreprise universitaire d'études et de publications.

Amuakwa-Mensah, F. and Nelson, A. A. (2014). Retention of medical doctors in Ghana through local postgraduate training. *Journal of Education and Practice*, 5(5). Retrieved from http://pub.epsilon.slu.se/11597/11/amukava_mensah_f_ayesua_ama_n_150116.pdf

Aneman, A., Frost, S., Parr, M., et al. (2015). Characteristics and outcomes of patients admitted to ICU following activation of the medical emergency team: Impact of introducing a two-tier response system. *Critical Care Medicine*, 43(4), 765–773.

Ansell, C. and Gash, A. (2008). Collaborative governance in theory and practice. *Journal of Public Administration Research and Theory*, 18(4), 543–571.

Antwi, J. and Phillips, D. (2012). Wages and health worker retention in Ghana: Evidence from public sector wage reforms. World Bank. Retrieved from https://openknowledge.worldbank.org/bitstream/handle/10986/13581/691070WP00PUBL0GhanaMigrationSalary.pdf?sequence=1

Arce, H. (1998). Hospital accreditation as a means of achieving international quality standards in health. *International Journal for Quality in Health Care*, 10(6), 469–472.

Arce, H. (1999). Accreditation: The Argentine experience in the Latin American Region. *International Journal for Quality in Health Care*, 11(5), 425–428.

Arozullah, A. M., Henderson, W. G., Khuri, S. F., et al. (2003). Postoperative mortality and pulmonary complication rankings: how well do they correlate at the hospital level? *Medical Care*, 41(8), 979–991.

Association of Finnish Local and Regional Authorities. (2017a). Finnish municipalities and regions. Retrieved from http://www.localfinland.fi/expert-services/finnish-municipalities-and-regions-0

Association of Finnish Local and Regional Authorities. (2017b). Specialized healthcare services (Erikoissairaanhoito, in Finnish). Retrieved from http://www.kuntaliitto.fi/asiantuntijapalvelu/sosiaali-ja-terveysasiat/erikoissairaanhoito.

Ataguba, J. and Kalisa, I. R. (2014). The analysis of the 2013 household survey of Community Based Health Insurance enrolees and uninsured households in Rwanda. Unpublished document.

Atun, R., Menabde, N., Saluvere, K., et al. (2006). Introducing a complex health innovation: Primary health care reforms in Estonia (multimethods evaluation). *Health Policy*, 79(1), 79–91.

Australian Agency for International Development. (2008). A situational analysis of the Fiji Health Sector. Suva, Fiji: Australian Agency for International Development.

Austrian Ministry of Health. (2015a). Herz-kreislauf-erkrankungen in Österreich. Retrieved from http://bmg.gv.at/cms/home/attachments/8/7/1/CH1075/CMS1421311013881/hke_bericht_2015.pdf

Austrian Ministry of Health. (2015b). A-IQI: 2014 Austrian inpatient quality indicators. Vienna: Austrian Ministry of Health.

Austrian Ministry of Health. (2016). Stroke-units in Austria. Retrieved from https://www.gesundheit.gv.at/Portal.Node/ghp/public/content/Stroke_Unit_LN.html

Ayres, I. and Braithwaite, J. (1992). *Responsive Regulation*. New York, NY: Oxford University Press.

Azzopardi Muscat, N. and Brand, H. (2014). Ten years on: Time for a public health celebration or sober reflection? *The European Journal of Public Health*, 24(3), 351–352.

Azzopardi Muscat, N., Calleja, N., Calleja, A., et al. (2014). Malta: Health systems review. *Health Systems in Transition*, 16(1), 1–101.

Bacon, N. and Samuel, P. (2012). *Partnership in NHSScotland 1999–2011*. Swindon, UK: ESRC.

Bailey, J. E., Pope, R. A., Elliott, E. C., et al. (2013). Health information exchange reduces repeated diagnostic imaging for back pain. *Annals of Emergency Medicine*, 62(1), 16–24.

Baines, R., Langelaan, M., de Bruijne, M., et al. (2015). How effective are patient safety initiatives? A retrospective patient record review study of changes to patient safety over time. *BMJ Quality & Safety*, 24(9), 561–571.

Bajaj, A., Schernhammer, E. S., Haidinger, G., et al. (2010). Trends in mortality from stroke in Austria, 1980–2008. *Wiener Klinische Wochenschrift*, 122(11–12), 346–353.

Bal, R. and Zuiderent-Jerak, T. (2011). The practice of markets. Are we drinking from the same glass? *Health Economics, Policy and Law*, 6(1), 139–145.

Bardfield, J. (2015). A quality improvement approach to capacity building in low and middle income countries. *AIDS*, 29(Suppl. 2), S179–S186.

Basinga, P., Gertler, P. J., Binagwaho, A., et al. (2011). Effect on maternal and child health services in Rwanda of payment to primary healthcare providers for performance: An impact evaluation. *The Lancet*, 377(9775), 1421–1428.

Bates, I., Manyasi, G., and Medina Lara, A. (2007). Reducing replacement donors in Sub-Saharan Africa: Challenges and affordability. *Transfusion Medicine*, 17(6), 434–442.

Baumann, A., Audibert, G., Claudot, F., et al. (2009). Ethics review: End of life legislation—The French model. *Critical Care*, 13(1), 204.

Behr, L., Grit, K., Bal, R., et al. (2015). Framing and re-framing critical incidents in hospitals. *Health, Risk & Society*, 17(1), 81–97.

Ben-Assuli, O., Shabtai, I., and Leshno, M. (2013). The impact of EHR and HIE on reducing avoidable admissions: Controlling main differential diagnoses. *BMC Medical Informatics and Decision Making*, 13, 49.

Benavente, F. (n.d.). Balanced scorecard: Una herramienta eficaz para la métrica de la estrategia en un Hospital Autogestionado. Ministerio de Salud, Government of Chile. Retrieved from http://www.minsal.cl/portal/url/item/b6456c5e-21594a21e0400101650152a0.pdf

Benning, A., Dixon-Woods, M., Nwulu, U., et al. (2011). Multiple component patient safety intervention in English hospitals: controlled evaluation of second phase. *BMJ*, 342. Retrieved from http://dx.doi.org/10.1136/bmj.d199

Berg, M., Schellekens, W., and Bergen, C. (2005). Bridging the quality chasm: Integrating professional and organizational quality. *International Journal for Quality in Health Care*, 17(1), 75–82.

Berwick, D. (2003). Improvement, trust, and the healthcare workforce. *Quality and Safety in Health Care*, 12(6), 448–452.

Berwick, D. M., Nolan, T. W., and Whittington, J. (2008). The triple aim: Care, health, and cost. *Health Affairs (Millwood)*, 27(3), 759–769.

Bhatia, H. S. (1983). *Ageing and Society: A Sociological Study of Retired Public Servants*. Udaipur, India: Arya's Book Centre.

Bigelow, D. A., Olson, M. M., Smoyer, S., et al. (1991). Quality of Life Questionnaire, respondent self-report version. Portland, OR: Oregon Health Sciences University.

Binagwaho, A., Hartwig, R., Ingeri, D., et al. (2012). Mutual health insurance and the contribution to improvements in child health in Rwanda. *Passauer Diskussionspapiere: Volkswirtschaftliche Reihe*, 66(12). Retrieved from https://www.econstor.eu/bitstream/10419/66213/1/727623443.pdf

Birkmeyer, J. D., Dimick, J. B., and Birkmeyer, N. J. (2004). Measuring the quality of surgical care: Structure, process, or outcomes? *Journal of the American College of Surgeons*, 198(4), 626–632.

Bojanic, A., Bojanic, K., and Likic, R. (2015). Brain drain: Final year medical students' intentions of training abroad. *Postgraduate Medical Journal*, 91, 315–321.

Bourdieu, P. (1986). The forms of capital. In J. Richardson (Ed.), *Handbook of Theory and Research for the Sociology of Education* (pp. 241–258). New York, NY: Greenwood.

Brainin, M. (2006). Time is brain. Upgrade 1.06. Retrieved from http://www.donau-uni.ac.at/imperia/md/content/upgrade/upgrade_1_06_brainin.pdf

Brainin, M. and Klingler, D. (1992). Schlaganfallversorgung in Österreich: Ergebnisse einer Erhebung für das Jahr 1990. *Neuropsychiatrie*, 6, 105–111.

Brainin, M. and Lang, W. (2008). Stroke-units in Austria: Structure, performance and results. *Wiener Medizinische Wochenschrift*, 158(15–16), 407–410.

Braithwaite, J., Matsuyama, Y., Mannion, R., et al. (Eds.). (2015). *Healthcare Reform, Quality and Safety: Perspectives, Participants, Partnerships and Prospects in 30 Countries*. Farnham, UK: Ashgate Publishing.

Britnell, M. (2015). *In Search of the Perfect Health System*. Basingstoke, UK: Palgrove.

Burns, A., Bowers, L., Pak, N., et al. (2010). The excess cost associated with health-care associated bloodstream infections at Auckland City Hospital. *New Zealand Medical Journal*, 123(1324), 17–24.

Busse, R. (2014). Integrated care experiences and outcomes in Germany, The Netherlands, and England. *Health Affairs*, 33(9), 1549–1558.

Busse, R., Geissler, A., Quentin, W., et al. (Eds.). (2011). *Diagnosis-Related Groups in Europe: Moving towards Transparency, Efficiency and Quality in Hospitals*. Berkshire, UK: Open University Press. Retrieved from http://www.euro.who.int/__data/assets/pdf_file/0004/162265/e96538.pdf

Busuttil, C. (2005). Fears of brain drain among doctors. *Times of Malta*. March. Retrieved from http://www.timesofmalta.com/articles/view/20050305/local/fears-of-brain-drain-among-doctors.97309

Canadian Institute for Health Information. (2011). Health care in Canada, 2011: A focus on senior and aging. Retrieved from secure.cihi.ca/free_products/HCIC_2011_seniors_report_en.pdf

Cancer Centrum. (2015). Standardiserade vårdförlopp i cancervården [Standardised care processes in cancer care]. Retrieved from http://www.cancercentrum.se/samverkan/vara-uppdrag/kunskapsstyrning/kortare-vantetider/vardforlopp/

Cardona-Morrell, M. and Hillman, K. (2015). Development of a tool for defining and identifying the dying patient in hospital: Criteria for Screening and Triaging to Appropriate aLternative care (CriSTAL). *BMJ Supportive & Palliative Care.*

Carlson, J. J. (2011). Current status and trends in performance-based schemes between health care payers and manufacturers. *Value in Health*, 14(7), A359–A360.

Carnwell, R. and Carson, A. (2009). The concepts of partnership and collaboration. In R. Carnwell and J. Buchanan (Eds.). *Effective Practice in Health, Social Care and Criminal Justice: A Partnership Approach* (pp. 3–21). Maidenhead, UK: Open University Press.

Cassels, A. (1995). Health sector reform: key issues in less developed countries. Geneva, Switzerland: World Health Organization.

Cassileth, B. R., Vlassov, V. V. and Chapman, C. C. (1995). Health care, medical practice, and medical ethics in Russia today. *Journal of the American Medical Association*, 273(20), 1569–1573.

Census and Statistics Department [Hong Kong]. (2015a). Thematic household survey report (No. 58). Hong Kong: Census and Statistics Department [Hong Kong].

Census and Statistics Department [Hong Kong]. (2015b). Hong Kong population projection 2015–2064. Hong Kong: Census and Statistics Department [Hong Kong].

Central Statistics Organization. (2014). National risk and vulnerability assessment, 2011–12. Afghan living conditions survey. Kabul, Afghanistan: Central Statistics Organization.

Centro de Estudios para el Desarrollo Institucional. (2002). El funcionamiento del sistema de salud Argentino en un contexto federal. Retrieved from http://faculty.udesa.edu.ar/tommasi/cedi/dts/dt77.pdf

Chalkidou, K., Tunis, S., Lopert, R., et al. (2009). Comparative effectiveness research and evidence-based health policy: Experience from four countries. *The Milbank Quarterly*, 87(2), 339–367.

Chami, M. and Mikhael, M. (2015). The saga of the Lebanese healthcare sector: Reforms on the run amid persistent challenges. Blominvest Bank. Retrieved from http://blog.blominvestbank.com/the-saga-of-the-lebanese-healthcare-sector-reforms-on-the-run-amid-persistent-challenges/

Chan, P. S., Jain, R., Nallmothu, B. K., et al. (2010). Rapid response teams: A Systematic review and meta-analysis. *Archives of Internal Medicine*, 170(1), 18–26.

Chaubey, P. C. and Vij, A. (1999). Planning consideration of comprehensive geriatric care in India. *Journal of Academic Hospital Medicine*, 11, 22–24.

Chen, H. (2013). Management and maintenance of self-service registration and payment system in hospital. *Computer CD Software and Applications*, 16(10), 32–33.

Chen, J., Bellomo, R., Flabouris, A., et al. (2009a). The relationship between early emergency team calls and serious adverse events. *Critical Care Medicine*, 37(1), 148–153.

Chen, J., Flabouris, A., Bellomo, R., et al. (2009b). Baseline hospital performance and the impact of medical emergency teams: Modelling vs. conventional subgroup analysis. *Trials*, 10, 117.

Chen, J., Ou, L., Hillman, K., et al. (2014). Cardiopulmonary arrest and mortality trends, and their association with rapid response system expansion. *Medical Journal of Australia*, 201(3), 167–170.

Chen, L., Ma, Z., and Guo, Zh. (2010). Talk about the security and management construction of health information system. *China Medical Devices Information*, 16(3), 21–25.

Chen, Z. (2012). Healthy China 2020: Strategy Research Report. Beijing: China: People's Medical Publishing House.

China Industry Research. (2015). China's medical information market: Depth investigation and analysis and prospects report, 2015–2020. China Industry Research.

Chinese Medical Doctor Association. (2015). White paper: Professional situation for medical doctors. Retrieved from http://www.cmda.net/xiehuixiangmu/falvshiwubu/tongzhigonggao/2015-05-28/14587.html

Clarke, E. (2003). The brain drain of health workers in Ghana. Paper presented at 27th International Conference on Occupational Health, Iguassu Falls, Brazil. February. Retrieved from http://www.equinetafrica.org/sites/default/files/uploads/documents/CLAHres.pdf

Cohen, M. E., Liu, Y., Ko, C. Y., et al. (2016). Improved surgical outcomes for ACS NSQIP hospitals over time: Evaluation of hospital cohorts with up to 8 years of participation. *Annals of Surgery*, 263(2), 267–273.

Coiera, E. (2009). Building a national health IT system from the middle out. *Journal of the American Medical Informatics Association*, 16(3), 271–273.

Collen, M. F. (2012). *Computer Medical Databases: The First Six Decades (1950–2010)*. London: Springer.

Commission Expert Group on Rare Diseases. (2016). Recommendations to support the integration of rare diseases into social services and social policies. Retrieved from http://ec.europa.eu/health/rare_diseases/docs/recommendations_socialservices_policies_en.pdf

Constitution of the Republica Bolivariana de Venezuela. (1999). Articulo 83. Retrieved from http://venezuela.justia.com/federales/constitucion-de-la-republica-bolivariana-de-venezuela/titulo-iii/capitulo-v/#articulo-83

Coombe, D. (1982). *A Review of the Administrative Aspects of the Management of Health Services in Fiji*. Suva, Fiji: Government Printer.

Coulter, A. and Collins, A. (2011). *Making Shared Decision-Making a Reality: No Decision about Me, without Me*. London: Kings Fund.

Council of Europe. (2009). Policy guidelines on integrated national strategies for the protection of children from violence. Retrieved from http://srsg.violenceagainstchildren.org/sites/default/files/political_declarations/COERecommendationprotectionofchildrenENG.pdf

Counties Manukau Health. (2013). Population profile. Retrieved from http://www.countiesmanukau.health.nz/about-us/our-region/population-profile/

Cretikos, M., Chen, J., Hillman, K., et al. (2007). The objective medical emergency team activation criteria: A case-control study. *Resuscitation*, 73(1), 62–72.

Crisp, N. (2015). The future for health in Portugal: Everyone has a role to play. *Health Systems and Reform*, 1(2), 98–106.

Cross, H. E., Sayedi, O., Irani, L., et al. (2017). Government stewardship of the for-profit private health sector in Afghanistan. *Health Policy and Planning*, 32(3), 338–348.

Cunill Grau, N., Fernández, M. and Vergara, M. (2011). Gobernanza sistémica para un enfoque de derechos en salud. Un análisis a partir del caso chileno. *Salud colectiva*, 7, 21–23.

Custer, B., Johnson, E. S., Sullivan, S. D., et al. (2004). Quantifying losses to the donated blood supply due to donor deferral and miscollection. *Transfusion*, 44(10), 1417–1426.

Damrauer, S. M., Gaffey, A. C., DeBord Smith, A., et al. (2015). Comparison of risk factors for length of stay and readmission following lower extremity bypass surgery. *Journal of Vascular Surgery*, 62(5), 1192–1200.

DANIDA (Denmark's International Development Agency). (2016). Ghana–Denmark 1994–2016: A healthy partnership: An account of 22 years of life-saving cooperation in the health sector. Retrieved from http://um.dk/en/~/media/Ghana/Documents/Ghana%20E-Paper%20UK%20health.pdf

de Blok, C., Koster, E., Schilp, J., et al. (2013). Implementatie VMS veiligheidsprogramma: Evaluatieonderzoek in Nederlandse ziekenhuizen. Utrecht: NIVEL.

de la Rosa, G., Domínguez-Gil, B., Matesanz, R., et al. (2012). Continuously evaluating performance in deceased donation: The Spanish quality assurance program. *American Journal of Transplantation*, 12(9), 2507–2513.

Degos, L., Romaneix, F., Michel, P., et al. (2008). Can France keep its patients happy? *BMJ*, 336(7638), 254–257.

Deguara, L. and Azzopardi Muscat, N. (2002). Malta, the European Union and the medical profession: The EU accession process: How EU membership will influence the Maltese medical profession. *Malta Medical Journal*, 14(1), 9–11.

Deilkås, E., Bukholm, G., Lindstrøm, J. C., and Haugen, M. (2015a). Monitoring adverse events in Norwegian hospitals from 2010 to 2013, *BMJ Open*, 5(12), e008576.

Deilkås, E. and Hofoss, D. (2008). Psychometric properties of the Norwegian version of the Safety Attitudes Questionnaire (SAQ), Generic version (Short Form 2006). *BMC Health Services Research*, 8, 191.

Deilkås, E. and Hofoss, D. (2010). Patient safety culture lives in departments and wards: Multilevel partitioning of variance in patient safety culture. *BMC Health Services Research*, 10, 85.

Deilkås, E., Ingebrigtsen, T., and Ringard, Å. (2015b). Norway. In J. Braithwaite, Y. Matsuyama, R. Mannion, et al. (Eds.). *Healthcare Reform, Quality and Safety: Perspectives, Participants, Partnerships and Prospects in 30 Countries* (pp. 261–272). Farnham, UK: Ashgate Publishing.

Delgado-García, G. (1996). Etapas del desarrollo histórico de la salud pública revolucionaria cubana. *Revista Cubana salud pública*, 22, 48–54.

Department of Health [UK]. (1997). The new NHS: Modern, dependable. London: The Stationary Office.

Department of Health, Social Services and Public Safety [Northern Ireland]. (2011). Quality 2020: A ten year strategy to protect and improve quality in health and social care in Northern Ireland. Retrieved from https://www.health-ni.gov.uk/sites/default/files/publications/dhssps/q2020-strategy.pdf

Department of Health, Social Services and Public Safety [Northern Ireland]. (2012). A strategy for maternity care in Northern Ireland, 2012–2018. Retrieved from https://www.health-ni.gov.uk/sites/default/files/publications/dhssps/maternitystrategy.pdf

Department of Health, Social Services and Public Safety [Northern Ireland]. (2014). Supporting leadership for quality improvement and safety: An attributes framework for health and social care. Retrieved from http://www.nursingandmidwiferycareersni.hscni.net/media/1259/q2020_attributes_framework.pdf

Department of Statistics [Jordan]. (2016). Jordan population and housing census report, 2015. Retrieved from http://census.dos.gov.jo/wp-content/uploads/sites/2/2016/02/Census_results_2016.pdf

Department of Treasury [Papua New Guinea]. (2015). Final budget outcome (FBO) 2011–2015. http://www.treasury.gov.pg

Dimick, J. B., Chen, S. L., Taheri, P. A., et al. (2004). Hospital costs associated with surgical complications: A report from the private-sector National Surgical Quality Improvement Program. *Journal of the American College of Surgeons*, 199(4), 531–537.

Dixon-Woods, M., Bosk, C. L., Aveling, E. L., et al. (2011). Explaining Michigan: Developing an ex post theory of a quality improvement program. *The Milbank Quarterly*, 89(2), 167–205.

Doetinchem, O., Carrin, G. and Evans, D. (2010). Thinking of introducing social health insurance? Ten questions. Geneva, Switzerland: World Health Organization. Retrieved from http://www.who.int/healthsystems/topics/financing/healthreport/26_10Q.pdf

Donald, I. P. and Berman, P. (2015). Geriatric outpatient clinics: An audit. Retrieved from http://ageing.oxfordjournals.org

Donaldson, B. (2004). A background for national quality policies in health systems. *International Journal for Quality in Health Care*, 16(1), 91–92.

Donaldson, B., O'Connor, E. and Fortune, T. (2015). Guidance on designing healthcare external evaluation programmes including accreditation. International Society for Quality in Health Care. Retrieved from http://www.isqua.org/accreditation-iap/reference-materials

Donner Sang Compter. (n.d). Retrieved from http://www.dsclebanon.org/en/mission/

Douglas, I. (2015). Investing in quality: Healthcare in the UAE. *The Economist*. Retrieved from http://www.wahacapital.ae/files/publications/Investing-in-quality-WEB.pdf

Dovlo, D. (2003). The brain drain and retention of health professionals in Africa [A case study prepared for a regional raining conference on improving tertiary education in Sub-Saharan Africa: Things That Work!]. Retrieved from http://siteresources.worldbank.org/INTAFRREGTOPTEIA/Resources/dela_dovlo.pdf

Dovlo, D., and Nyonator, F. (1999). Migration of graduates of the University of Ghana Medical School: A preliminary rapid appraisal. *Human Resources for Health Development Journal*, 3(1), 34–37.

Drakeford, M. (2014). Written statement: delivering prudent healthcare in Wales [Minister for Health and Social Services, Wales]. Retrieved from http://gov.wales/about/cabinet/cabinetstatements/previous-administration/2014/prudenthealthcare/?lang=en

Dückers, M. (2009). Longitudinal analysis on the development of hospital quality management systems in the Netherlands. *International Journal for Quality in Health Care*, 21(5), 330–340.

Dunn, I. (1997). Divisional hospital management, World Health Organization Mission Report. Suva Fiji: WHO.

The Economist. (2015). Crime in Venezuela: Justice decayed. 27 August. Retrieved from http://www.economist.com/news/americas/21662569-government-wrongly-blames-colombia-its-high-murder-rate-justice-decayed

El Universal. (2014). Cabildo Metropolitano evaluará funcionamiento de Barrio Adentro. Retrieved from http://www.eluniversal.com/caracas/140506/cabildo-metropolitano-evaluara-funcionamiento-de-barrio-adentro

Elgazar, H., Raad, F., Arfa, C., et al. (2010). Who pays? Out-of-pocket health spending and equity implications in the Middle East and North Africa. World Bank. Retrieved from http://documents.worldbank.org/curated/en/464431468276384167/pdf/580140revised0155B01PUBLIC10WhoPays.pdf

El-Tohamy, A. and Al Raoush, A. (2015). The impact of applying total quality management principles on the overall hospital effectiveness: An empirical study on the HCAC accredited governmental hospitals in Jordan. *European Scientific Journal*, 11(10), 63–76. Retrieved from http://eujournal.org/index.php/esj/article/viewFile/5409/5310

Eng, C., Pedulla, J., Eleazer, G. P., et al. (1997). Program of All-Inclusive Care for the Elderly (PACE): An innovative model of integrated geriatric care and financing. *The American Geriatrics Society*, 45(2), 223–232.

Engholm, G., Ferlay, J., Christensen, N., et al. (2016). NORDCAN: Cancer incidence, mortality, prevalence and survival in the Nordic Countries (Version 7.2). Association of the Nordic Cancer Registries, Danish Care Society. Retrieved from http://www.ancr.nu

Englesbe, M. J. (2010). A statewide assessment of surgical site infection following colectomy: the role of oral antibiotics. *Annals of Surgery*, 252(3), 514–519.

Essen, A. and Lindblad, S. (2013). Innovation as emergence in healthcare: Unpacking change from within. *Social Science & Medicine*, 93, 203–211.

Estonian Health Insurance Fund. (2016). Uuringud ja analüüsid. Retrieved from https://haigekassa.ee/et/haigekassa/uuringud

Etzioni, D. A., Wasif, N., Dueck, A. C., et al. (2015). Association of hospital participation in a surgical outcomes monitoring program with inpatient complications and mortality. *JAMA*, 313(5), 505–511.

Europatientrights.org. (n.d.). National patient rights legislation: France. Retrieved from http://europatientrights.eu/countries/signed/france/france.html

European Commission, Public Health. (2016). Presentation by Italian Medicines Agency at the 4th Meeting of the Commission Expert Group on Safe and Timely Access to Medicines for Patients (STAMP). Retrieved from http://ec.europa.eu/health/documents/pharmaceutical-committee/stamp/index_en.htm

European Union. (2011). Directive 2011/24/EU of the European Parliament and of the Council of 9 March 2011 on the application of patients' rights in cross-border healthcare. *Official Journal of the European Union*, 4 April, L88, 45.

Faridfar, N., Alimohammadzadeh, K., and Seyedin, H. (2016). The impact of health system reform on clinical, paraclinical and surgical indicators as well as patients' satisfaction in Rasoul-e-Akram hospital. *Razi Journal of Medical Sciences*, 22(140), 92–99.

Farmer, P. E., Nutt, C. T., Wagner, C. M., et al. (2013). Reduced premature mortality in Rwanda: lessons from success. *BMJ*, 346, 20–22.

Federal Ministry of Health [Nigeria]. (2014). National Health Act, 2014: Explanatory Memorandum. Retrieved from: http://www.nassnig.org/document/download/7990

Feeney, C. L., Roberts N. J., and Partridge, M. R. (2005). Do medical outpatients want out of hours' clinics? *BMC Health Services Research*, 5(1), 47.

Feigin, V., Krishnamurthi, R., Bhattacharjee, R., et al. (2015). New strategy to reduce the global burden of stroke. *American Heart Association*, 46(6), 1740–1747.

Felce, D. and Perry, J. (1995). Quality of life: its definition and measurement. *Research in Development Disabilities*, 16(1), 51–74.

Ferré, F., de Belvis, A. G., Valerio, L., et al. (2014). Italy: Health System Review. *Health Systems in Transition*, 16(4), 1–172.

Fink, A. S. Campbell, D. A., Jr., Mentzer, R. M., Jr., et al. (2002). The National Surgical Quality Improvement Program in non-veterans administration hospitals: Initial demonstration of feasibility. *Annals of Surgery*, 236(3), 344–353.

Finnish Government. (2015). Finland, a land of solutions. Prime Minister Juha Sipilä's Programme. Retrieved from http://valtioneuvosto.fi/docu-ments/10184/1427398/Ratkaisujen+Suomi_EN_YHDISTETTY_netti.pdf/8d2e1a66-e24a-4073-8303-ee3127fbfcac

Food and Health Bureau [Hong Kong]. (n.d.). Hong Kong's domestic health accounts (HKDHA)—Estimate of domestic health expenditure, 1989/90–2012/13. Retrieved from http://www.fhb.gov.hk/statistics/en/dha.htm

Fox News Latino. (2014). Venezuela Faces Health Crisis Amid Shortage of HIV/Aids Medication. *Fox News Latino*. May 14. Retrieved from http://latino.foxnews.com/latino/health/2014/05/14/venezuela-faces-health-crisis-amid-shortage-hivaids-medication/

Franchini, M. and Mannucci, P. M. (2012). Past, present and future of hemophilia: A narrative review. *Orphanet Journal of Rare Diseases*, 7(24).

Franco, L. M. (2011). Effectiveness of collaborative improvement: Evidence from 27 applications in 12 less-developed and middle-income countries. *BMJ Quality & Safety*, 20, 658–665.

Frenk, J. and Gómez-Dantés, O. (2009). Ideas and ideals: Ethical basis of health reform in Mexico. *The Lancet*, 373(9673), 1406–1408.

Frenk, J., González-Pier, E., Gómez-Dantés, O., et al. (2006). Comprehensive reform to improve health system performance in Mexico. *The Lancet*, 368(9546), 1524–34.

Gakidou, E., Lozano, R., González-Pier, E., et al. (2006). Assessing the effect of the 2001–2006 Mexican health reform: an interim report card. *The Lancet*, 368(9550), 1920–1935.

Gao, L. (2011). Design and implementation of Medicare self-service system. *China CIO News*, 11, 51–52.

García-Pérez, M. A., Amaya, C., and Otero, Á. (2007). Physicians' migration in Europe: An overview of the current situation. *BMC Health Services Research*, 7(1), 201.

Garling, P. (2008). Final report of the special commission of inquiry into acute care services in NSW public hospitals. Sydney, Australia: Department of Attorney General and Justice.

Garrison, L. P., Jr., Towse, A., Briggs, A., et al. (2013). Performance-based risk-sharing arrangements-good practices for design, implementation, and evaluation: report of the ISPOR good practices for performance-based risk-sharing arrangements task force. *Value in Health*, 16(5), 703–719.

German Technical Cooperation Agency. (2010). Quality improvement for health care providers: With friendly guidance and support. Ministry of public health and population, Republic of Yemen. Retrieved from https://www.giz.de/exper-tise/downloads/giz2010-en-ygrhp-quality-improvement.pdf

German Technical Cooperation Agency (GTZ). (2011). Improving health care system-wide: A publication in the German Health Practice Collection [Online]. Retrieved from http://health.bmz.de/what_we_do/Quality-management/Quality-Improvement/index.jsp

German Technical Cooperation Agency. (2012). Improving health care system-wide: approaches in Morocco and Yemen. Retrieved from http://health.bmz.de/what_we_do/Quality-management/Quality-Improvement/index.jsp

Gesundheit Österreich GmbH. (2016). Ergebnisqualität, dokumentation und berichterstattung [Outcome quality, documentation and reporting]. Retrieved from http://www.goeg.at/de/Bereich/Stroke-Unit-Register.html

Ghazal, M. (2006). Population stands at around 9.5 million, including 2.9 million guests. *The Jordan Times*. Retrieved from http://www.jordantimes.com/news/local/population-stands-around-95-million-including-29-million-guests

Gillespie, P. (2016, January 20). 5 reasons why Venezuela's economy is in a "meltdown". *CNN Money*. Retrieved from http://money.cnn.com/2016/01/18/news/economy/venezuela-economy-meltdown/

Gliklich, R. E. and Dreyer, N. A. (Eds.). (2010). Registries for evaluating patient outcomes: A user's guide (2nd ed). AHRQ Publication No.10-EHC049. Rockville, MD: Agency for Healthcare Research and Quality.

Global Health Technical Assistance Project. (2009). Afghanistan private sector health survey 2008. Washington, DC: Global Health Technical Assistance (GHTA) Project.

Goddard, M. and Smith, P. C. (1998). Equity of access to health care. York, UK: Centre for Health Economics, University of York. Retrieved from https://www.york.ac.uk/che/pdf/op32.pdf

Goel, P. K., Garg, S. K., Singh, J. V., et al. (2003). Unmet needs of the elderly in a rural population of Meerut. *Indian Journal of Community Medicine*, 28(4), 165–166.

Goeschel, C. A., Weiss, W. M., and Pronovost, P. J. (2012). Using a logic model to design and evaluate quality and patient safety improvement programs. *International Journal for Quality in Health Care*, 24(4), 330–337.

Gouda, P., Kitt, K., Evans, D. S., et al. (2015). Ireland's medical brain drain: Migration intentions of Irish medical students. *Human Resources for Health*, 13(1), 3–3.

Goudarzian, A. H., Sharif-Nia, H., Jafari, H., et al. (2016). Inpatient satisfaction with health system transformation project in Mazandaran educational hospitals. *Journal of Mazandaran University of Medical Sciences*, 26(136), 190–195.

Government of Fiji. (1979). The report of the Select Committee on the Fiji Health Service (Parliamentary Paper No. 28). Suva, Fiji: Government of Fiji.

Government of Fiji. (1996). The economy and efficiency review of the Colonial War Memorial Hospital. Suva, Fiji: Government of Fiji.

Government of Fiji. (1997). Report of the Senate Select Committee of the Fiji Health Service (Parliamentary Paper No.44 of 1997). Suva, Fiji: Government of Fiji.

Government of Fiji. (2013). Constitution of the Republic of the Fiji Islands. Suva, Fiji: Government of Fiji.

Government of Papua New Guinea. (2007). The Provincial Health Authority Act, No 9 of 2007.

Government of Papua New Guinea. (2015). Independent review of the Provincial Health Authority management structures.

Government of Malaysia. (1990). The Midwives Act 1966: Midwives regulations 1990. In *His Majesty's Government Gazette* (No. 15). Kuala Lumpur: Government Printers.

Government of Republic of Serbia. (2005). National strategy for the prevention and protection of children from violence. Belgrade, Serbia: Government of Republic of Serbia.

Gray, J., Proudfoot, S., Power, M., et al. (2015). Target CLAB Zero: A national improvement collaborative to reduce central line-associated bacteraemia in New Zealand intensive care units. *New Zealand Medical Journal*, 128(1421), 13–21.

Grech, K., Podesta, M., Calleja, A., et al. (2015). Performance of the Maltese health system. Valletta, Malta: Ministry for Energy and Health.

Green A., Ross D., and Mirzoev T. (2007). Primary health care and England: The coming of age of Alma Ata? *Health Policy*, 80(1), 11–31.

Greene, A., Pagliari, C., Cunningham, S., et al. (2009). Do managed clinical networks improve quality of diabetes care? Evidence from a retrospective mixed methods evaluation. *Quality and Safety in Healthcare*, 9(18), 456–461.

Griffin, F. and Resar, R. (2009). IHI global trigger tool for measuring adverse events. Cambridge, MA: IHI Innovation series.

The Gulf Health Council for Cooperation Council States. (2009). Group purchasing in 30 years. Retrieved from http://www.sgh.org.sa

The Gulf Health Council for Cooperation Council States. (2013a). Manual for group purchasing. Retrieved from http://www.sgh.org.sa

The Gulf Health Council for Cooperation Council States. (2013b). Working together for better health: Technical cooperation among the Gulf states in the field of health. Retrieved from http://www.sgh.org.sa

Guo, X., Xiao, F., Huang, Z., et al. (2012). Design and application of self-service registration system in outpatient department and emergency department. *Military Medical Journal of South China*, 26(1), 61–62.

Guptill, J. (2005). Knowledge management in health care. *Journal of Health Care Finance*, 31(3), 10–14.

Guthrie, B., Davies, H., Greig, G., et al. (2010). Delivering health care through managed clinical networks (MCNs): Lessons from the North. Southampton: NIHR Evaluation, Trials and Studies Coordinating Centre.

Häkkinen, U., Rosenqvist, G. T., Iversen T., et al. (2015). Outcome, use of resources and their relationship in the treatment of AMI, stroke and hip fracture at European hospitals. *Health Economics*, 24(Suppl. 2), 116–139.

Hall, B. L., Hamilton, B. H., Richards, K., et al. (2009). Does surgical quality improve in the American College of Surgeons National Surgical Quality Improvement Program: An evaluation of all participating hospitals. *Annals of Surgery*, 250(3), 363–376.

Ham, C., Heenan, D., Longley, M., et al. (2013). *Integrated Care in Northern Ireland, Scotland and Wales: Lessons for England*. London: King's Fund.

Hannan, E. L. and Chassin, M. R. (2005). Publicly reporting quality information. *JAMA*, 293(24), 2999–3000; author reply 3000–2991.

Hansen, R. P. (2008). Delay in the diagnosis of cancer (Unpublished doctoral thesis). Research Unit and Department of General Practice, Faculty of Health Sciences, University of Aarhus.

Hashemi, B., Baratloo, A., Forouzafar, M. M., et al. (2015). Patient satisfaction before and after executing health sector evolution plan. *Iranian Journal of Emergency Medicine*, 2(3), 127–133.

Health Authority [Abu Dhabi]. (2014). Health statistics. Retrieved from http://www.haad.ae/HAAD/LinkClick.aspx?fileticket=LrAOka_Zx3Q%3d&tabid=349

Health Care Accreditation Council. (2011). Primary health care and family planning centers accreditation standards. Amman, Jordan: Health Care Accreditation Council.

Health Care Accreditation Council. (2013). Hospital accreditation standards. Amman, Jordan: Health Care Accreditation Council.

The Health Foundation. (n.d.). MAGIC: Shared decision making. Retrieved from http://www.health.org.uk/programmes/magic-shared-decision-making

Health Quality and Safety Commission New Zealand. (2015). CLAB graduates from quality and safety markers after "remarkable" bundle success. Retrieved from http://www.hqsc.govt.nz/our-programmes/health-quality-evaluation/news-and-events/news/2062/

HEALTHQUAL International. (2015). HEALTHQUAL performance measurement report. Retrieved from http://www.healthqual.org/healthqual-performance-measurement-report-2015

HEALTHQUAL International. (2016). Adaptive implementation in the absence of formal design. Retrieved from http://www.healthqual.org/adaptive-implementation-absence-formal-design-healthqual-international

Healy J., Sharman E., and Lokuge, B. (2006). Australia: health system review. *Health Systems in Transition*, 8(5), 1–158.

Heart and Stroke Foundation. (2014). 2014 Stroke report: Together against a rising tide: Advancing stroke systems of care. Retrieved from http://www.heartand-stroke.com/atf/cf/%7B99452D8B-E7F1-4BD6-A57D-B136CE6C95BF%7D/HSF_SMReport2014E_Final.pdf

Heidarian, N. and Vahdat. Sh. (2015). The impact of health transformation plan on inpatients' out of pocket payment in Isfahan hospitals. *Journal of Medical Council of Iran*, 33(3), 187–194.

Helsedirektoratet. (2016). Pakkeforløp for kreft. Retrieved from https://helsedirek-toratet.no/kreft/pakkeforlop-for-kreft

Herberts, P. and Malchau, M. (2000). Long-term registration has improved the quality of hip replacement A review of the Swedish THR Register comparing 160,000 cases. *Acta Orthopaedica Scandinavica*, 71(2), 111–121.

High Health Council and World Health Organization. (2016). Al-Istratijiah Al-Wataniah Lil Kita'a Al-Sahi fi Al-Ordon. Amman, Jordan: High Health Council and World Health Organization.

Hildebrandt, H., Stunder, B., and Schulte, T. (2012). Triple Aim in Kinzigtal, Germany: Improving population health, integrating health care and reducing costs of care—Lessons for the UK? *Journal of Integrated Care*, 20(4), 205–222.

Hillman, K., Braithwaite, J., and Chen, J. (2011). Healthcare systems and their (Lack of) integration. In M. DeVita, K. Hillman, and R. Bellomo (Eds.). *Textbook of Rapid Response Systems: Concept and Implementation* (pp. 79–86). New York, NY: Springer.

Hillman, K., Chen, J., Cretikos, M., et al. (2005). Introduction of the medical emergency team (MET) system: A cluster-randomised controlled trial. *The Lancet*, 365(9477), 2091–2097.

Hillman, K., Rubenfeld, G., and Braithwaite, J. (2015). Time to shut down the acute care conveyor belt? *Medical Journal of Australia*, 203(11), 429–430.

Hjort, P. F. (2007). *Uheldige hendelser i helsetjenesten—en lære-, tenke- og faktabok*. Oslo, Norway: Gyldendal Akademisk.

Ho, J. (2006). Telephone Nursing Consultation Service: Improving the health of high risk elders in the community with a collaborative community health care program June 8–9. Paper presented at the Hospital Authority Convention, Hong Kong.

Hofmarcher, M. M. (2010). Excess capacity and planning: Kain tortures Abel. *Health Policy Monitor*. Retrieved from http://hpm.org/en/Surveys/GOEG_Austria/15/Excess_Capacity_and_Planning__Kain_tortures_Abel.html

Hofmarcher, M. M. (2013). Austria: Health system review. *Health Systems in Transition*, 15(7), 1–331.

Hofmarcher, M. M. (2014). The Austrian health reform 2013 is promising but requires continuous political ambition, *Health Policy*, 118(1), 8–13.

Hollenbeak, C. S., Boltz, M. M., Wang, L., et al. (2011). Cost-effectiveness of the National Surgical Quality Improvement Program. *Annals of Surgery*, 254(4), 619–624.

Hollnagel, E., Braithwaite, J., and Wears, R. L. (Eds.). (2013). *Resilient Health Care*. Farnham, UK: Ashgate Publishing.

Hospital Authority [Hong Kong]. (2014). Update on the development of the Community Health Call Centre (HAB-P206). Hong Kong: Hospital Authority [Hong Kong].

Hospital Authority [Hong Kong]. (2015). Hospital authority statistical report 2013/14. Hong Kong: Hospital Authority [Hong Kong].

Hospital de Especialidades Abel Gibert Pontón. (2016). Guayaquil. Retrieved from http://www.hagp.gob.ec.

Hospital de Especialidades Teodoro Maldonado Carbo. (2016). Guayaquil. Retrieved from http://www.htmc.gob.ec.

House of Commons Health Select Committee. (2007). The National Institute for Health and Clinical Excellence. London: The Stationery Office.

Hsing, A. W. and Ioannidis, J. A. (2015). Nationwide population science: Lessons from the Taiwan National Health Insurance Research Database. *JAMA Internal Medicine*, 175(9), 1527–29. Retrieved from http://www.hqsc.govt.nz/our-programmes/health-quality-evaluation/news-and-events/news/2062/

Huang, S. K., Wang, P. J., Tseng, W. F., et al. (2015). NHI-PharmaCloud in Taiwan: A preliminary evaluation using the RE-AIM framework and lessons learned. *International Journal of Medical Informatics*, 84(10), 817–25.

Hughes, C., Pain, C., Braithwaite, J., et al. (2014). "Between the flags": Implementing a rapid response system at scale. *BMJ Quality & Safety*, 23(9), 714–717.

Hui E., Lee, I., Tang, M., et al. (2014). Outcomes of an integrated care model for high risk older patients discharged from acute hospitals in Hong Kong. *International Journal of Integrated Care*, 14(6). Retrieved from http://doi.org/10.5334/ijic.1668

Hvitfeldt, H., et al. (2009). Feed forward systems for patient participation and provider support: Adoption results from the original US context to Sweden and beyond. *Quality Management in Health Care*, 18(4), 247–256.

Hyppönen, H., Hämäläinen, P., and Reponen, J. (Eds.) (2015). eHealth and eWelfare of Finland: Checkpoint 2015. Helsinki: National Institute for Health and Welfare (THL). Report 18/2015.

Information Technology Authority, Sultanate of Oman. (c.2013). Brief summary of e.Oman achievements. Retrieved from http://www.itu.int/net/wsis/review/inc/docs/submissions/WSIS10-HLE-OC_OfficialSubmissions-ITA.Oman.Add.pdf

Information Technology Authority, Sultanate of Oman. (2014). Sultanate of Oman progress report on the Information Society 2003–2013. Information Technology Authority, Sultanate of Oman.

Innes, J. E. and Booher, D. E. (2010). *Planning with Complexity*. Abingdon, UK: Routledge.

Institute for Health Metrics and Evaluation. (2010). Global burden of diseases, injuries, and risk factors study 2010: Austria. Retrieved from http://www. healthdata.org/sites/default/files/files/country_profiles/GBD/ihme_gbd_country_report_austria.pdf

Institute for Healthcare Improvement. (2003). The breakthrough series: IHI's collaborative model for achieving breakthrough improvement. IHI Innovation Series white paper. Boston: Institute for Healthcare Improvement.

Institute for Healthcare Improvement. (2006). Getting started kit: Prevent central line infections. How-to guide. Boston: Institute for Healthcare Improvement.

Institute of Medicine. (2007). *The Learning Healthcare System: Workshop Summary*. Washington, DC: National Academies Press.

Institute of Medicine. (2014). *The Learning Health System Series: Continuous Improvement and Innovation in Health and Health Care*. Washington, DC: National Academies Press.

International Monetary Fund. (2001). Ghana: Enhanced Heavily Indebted Poor Countries (HIPC) Initiative–Preliminary document. Retrieved from https://www.imf.org/external/np/hipc/2001/gha/ghapd.pdf

Islam, A. (2002). Health sector reform in Pakistan: Why is it needed? *The Journal of the Pakistan Medical Association*, 52(3), 95–100.

Jha, A. K., Doolan, D., Grandt, D., et al. (2008). The use of health information technology in seven nations. *International Journal of Medical Informatics*, 77(12), 848–54.

Jian, W. S., Syed-Abdul, S., Sood, S. P., et al. (2012). Factors influencing consumer adoption of USB-based Personal Health Records in Taiwan. *BMC Health Services Research*, 12(1), 277–284.

Johns Hopkins University. (2008). Afghanistan health survey 2006: Estimates of priority health indicators for rural Afghanistan. Baltimore, MD: Bloomberg School of Public Health and Indian Institute of Health Management Research.

Joint Commission International. (2013). JCI accreditation standards for hospitals. Joint Commission Resources. Retrieved from http://www.jointcommissioninternational.org/assets/3/7/Hospital-5E-Standards-Only-Mar2014.pdf

Joint Commission International. (2016). JCI-accredited organizations. Retrieved from http://www.jointcommissioninternational.org/about-jci/jci-accredited-organizations/

Joint United Nations Programme on HIV/AIDS [UNAIDS]. (2015). HIV and AIDS estimates. Retrieved from http://www.unaids.org/en/regionscountries/countries/namibia

Jones, D., Bagshaw, S., Barrett, J., et al. (2012). The role of the medical emergency team in end-of-life care: A multicenter, prospective, observational study. *Critical Care Medicine*, 40(1), 98–103.

Jones, D. A., DeVita, M. A., and Bellomo, R. (2011). Rapid-response teams. *New England Journal of Medicine*, 365(2), 139–146.

Jones, R. (2008). Hugo Chavez's health-care programme misses its goals. *The Lancet*, 371(9629), 1988.

JSI Research & Training Institute, Inc. (n.d.). Male health workers increase access to family planning in Sokoto. Retrieved from http://www.jsi.com/JSIInternet/Inc/Common/_download_pub.cfm?id=15901&lid=3

Kalda, R. and Lember, M. (2000). Setting national standards for practice equipment. Presence of practice equipment in Estonian practices before and after introduction of guidelines with feedback. *International Journal of Quality in Health Care*, 12(1), 59–63.

Kalda, R., Maaroos, H.-I., and Lember, M. (2000). Motivation and satisfaction among Estonian family doctors working in different settings. *European Journal of General Practice*, 6(1), 15–19.

Kalda, R. and Västra, K. (2013). The effect of continuous monitoring of hypertension and type 2 diabetes mellitus on the number of visits to medical specialists and hospitalization: A retrospective study. *Medicina (Kaunas)*, 49(11), 490–496.

Kallio, A. (2015). eHealth and eSocial in Finland, now and in 2020. Presentation. May. Retrieved from http://ec.europa.eu/health/ehealth/docs/ev_20150512_co53_en.pdf

Kaplan, R. and Norton, D. (2000). *Cuadro de mando integral*. Barcelona: Harvard Business School Press.

Karim, R. and Ali, S. H. M. (2013). Maternal health in Malaysia: progress and potential. *The Lancet*, 381(9879), 1690–1691.

Kayral, İ. (2014). Perceived service quality in healthcare organizations and a research in Ankara by hospital type. *Journal of Ankara Studies*, 2(1), 22–34.

Kennon, B., Leese, G., Cochrane, L., et al. (2012). Reduced incidence of lower-extremity amputations in people with diabetes in Scotland: A nationwide study. *Diabetes Care*, 35, 2588–2590.

Khammash, T. (2012). The health sector of Jordan. Amman, Jordan: Jordinvest. Retrieved from http://network-medical.me/wp-content/uploads/2015/04/jordan.pdf

Khoja, T. and Bawazir, S. (2005). Group purchasing of pharmaceuticals and medical supplies by the Gulf Cooperation Council states. *Eastern Mediterranean Health Journal*, 11(1–2), 217–225.

Khunou, S. F. (2009, January). Traditional leadership and independent Bantustans of South Africa: some milestones of transformative constitutionalism beyond Apartheid. *PER: Potchefstroomse Elektroniese Regsblad*, 12(4), 81–122.

Khuri, S. F. Daley, J., Henderson, W., et al. (1995). The National Veterans Administration surgical risk study: Risk adjustment for the comparative assessment of the quality of surgical care. *Journal of the American College of Surgeons*, 180(5), 519–531.

Khuri, S. F., Henderson, W. G., Daley, J., et al. (2008). Successful implementation of the Department of Veterans Affairs' National Surgical Quality Improvement Program in the private sector: The patient safety in surgery study. *Annals of Surgery*, 248(2), 329–36.

King, G., Gakidou, E., Imai, K., et al. (2009). Public policy for the poor? A randomised assessment of the Mexican universal health insurance programme. *The Lancet*, 373(9673), 1447–1454.

Klein, R. (2013). *The New Politics of the NHS*. Oxford, UK: Radcliffe Medical Publishing.

Knaul, F. M., González-Pier, E., Gómez-Dantés, O., et al. (2012). The quest for universal health coverage: Achieving social protection for all in Mexico. *The Lancet*, 380(9849), 1259–1279.

Ko Awatea. (2011). National programme to prevent central-line associated bacteraemia (Project Charter: October 2011 to April 2013). Retrieved from http://koawatea.co.nz/wp-content/uploads/2012/07/Project-Charter-CLAB-participants-v6-04.11.11.pdf

Ko Awatea and Counties Manukau Health. (2015). We are Ko Awatea. Auckland: Ko Awatea and Counties Manukau Health. Retrieved from http://koawatea. co.nz/about/

Ko Awatea and Health Quality and Safety Commission [New Zealand] (n.d.). *Target CLAB zero*. Wellington: Ko Awatea and Health Quality and Safety Commission [New Zealand]. Retrieved from http://www.hqsc.govt.nz/our-programmes/infection-prevention-and-control/publications-and-resources/ publication/484/

Koenig, M. E. D. (2012). What is KM? Knowledge management explained. *KMWorld*. May 4. Retrieved from http://www.kmworld.com/Articles/Editorial/ What-Is-../What-is-KM-Knowledge-Management-Explained-82405.aspx

Kohn, L. T., Corrigan, J. M., and Donaldson, M. S. (Eds.). (2000). *To Err Is Human: Building a Safer Health System*. Washington, WA: National Academy Press.

Koornneef, E., Robben, P., Al Seiari, M., et al. (2012). Health system reform in the Emirate of Abu Dhabi, United Arab Emirates. Retrieved from http://www. healthpolicyjrnl.com/article/S0168-8510(12)00249-7/abstract

Kronfol, N. M. (2012). Delivery of health services in Arab Countries: A review. *Eastern Mediterranean Health Journal*, 18(12). Retrieved from http://www.emro.who. int/emhj-volume-18-2012/issue-12/08.html

Kruk, M. E., Myers, M., Tornorlah Varpilah, S., et al. (2015). What is a resilient health system? Lessons from Ebola. *The Lancet*, 385(9980), 1910–1912.

Kruk, M. E., Porignon D., Rockers P. C., et al. (2010). The contribution of primary care to health and health systems in low-and middle-income countries: a critical review of major primary care initiatives. *Social Science & Medicine*, 70(6), 904–911.

Kurowski, C., Chandra, A., Finkel, E., et al. (2015). The state of health care integration in Estonia. Summary report. The World Bank Group. Retrieved from https:// www.haigekassa.ee/sites/default/files/Maailmapanga-uuring/summary_ report_hk_2015.pdf

La Forgia, G. and Nagpal, S. (2012). Government-sponsored health insurance in India: Are you covered? (Directions in Development, No. 72238): World Bank. Retrieved from http://documents.worldbank.org/curated/en/644241468042840697/pdf /722380PUB0EPI008029020120Box367926B.pdf

La Patilla. (2014). El 80% de los módulos de Barrio Adentro del País está cerrado. Retrieved from http://www.lapatilla.com/site/2014/12/08/ el-80-de-los-modulos-de-barrio-adentro-del-pais-esta-cerrado/

Labour and Welfare Bureau and Hospital Authority [Hong Kong]. (2011). Integrated Discharge Support Programme for elderly patients (LC Papers No. CB(2)1411/10-11(01)). Hong Kong: Legislative Council Panel on Welfare Services.

Lai, T., Johansen, A. S., Breda, J., et al. (2015). Better non-communicable disease outcomes: challenges and opportunities for health systems. Country Assessment. Estonia. Copenhagen, Denmark: WHO.

The Lancet. (2008). Health-system reform in China [Editorial]. *The Lancet*, 372(9648), 1437.

The Lancet. (2011). Japan: Universal Health Care at 50 years [Editorial]. *The Lancet*, 378(9796), 1049.

The Lancet. (2015). How to attain the ambitious goals for health reform in China [Editorial]. *The Lancet*, 386(10002), 1419.

Landrigan, C. P., Parry, G. J., Bones, C. B., et al. (2010). Temporal trends in rates of patient harm resulting from medical care. *New England Journal of Medicine*, 363(22), 2124–2134.

Lang, R. (2011). Future challenges to the provision of healthcare' in the 21st century. Paper presented at the Consortium of Institutes of Higher Education in Health and Rehabilitation in Europe annual conference. April. Lisbon, Portugal. Retrieved from http://www.ucl.ac.uk/lc-ccr/downloads/presentations/R_LANG_COHEHRE_LISBON_PRESENTATION.pdf

Langaas, H. (2006). Pasientsikkerhet ved norske sykehus Rapport fra en arbeidsgruppe oppnevnt for å gi anbefalinger om framtidig meldesystem for utilsiktede hendelser i spesialisthelsetjenesten. Norway: Ministry of Health and Care Services.

Langley, G. L., Moen, R., Nolan, K. M., et al. (2009). *The Improvement Guide: A Practical Approach to Enhancing Organizational Performance.* San Francisco: Jossey-Bass.

Larsson, S. (2012). Use of 13 disease registries in 5 countries demonstrates the potential to use outcome data to improve health care's value. *Health Affairs*, 31(1), 220–227.

Lashari, T. (2004). *Pakistan's National Health Policy: Quest for a Vision.* Islamabad, Pakistan: Network Publications.

Leape, L. L., Berwick, D. M., and Bates, D. W. (2002). What practices will most improve safety? Evidence-based medicine meets patient safety. *Journal of the American Medical Association*, 288(4), 501–507.

Leatherman, A., Ferris, T., Berwick, D., et al. (2010). The role of quality improvement in strengthening health systems in developing countries. *International Journal for Quality in Health Care*, 22(4), 237–243.

Lember, M. (2002). A policy of introducing a new contract and funding system of general practice in Estonia. *International Journal of Health Planning and Management*, 17(1), 41–53.

Lember, M., Kosunen, E., and Boerma, W. (1998). Task profiles of district doctors in Estonia and general practitioners in Finland. *Scandinavian Journal of Primary Health Care*, 16(1), 56–62.

Li, K. (2012). Deepening the reform of health care (English edition). *Qiushi Journal*, 4(1), Retrieved from http://english.qstheory.cn/leaders/201204/t20120401_149156.htm

Li, Y. C., Lee, P. S., Jian, W. S., et al. (2009). Electronic health record goes personal world-wide. *Yearbook of Medical Informatics*, 2009, 40–43.

Li, Y. C., Yen, J. C., Chiu, W. T., et al. (2015). Building a national electronic medical record exchange system–Experiences in Taiwan. *Computer Methods and Programs in Biomedicine*, 121(1), 14–20.

Li, Y-C. J. (n.d.). Taiwan HIT case study. Secondary Taiwan HIT case study. Retrieved from http://www.pacifichealthsummit.org/downloads/hitcasestudies/economy/taiwanhit.pdf

Lin, F. O., Luk, J. K., Chan, T. C., et al. (2015). Effectiveness of a discharge planning and community support program in preventing readmission of high-risk older patients. *Hong Kong Medical Journal*, 21(3), 208–216.

Liu, D. (2012). Exploration and development of self-service registration system. *Silicon Valley*, 18, 100.

Lloyd, A., Joseph-Williams, N., Edwards, A., et al. (2013). Patchy "coherence": Using normalization process theory to evaluate a multi-faceted shared decision making implementation program (MAGIC). *Implementation Science*, 8, 102.

Lo, S. V. (2013). Challenges ahead in healthcare management. Paper presented at the Hospital Authority Convention, Hong Kong. May 16.

Lohman, D. (2015). Venezuela's health care crisis. *The Washington Post*. April 29. Retrieved from https://www.hrw.org/news/2015/04/29/venezuelas-health-care-crisis

Lowell, B. L. and Findlay, A. (2001). Migration of highly skilled persons from developing countries: Impact and policy responses: Synthesis report. Geneva: International Labour Office. Retrieved from http://ilo.org/wcmsp5/groups/public/---ed_protect/---protrav/---migrant/documents/publication/wcms_201706.pdf

Lu, C. (2012). Towards universal health coverage: An evaluation of Rwanda mutuelles in its first eight years. *Plos One*, 7(6). Retrieved from http://journals.plos.org/plosone/article?id=10.1371/journal.pone.0039282

Lu, Zh. (2014). Design and application of hospital information system. *China Science and Technology Information*, 8, 162–163.

Maaroos, H. I. (2004). Family medicine as a model of transition from academic medicine to academic health care: Estonia's experience. *Croatian Medical Journal*, 45(5), 563–566.

Maaroos, H. I. and Meiesaar, K. (2004). Does equal availability of geographical and human resources guarantee access to family doctors in Estonia? *Croatian Medical Journal*, 45(5), 567–572.

Maharaj, R., Raffaele, I., and Wendon, J. (2015). Rapid response systems: A systematic review and meta-analysis. *Critical Care*, 19, 254.

Malhotra, A., Maughan, D., Ansell, J., et al. (2015). Choosing wisely in the UK: The Academy of Medical Royal Colleges' initiative to reduce the harms of too much medicine. *BMJ*, 350, h2308.

Malta Independent. (2006). Medical brain drain starting at a younger age. 3 September. Retrieved from http://www.independent.com.mt/articles/2006-09-03/news/medical-brain-drain-starting-at-a-younger-age-96223/

Malta Independent. (2010). Doctors complete first specialist course in family medicine. 12 August. Retrieved from http://www.independent.com.mt/articles/2010-08-12/news/doctors-complete-first-specialist-course-in-family-medicine-278665

Marantidou, O., Loukopoulou, L., Zervou, E., et al. (2007). Factors that motivate and hinder blood donation in Greece. *Transfusion Medicine*, 17(6), 443–450.

Marchildon, G. (2013). Canada: Health system review. *Health Systems in Transition*, 15(1), 1–211.

Martin, G. S. (2008). The essential nature of healthcare databases in critical care medicine. *Critical Care*, 12(5), 176.

Martínez, J. and Martineau, T. (2002). Human resources in the health sector: An international perspective. DFID Health Systems Resource Centre. Retrieved from http://www.heart-resources.org/wp-content/uploads/2012/10/Human-resources-in-the-health-sector.pdf

Martins, A. C. M., Lima, C. R. A., Santos, I. S., et al. (2014). Relatório de pesquisa sobre os recursos físicos de saúde no Brasil. Rio de Janeiro: Fiocruz Institute. Retrieved from http://saudeamanha.fiocruz.br/relatórios-de-pesquisa

Mascherek, A., Bezzola, P., Gehring, K., et al. (2016). Effect of a two-year national quality improvement program on surgical checklist implementation. *Zeitschrift für Evidenz, Fortbildung und Qualität im Gesundheitswesen*, 114, 39–47.

Matesanz, R. (1998). Cadaveric organ donation: Comparison of legislation in various countries of Europe. *Nephrology Dialysis Transplantation*, 13, 1632–1635.

Matesanz, R. (2013). Factors influencing the adaptation of the Spanish Model of organ donation. *Transplant International*, 16(6), 736–741.

Matesanz, R., Domínguez-Gil, B., Coll, E., et al. (2011). Spanish experience as a leading country: What kind of measures were taken? *Transplant International*, 24, 333–343.

Matesanz, R., Marazuela, R., Domínguez-Gil, B., et al. (2009). The 40 donors per million population plan: An action plan for improvement of organ donation and transplantation in Spain. *Transplantation Proceedings*, 41(8), 3453–3456.

Matesanz, R. and Miranda, B. (1996). Organ donation-the role of the media and public opinion. *Nephrology Dialysis Transplantation*, 11(11), 2127–2128.

Matesanz, R., Soratti, C., and Pérez Rosales, M. D. (2015). Regional perspective: The Iberoamerican Network/Council on Donation and Transplantation. *Transplantation*, 99(9), 1739–1742.

May, R. J. (2007). *Policy Making and Implementation: Studies from Papua New Guinea*. Canberra, Australia: ANU Press. Retrieved from https://press. anu.edu.au/publications/series/state-society-and-governance-melanesia/ policy-making-and-implementation

McCaffery, K. J., Jansen, J., Scherer, L. D., et al. (2016). Walking the tightrope: Communication overdiagnosis in modern healthcare. *BMJ*, 352, i348.

McDermott, A., Steel, D., McKee, L., et al. (2015). Scotland "bold and brave"? Conditions for creating a coherent national healthcare quality strategy. In S. Boch Waldorff et al. (Eds.). *Managing Change: From Health Policy to Practice*. London: Palgrave Macmillan.

McKnight, J. A. (2015). The Scottish Diabetes Improvement Plan, 2014. *British Journal of Diabetes and Vascular Disease*, 15(3), 131–134.

Medical Credit Fund, Africa. (2015). Financial medical quality Improvement in Africa. Retrieved from http://www.medicalcreditfund.org/news/2015/11/ nigeria's-ogun-state-continues-to-expand-araya-health-insurance-scheme/

Meiesaar, K. and Lember, M. (2004). Efficiency and sustainability of using resources in Estonian primary health care. *Croatian Medical Journal*, 45(5), 573–577.

Merilind, E., Salupere, R., Västra, K., et al. (2015). The influence of performance-based payment on childhood immunisation coverage. *Health Policy*, 119(6), 770–777.

Michel, P., Quenon, J. L., Djihoud, A., et al. (2008). French national survey of inpatient adverse events prospectively assessed with ward staff. *Quality and Safety in Health Care*, 16(5), 369–377.

Middleton, L., Mason, D., Villa, L., et al. (2014). Evaluation of the 20,000 days campaign: A report for counties Manukau District Health Board. Wellington, New Zealand: Health Services Research Centre. Retrieved from http://www.victoria.ac.nz/ sog/researchcentres/health-services-research-centre/publications/reports

Middleton, L., Villa, L., Mason, D., et al. (2015). 20,000 days and beyond: Evaluation of CMDHB's quality improvement campaigns. Wellington, New Zealand: Health Services Research Centre. Retrieved from http://www.victoria.ac.nz/ sog/researchcentres/health-services-research-centre/publications/reports

Ministerio de Salud (MINSAL). (2005). Decreto 38: Reglamento orgánico de los establecimientos de Salud de menor complejidad y de autogestión en red. Retrieved from http://www.hep.cl/transparencia/normativa/decreto_38.pdf

Ministry for Justice, Culture and Local Government. (2003). Health Care Professions Act (Act X11 of 2003) (Cap. 464). Retrieved from http://www.pharmine. org/wp-content/uploads/2014/05/Health-Care-Professions-Act-CAP-464-Nov-2003.pdf

Ministry of Employment and the Economy [Finland]. (2016). Innovating together: Growth strategy for health sector research and innovation activities: The roadmap for 2016–2018. Retrieved from http://urn.fi/URN:ISBN:978-952-327-142-5

Ministry of Finance and Economic Planning [Rwanda]. (2000). Rwanda Vision 2020. Retrieved from http://www.sida.se/globalassets/global/countries-and-regions/africa/rwanda/d402331a.pdf

Ministry of Finance and Economic Planning [Rwanda]. (2013). Economic Development and Poverty Reduction Strategy II: 2013–2018. Retrieved from http://www.minecofin.gov.rw/fileadmin/templates/documents/NDPR/EDPRS_2.pdf

Ministry of Health [China]. (2009). China medical quality champions strategy. Retrieved from http://www.gov.cn/gzdt/2009-05/20/content_1320385.htm

Ministry of Health [Fiji]. (2008). *Annual Report*. Suva, Fiji: Government Publishers. Retrieved from http://www.health.gov.fj/PDFs/Annual%20Report/Annual%20Report%202008.pdf

Ministry of Health [Fiji]. (2010). *Decentralisation of the Outpatient Services from CWM Hospital to the Health Centres in the Suva Sub Division*. Suva, Fiji: Government Publishers.

Ministry of Health [Fiji]. (2011a). *Cabinet Memorandum: Report of the Decentralisation of the General Outpatient Department Services*. Suva, Fiji: Government Publishers.

Ministry of Health [Fiji]. (2011b). *Memorandum: Decentralisation Meeting*. Suva, Fiji: Government Publishers.

Ministry of Health [Fiji]. (2011c). *Annual Report*. Suva, Fiji: Government Publishers. Retrieved from http://www.health.gov.fj/PDFs/Annual%20Report/Annual%20Report%202011.pdf

Ministry of Health [Fiji]. (2011d). *Decentralisation Update as of April 2011*. Suva, Fiji: Government Publishers.

Ministry of Health [Ghana]. (2013). Human resources for health: Strategies and implementation plans. Ghana: Ministry of Health.

Ministry of Health [Jordan]. (2008). Al Khutah Al Istratijiah Li Wizaret Al-Saha [The Ministry of Health's Strategic Plan 2013–2017]. Amman, Jordan: Ministry of Health.

Ministry of Health [Jordan]. (2016). Health statistics and indicators. Retrieved from http://www.moh.gov.jo/EN/Pages/HealthStatisticsandIndicators.aspx

Ministry of Health [New Zealand]. (2016). New Zealand health strategy: Future direction: All New Zealanders live well, stay well, get well. Wellington, New Zealand: Ministry of Health. Retrieved from http://www.health.govt.nz/system/files/documents/publications/new-zealand-health-strategy-futuredirection-2016-apr16.pdf

Ministry of Health [Oman]. (2014). Annual health report. Muscat, Oman: Ministry of Health.

Ministry of Health [Oman]. (n.d.). Health Care Information System (Al Shifa). Retrieved from http://unpan1.un.org/intradoc/groups/public/documents/un-dpadm/unpan039615.pdf

Ministry of Health [Republic of Serbia]. (2009). Special health service protocol for the protection of children from abuse and neglect. Belgrade, Serbia: Ministry of Health.

Ministry of Health [Rwanda]. (2012). Annual report: Community based health insurance. Retrieved from http://www.moh.gov.rw/fileadmin/templates/Docs/CBHI-Annual-Report-2011-2012f-3__1_.pdf

Ministry of Health [Rwanda]. (2014). Health sector policy. Retrieved from http://www.moh.gov.rw/fileadmin/templates/policies/Health_Sector_Policy_2014.pdf

Ministry of Health [Turkey]. (2003). Health Transformation Program (HTP). Ankara, Turkey: Ministry of Health.

Ministry of Health [Turkey]. (2011). Standards of accreditation in health. Retrieved from https://kalite.saglik.gov.tr/content/files/duyurular_2011/2011/04_ocak_2011/sasrehber.pdf

Ministry of Health [Turkey]. (2015a). Announcements of Accreditation System of Health (AASH), 2013–2015. Ankara, Turkey: Department of Quality and Accreditation in Health.

Ministry of Health [Turkey]. (2015b). Performance, Quality and Patient Safety Agency. Ankara, Turkey: General Directorate of Health Services.

Ministry of Health [Turkey]. (2015c). *Health Statistics Yearbook: 2014*. Ankara, Turkey: Ministry of Health.

Ministry of Health and Care Services [Norway]. (2015). Innovation in the care services. Retrieved from https://www.regjeringen.no/en/dokumenter/nou-2011-11/id646812/

Ministry of Health and Medical Services [Fiji]. (2015a). *Annual report 2014*. Suva, Fiji: Government Publishers. Retrieved from http://www.health.gov.fj/PDFs/Annual%20Report/Annual%20Report%202014.pdf

Ministry of Health and Medical Services [Fiji]. (2015b). *Fiji Health Accounts National Health Expenditure 2011–2014*. Suva, Fiji: Government Publishers.

Ministry of Health and Medical Services [Fiji]. (2016). *National Strategic Plan 2016–2020 Executive Version*. Suva, Fiji: Government Publishers.

Ministry of Health and Social Services [Namibia]. (2014). Quality management assessment report. Retrieved from http://www.mhss.gov.na/files/downloads/fa1_Quality%20Management%20Systems%20Assessment%20Report%202014.pdf

Ministry of Health and Social Services [Namibia]. (2015). *Operation Theatre Manual: Infection Prevention and Control Guidelines* (2nd ed.). Windhoek, Namibia: Ministry of Health and Social Services.

Ministry of Health and Social Services [Namibia]. (n.d.). Quality management directorate. Unpublished.

Ministry of Health, Labour, and Welfare [Japan]. (2014). Long term care insurance statistics. Retrieved from http://www.mhlw.go.jp/toukei/list/45-1b.html

Ministry of Labour, Employment and Social Policy [Republic of Serbia]. (2005). General protocol on protection of children from abuse and neglect. Belgrade, Serbia: Ministry of Labour, Employment and Social Policy.

Ministry of National Health Services, Regulations, and Coordination, Government of Pakistan. (n.d.). Achievements. Retrieved from http://nhsrc.gov.pk/

Ministry of National Planning [Fiji]. (2009). Roadmap for democracy and sustainable socio-economic development 2009–2014: A better fiji for all. Suva, Fiji: The Ministry of National Planning.

Ministry of Planning and International Cooperation [Jordan]. (2015). Al-Ordon 2025 Ro'ya wa Istratijiah watanya [Jordan 2025 Vision and National Strategy]. Amman, Jordan: Ministry of Planning and International Cooperation.

Ministry of Public Health [Afghanistan]. (2009). Afghanistan National Private Health Sector Policy, 2009–2014. Kabul, Afghanistan: Ministry of Public Health.

Ministry of Public Health [Afghanistan]. (2013). Afghanistan national health accounts with subaccounts for reproductive health 2011–2012. Kabul, Afghanistan: Ministry of Public Health.

Ministry of Public Health [Afghanistan]. (2015). Vision for Health 2011–2015: Vision Statement for the MoPH in the year 2015. Kabul, Afghanistan: Ministry of Public Health.

Ministry of Public Health [Ecuador]. (2012). Estatuto orgánico de gestión organizacional por procesos de los hospitales del Ministerio de Salud Pública (Acuerdo Ministerial 1537). Quito, Ecuador: Ministry of Public Health.

Ministry of Public Health and Population [Yemen]. (2000). Health sector reform in the Republic of Yemen. Retrieved from http://www.mophp-ye.org/docs/HSR_Strategy.pdf

Ministry of Social Affairs and Health [Finland]. (2002). Decision in principle by the Council of State on securing the future of health care. Retrieved from https://www.julkari.fi/handle/10024/114676

Mitchell, J., Nicklin, W., and MacDonald, B. (2014). Interorganizational networks: Fundamental to the Accreditation Canada program. *Healthcare Management Forum*, 27, 139–142.

Moeller, J. (2001). The EFQM Excellence Model. German experiences with the EFQM approach in health care. *International Journal for Quality in Health Care*, 13(1), 45–49.

Mohammed, J., Ashton, T., and North, N. (2016a). Wave upon wave: Fiji's experiments in decentralising its healthcare system. *Asia-Pacific Journal of Public Health*, 28(3), 232–243.

Mohammed, J., North, N., and Ashton, T. (2016b). Decentralisation of health services in Fiji: A decision space analysis. *International Journal of Health Policy and Management*, 5(3), 173–181.

Montilla, S., Xoxi, E., Russo, P., et al. (2015). Monitoring registries at Italian Medicines Agency: Fostering access, guaranteeing sustainability. *International Journal of Technology Assessment in Health Care*, 31(4), 210–213.

Moradi-Lakeh, M. and Vosoogh-Moghaddam, A. (2015). Health sector evolution plan in Iran: Equity and sustainability concerns. *International Journal of Health Policy and Management*, 4(10), 637–640.

Mosadeghrad, A. M. (2014a). Factors influencing health care service quality. *International Journal of Health Policy and Management*, 3(2), 77–89.

Mosadeghrad, A. M. (2014b). Patient choice of a hospital: Implications for health policy and management. *International Journal of Health Care Quality Assurance*, 27(2), 152–164.

Müezzinoğlu, M. (2014). Minister of Health of Republic of Turkey, Presidency of Health Institutes of Turkey workshop speech, presented at İstanbul, Turkey.

Mulgan, G., Tucker, S., Ali, R., et al. (2007). Social innovation: What it is, why it matters and how it can be accelerated. Retrieved from http://eureka.bodleian.ox.ac.uk/761/

Muñoz, F., Lopez-Acuña D., Halverson P., et al. (2000). Las funciones esenciales de la salud pública: un tema emergente en las reformas del sector de la salud. *Revista Panamericana de Salud Pública*, 8(1–2), 126–134.

Muntaner, C., Guerra, R., Rueda, S., et al. (2006). Challenging the neoliberal trend: The Venezuelan health care reform alternative. *Canadian Journal of Public Health*, 97(6), I19–I24.

Murray, C. J. L. and Frenk, J. (2000). A framework for assessing the performance of health systems. *Bulletin of the World Health Organization*, 78(6), 717–731.

Mutume, G. (2003). Reversing Africa's "brain drain": New initiatives tap skills of African expatriates. *Africa Recovery*, 17(2), 1. Retrieved from http://www.un.org/en/africarenewal/vol17no2/172brain.htm

Nabitz, U., Klazinga, N., and Walburg, J. (2000). The EFQM excellence model: European and Dutch experiences with the EFQM approach in health care. European Foundation for Quality Management. *International Journal for Quality in Health Care*, 12(3), 191–201.

Nagano Prefecture Healthy Longevity Project Study Team. (2015). Report on Nagano Prefecture healthy longevity project and research program. Retrieved from http://www.pref.nagano.lg.jp/kenko-fukushi/kenko/kenko/documents/saisyueiyaku.pdf

Natarajan, V. S. (1987). Geriatrics: A new discipline. *Indian Journal of Community Guidance*, 4(1), 63–70.

National Department of Health [Papua New Guinea]. (2014). Sector performance annual review: Assessment of sector performance (2009–2013). Port Moresby, Papua New Guinea: National Department of Health.

National Department of Health [Papua New Guinea]. (2015). The mid term review and joint assessment of the Papua New Guinea National Health Plan (2011–2020). Port Moresby, Papua New Guinea: National Department of Health.

National Department of Health [Papua New Guinea]. (2016). Expenditure analysis for 2016. Port Moresby, Papua New Guinea: National Department of Health.

National Department of Health [South Africa]. (2011a). National core standards for health establishments in South Africa. Tshwane, South Africa: National Department of Health.

National Department of Health [South Africa]. (2011b). National health insurance in South Africa: Policy paper. Retrieved from http://www.gov.za/sites/www.gov.za/files/nationalhealthinsurance_2.pdf

National Department of Health [South Africa]. (2015). National health insurance for South Africa: Towards universal health coverage. *Government Gazette*, 606, (39506). Retrieved from http://www.gpwonline.co.za/Gazettes/Gazettes/39506_11-12_Health.pdf

National Department of Planning and Monitoring [Papua New Guinea]. (2004). Medium term development strategy. Port Moresby, Papua New Guinea: National Department of Planning and Monitoring.

National Health Act, 2014 [Federal Republic of Nigeria]. (2014). Retrieved from http://www.nphcda.gov.ng/Reports%20and%20Publications/Official%20Gazette%20of%20the%20National%20Health%20Act.pdf

National Health and Family Planning Commission [China]. (2015a). NHFPC medical institutions report. Retrieved from http://www.nhfpc.gov.cn/mohwsbwstjxxzx/s7967/201512/833751d6965c4fb1895b54e75ce0263d.shtml

National Health and Family Planning Commission [China]. (2015b). NHFPC medical service report. Retrieved from http://www.nhfpc.gov.cn/mohwsbwstjxxzx/s7967/201512/37c45c45707f4ab1982375156e1bc751.shtml

National Health Insurance Administration [Taiwan]. (2016). My health bank. Retrieved from http://www.nhi.gov.tw/English/webdata/webdata.aspx?menu=11&menu_id=590&WD_ID=590&webdata_id=4922

National Institute for Health and Clinical Excellence. (n.d.). Improving health and social care through evidence-based guidance. Retrieved from https://www.nice.org.uk/

National Institute for Health and Welfare [Finland]. (n.d.). The MUMM programme. Retrieved from https://www.thl.fi/en/web/thlfi-en/research-and-expertwork/projects-and-programmes/mumm-programme

National Institute of Health Research [Iran]. (2016). Health transformation plan factsheets. Retrieved from http://nihr.tums.ac.ir

National Institute of Population and Social Security Research [Japan]. (2012). Population projections for Japan. Retrieved from http://www.ipss.go.jp/site-ad/index_english/esuikei/gh2401e.asp

National Institute of Statistics of Rwanda. (2011). *Annual report, 2010*. Retrieved from http://www.statistics.gov.rw/publication/annual-report-2010

National Institute of Statistics of Rwanda. (2012). The evolution of poverty in Rwanda from 2000 to 2011: 2012 results from the household surveys. Retrieved from https://eeas.europa.eu/delegations/rwanda/documents/press_corner/news/poverty_report_en.pdf

National Planning Commission [South Africa]. (n.d). National Development Plan: Vision 2030. Retrieved from https://nationalplanningcommission.wordpress.com/the-national-development-plan/

National Primary Healthcare Development Agency [Nigeria]. (2015). Department of Primary Healthcare Systems Development. Retrieved from http://www.nphcda.gov.ng/index.php/department/phcsd

National Statistics Office [Malta]. (2014) Demographic Review, 2014. Retrieved from: https://nso.gov.mt/en/publications/Publications_by_Unit/Documents/C3_Population_and_Tourism_Statistics/Demographic_Review_2014.pdf

Ng, B. (2011). Establishment of an innovative CHCC in Hong Kong to prevent avoidable hospitalizations. *The Quarterly RACMA*. Retrieved from http://www.racma.edu.au/index.php?option=com_content&view=article&id=351:establishment-of-an-innovative-chcc-in-hong-kong-to-prevent-avoidable-hospitalisations&catid=146:the-quarterly-2011&Itemid=60

Ng, K. H. (2014). An innovative health service model to support discharged high risk elderly patients. Paper presented at the Seminar in a New Models for a Seamless Community Geriatric Care, Sharing Forum, October 16, Hong Kong.

Ng, M. F., Sha, K. Y. and Tong, B. C. (2011). Bridging the gap: Win-win from integrated discharge support for elderly patients. Paper presented at the Hospital Authority Convention, June 7, Hong Kong.

Nichols, M., Townsend, N., Luengo-Fernandez, R., et al. (2012). European cardiovascular disease statistics 2012. Brussels, Belgium: European Heart Network.

Nigeria Local. (2014). A complete list of ethnic groups in Nigeria. Retrieved from http://www.nigerialocal.com.ng/complete-list-ethnic-groups-nigeria/

Nirel, N., Rosen, B., Sharon, A., et al. (2010). The impact of an integrated hospital-community medical information system on quality and service utilization in hospital departments. *International Journal of Medical Informatics*, 79(9), 649–657.

Nirel, N., Rosen, B., Sharon, A., et al. (2011). The impact of an integrated hospital-community medical information system on quality of care and medical service utilisation in primary-care clinics. *Informatics for Health and Social Care*, 36(2), 63–74.

Niringiye, A. and Ayebale, C. (2012). Impact evaluation of the Ubudehe Programme in Rwanda: An examination of the sustainability of the Ubudehe Programme. *Journal of Sustainable Development in Africa*, 14(3), 141–153.

Nolte, E. and McKee, M. (2008). Measuring the health of nations: Updating an earlier analysis. *Health Affairs*, 27(1), 58–71.

Noronha, J. C., Grabois, V., and Gomes, A. Q. (2015). Brazil. In J. Braithwaite, Y. Matsuyama, R. Mannion, et al. (Eds.). *Healthcare Reform, Quality and Safety: Perspectives, Participants, Partnerships and Prospects in 30 Countries* (pp. 171–191). Farnham, UK: Ashgate Publishing.

Norton Rose Fullbright. (2015). China New Healthcare Reform 2020: Ten things to know. Retrieved from http://www.nortonrosefulbright.com/files/china-healthcare-reform_10-things-to-know-128860.pdf

Norwegian Directorate of Health. (2016). Pasientsikkerhetsprogrammet I trygge hender 24-7. Rapport fra Nasjonal Journalundersøkelse med Global Trigger Tool 2014. Olso, Norway: The Norwegian Directorate of Health.

The Norwegian Patient Safety Campaign (2013). Gjennomføring av journalundersøkelse med Global Trigger Tool (GTT) i den norske pasientsikkerhetskampanjen. Oslo, Norway: The Norwegian Patient Safety Campaign.

Nullis-Kapp, C. (2005). Efforts under way to stem "brain drain" of doctors and nurses. *Bulletin of the World Health Organization*, 83(2), 84–85.

Nyinawankunsi, J., Kunda, T., Ndizeye, C., et al. (2015). Increasing equity among community-based health insurance members in Rwanda. *African Health Monitor*, 20, 58–62. Retrieved from https://www.aho.afro.who.int/sites/default/files/ahm/reports/4406/ahm-20-10-increasing-equity-among-community-based-health-insurance-rwanda.pdf

Nyonator, F., Dovlo, D., and Sagoe, K. (2004). The health of the nation and the brain drain in the health sector. Paper presented at the UNDP Conference on Migration and Development, September, Ghana.

Odeyemi, I. (2014). Community-based health insurance programmes and the national health insurance scheme of Nigeria: Challenges to uptake and integration. *International Journal for Equity in Health*, 13(20). Retrieved from http://www.ncbi.nlm.nih.gov/pmc/articles/PMC3941795

OECD (Organisation for Economic Co-operation and Development). (2013). *Cancer Care: Assuring Quality to Improve Survival*. Paris: OECD.

OECD (Organisation for Economic Co-operation and Development). (2014a). *Health at a Glance: Europe 2014*. Paris: OECD. Retrieved from http://dx.doi.org/10.1787/health_glance_eur-2014-en

OECD (Organisation for Economic Co-operation and Development). (2014b). *Obesity Update*. Retrieved from http://www.oecd.org/health/Obesity-Update-2014.pdf

OECD (Organisation for Economic Co-operation and Development). (2015a). *Health at a Glance 2015: OECD Indicators*. Paris: OECD. Retrieved from http://dx.doi.org/10.1787/health_glance-2015-en

OECD (Organisation for Economic Co-operation and Development). (2015b). *Health Note: How does Health Spending in Turkey Compare?* Retrieved from https://www.oecd.org/els/health-systems/Country-Note-TURKEY-OECD-Health-Statistics-2015.pdf

OECD (Organisation for Economic Co-operation and Development). (2015c). *OECD Health Statistics 2015*. Retrieved from http://www.oecd.org/els/health-systems/health-data.htm.

OECD (Organisation for Economic Co-operation and Development). (2016). *OECD Reviews of Health Care Quality: United Kingdom 2016—Raising Standards*. Paris: OECD.

OECD (Organisation for Economic Co-operation and Development) and WHO (World Health Organization). (2011). *OECD Reviews of Health Systems*. Geneva, Switzerland: OECD Publishing.

Office of Health Standards Compliance [South Africa]. (2014). Vision, mission, values. Retrieved from http://www.ohsc.org.za/index.php/who-we-are/vision-mission-values

Office of Health Standards Compliance [South Africa]. (2015a). Annual performance plan 2015. Retrieved from http://ohsc.org.za/index.php/publications/ohsc-documents

Office of Health Standards Compliance. [South Africa]. (2015b). Strategic plan 2015. Retrieved from http://ohsc.org.za/index.php/publications/ohsc-documents

Olesen, F, Hansen, R. P., and Vedsted, P. (2009). Delay in diagnosis: The experience in Denmark. *British Journal of Cancer*, 101(Suppl. 2), S5–S8.

Ollenschlager, G. (2003). Guidelines International N. [International Guideline Network G-I-N (Guidelines International Network). Background and goals]. *Medizinische Klinik*, 98(7), 411–412.

Omoigui, N. A., Miller, D. P., Brown, K. J., et al. (1996). Outmigration for coronary bypass surgery in an era of public dissemination of clinical outcomes. *Circulation*, 93(1), 27–33.

Organización Panamericana de la Salud Oficina, Regional de la Organización Mundial de la Salud. (2006). Barrio Adentro: Derecho a la salud e inclusión social en Venezuela. Caracas, Venezuela: Organización Panamericana de la Salud.

Osborne, N. H., Nicholas, L. H., Ryan, A. M., et al. (2015). Association of hospital participation in a quality reporting program with surgical outcomes and expenditures for Medicare beneficiaries. *Journal of the American Medical Association*, 313(5), 496–504.

Øvretveit, J., Bate, P., Cleary, P., et al. (2002). Quality collaboratives: Lessons from research. *Quality and Safety in Health Care*, 11(4), 345–351.

Øvretveit, J. (2015). Melhoria da qualidade que agrega valor. Rio de Janeiro: Proqualis. Retrieved from http://proqualis.net/sites/proqualis.net/files/melhorias que agregam valor.pdf

Øvretveit, J. and Keel, (2014). Full evidence review of the Swedish Rheumatology Quality Register and Care and Learning System. Stockholm, Sweden: Medical Management Center, Karolinska Institutet.

Øvretveit, J., Keller, C., Hvitfeldt Forsberg, H., et al. (2013). Continuous innovation: The development and use of the Swedish rheumatology register to improve the quality of arthritis care. *International Journal for Quality in Health Care*, 25(2), 118–124.

OvV [Dutch Safety Board]. (2008). An incomplete administrative process: Cardiac surgery at St Radboud UMC. Investigation after reports of high mortality on September 28, 2005 (No. S2005GZ0929-1). April. The Hague, The Netherlands: OvV.

Pan American Health Organization. (2006). Mission Barrio Adentro: The right to health and social inclusion in Venezuela. Retrieved from http://www1.paho.org/English/DD/PUB/BA_ENG_TRANS.pdf

Pardo, D. (2014). The malaria mines of Venezuela. *BBC News*. August 24. Retrieved from http://www.bbc.com/news/health-28689066

Parry, G. and Power, M. (2016). To RCT or not to RCT? The ongoing saga of randomised trials in quality improvement. *BMJ Quality & Safety*, 25(4), 221–223.

Parry, G. J., Carson-Stevens, A., Luff, D. L., McPherson, M. E., and Goldmann, D. A. (2013). Recommendations for evaluation of health care improvement initiatives. *Academic Pediatrics*, 13(6), S23–S30.

Pathmanathan, I., and Dhairiam, S. (1990). Malaysia: Moving from infectious to chronic diseases. In E. Tarimo and A. Creese (Eds.). *Achieving Health for All by the Year 2000: Midway Reports of Country Experiences*. Geneva, Switzerland: World Health Organization.

Pathmanathan, I., Liljestrand, J., Martins, J. M., et al. (2003). Investing in maternal health: Learning from Malaysia and Sri Lanka: The World Bank. Retrieved from https://www.ssatp.org/sites/ssatp/files/pdfs/Topics/gender/259010REPLA CEM10082135362401PUBLIC1%5B2%5D.pdf

Pejovic-Milovancevic, M., Mincic, T., and Kalanj, D. (2012). *Handbook for the Application of Special Health Service Protocol for the Protection of Children from Abuse and Neglect*. Belgrade, Serbia: Institute of Mental Health.

Penchansky, R. and Thomas, J. W. (1981). The concept of access: Definition and relationship to consumer satisfaction. *Medical Care*, 19(2), 127–140.

Peyvandi, F., Garagiola, I., and Young, G. (2016). The past and future of haemophilia: Diagnosis, treatments, and its complications. *The Lancet*, 387(10037), 1–11.

PharmAccess Nigeria (2015). State-supported health insurance: Research & results day. Retrieved from http://hifund.org/uploads/State-Supported%20 Health%20Insurance%20-%20Research%20and%20Results%20Day%20-%20 Booklet%20Kwara%20conference%2021July2015.pdf

Piroozi, B., Moradi, G., Nouri, B., et al. (2016). Catastrophic health expenditure after the implementation of health sector evolution plan: A case study in the West of Iran. *International Journal of Health Policy and Management*, 5(7), 417–423.

Põlluste, K., Habicht, J., Kalda, R., et al. (2006). Quality improvement in the Estonian health system: Assessment of progress using an international tool. *International Journal of Quality in Health Care*, 18(6), 403–413.

Põlluste, K., Kasiulevi, V., Veide, S., et al. (2013). Primary care in Baltic countries: A comparison of progress and present systems. *Health Policy*, 109(2), 122–130.

Porter, M. and Teisberg, E. (2004). Redefiniendo la competencia en el sector salud. *Harvard Business Review*, 82(6), 56–69.

Probst, H. B., Hussain, Z. B., and Andersen, O. (2012). Cancer patient pathways in Denmark as a joint effort between bureaucrats, health professionals and politicians: A national Danish project. *Health Policy*, 105(1), 65–70.

Proudfoot, S. (2013). Target CLAB Zero National Collaborative to Prevent Central Line Associated Bacteraemia (Final Report September 2011 to August 2012). Wellington: Health Quality and Safety Commission and Ko Awatea. Retrieved from https://www.hqsc.govt.nz/assets/Infection-Prevention/Catheter-Related-Bloodstream-Infections/CLAB-final-report-June-2013.pdf

Public Sector Reform Management Unit. (2001). Functional and Expenditure Review of Health Services. Port Moresby: Interim report on Rural Health Services.

Qadir, I., Ahmed, M., and Sharif, H. (2012). *Risk Stratification in Cardiac Surgery in Pakistan*. Saarbrücken, Germany: Lap Lambert Academic Publishing.

Quartz, J., Wallenburg, I., and Bal, R. (2013). The performativity of rankings: On the organizational effects of hospital league tables (iBMG Working Paper W2103.2). Rotterdam: Institute of Health Policy and Management.

Ramamurti, P. V. and Jamuna, D. (1993). Development and research on ageing in India. In E. B. Palmore (Ed.), *Development and Research on Ageing: An International Handbook*. Westport, CT: Greenwood Press.

Rao Venkoba, A. (1984). *Health Care of the Rural Aged*. New Delhi, India: Indian Council of Medical Research.

Raval, M. V., Dillon, P. W., Bruny, J. L., et al. (2011). American College of Surgeons National Surgical Quality Improvement Program Pediatric: a phase 1 report. *Journal of the American College of Surgeons*, 212(1), 1–11.

Ravichandran, J. and Ravindran, J. (2014). Lessons from the confidential enquiry into maternal deaths, Malaysia. *British Journal of Obstetrics and Gynaecology*, 121(Suppl. 4), 47–52.

Ravindran, J. (1998). Has the advice been heeded? An audit of maternal deaths in Malaysia. *Journal of Obstetrics and Gynaecology Research*, 24(3), 8.

Ravindran, J. and Mathews, A. (1996). Maternal mortality in Malaysia 1991–1992: The paradox of increased rates. *Journal of Obstetrics & Gynaecology*, 16(2), 86–88.

Ravindran, J., Shamsuddin, K., and Selvaraju, S. (2003). Did we do it right? An evaluation of the colour coding system for antenatal care in Malaysia. *Medical Journal of Malaysia*, 58(1), 37–53.

Rawlins, M. (2009). The decade of NICE. *The Lancet*, 374(9686), 351–352.

Rechel, B., Dubois, C.-A., and McKee, M. (2006). The health care workforce in Europe. In *Research Report of the European Observatory on Health Systems and Policies (European Observatory on Health Care Systems and Policies Edition)*, pp. 147. Trownbridge, UK: The Cromwell Press.

Rechel, B. and McKee, M. (2009). Health reform in central and eastern Europe and former Soviet Union. *The Lancet*, 374(9696), 1186–1195.

Reilly, B., Brown, M. and Flower, S. (2014). The National Research Institute political governance and service delivery in Papua New Guinea: A Strategic review of current and alternative governance systems to improve service delivery. Retrieved from http://www.academia.edu/9082931/Systems_of_Political_Governance_and_Service_Delivery_in_Papua_New_Guinea

Report of the Global Observatory on Donation and Transplantation. (2013). Retrieved from http://www.transplant-observatory.org/Documents/Data%20Reports/Basic%20slides%202013.pdf

República Bolivariana de Venezuela. (2011). *Gaceta oficial de la República Bolivariana de Venezuela* (Número 39.823). Retrieved from https://informadormic.files.wordpress.com/2012/11/gaceta-39823-19dic11-ley-del-ejercicio-de-la-medicina.pdf

Republic of Serbia. (2014). Law on Health Documentation and Healthcare Records, *Official Gazette of the Republic of Serbia*, 123. Retrieved from http://www.paragraf.rs/propisi/zakon_o_zdravstvenoj_dokumentaciji_i_evidencijama_u_oblasti_zdravstva.html

Republic of South Africa. (2004). National Health Act, No. 61 of 2003, 2004. *Government Gazette*, 469 (26595). Cape Town, South Africa: Government Printer.

Republic of South Africa. (2013). National Health Act Amendment, No 12 of 2013. *Government Gazette*, 577(36702). Cape Town, South Africa: Government Printer.

Rezaei, S., Rahimi, A., Arab, M., et al. (2016). Effects of the new health reform plan on the performance indicators of Hamedan University hospitals. *Journal of School of Public Health and Institute of Public Health Research*, 14(2), 51–60.

Richards, D. and Smith, M. J. (2002). *Governance and Public Policy in the UK*. Oxford, UK: Oxford University Press.

Rigby, M., Hill, P., Koch, S., and Keeling. D. (2011). Social care informatics as an essential part of holistic health care: A call for action. *International Journal of Medical Informatics*, 80(8), 544–554.

Riley, W., Schwei, M., and Mccullough, J. (2007). The United States' potential blood donor pool: Estimating the prevalence of donor-exclusion factors on the pool of potential donors. *Transfusion*, 47(7), 1180–1188.

Ringard, Å., Sagan, A., Saunes, I., et al. (2013). Norway: Health systems review. *Health Systems in Transition*, 15(8), 1–195.

Robben, P., Grit, K., and Bal, R. (2015). Inspectie voor de gezondheidszorg. In F. J. H. Mertens, E. R. Muller, H. B. Winter (Eds.). *Toezicht inspecties en autoriteiten in Nederland*. Deventer, Netherlands: Wolters Kluwer.

Roberts, A. and Charlesworth, A. (2014). A decade of austerity in Wales? The funding pressures facing the NHS in Wales to 2025/26. London: Nuffield Trust. Retrieved from http://www.nuffieldtrust.org.uk/sites/files/nuffield/publication/140617_decade_of_austerity_wales.pdf

Roberts, G., Irava, W., Tuiketei, T., et al. (2011). The Fiji Islands health system review. *Health Systems in Transition*, 1(1), 1–150.

Robinson, T., Zaheer, Z., and Mistri, A. K. (2011). Thrombolysis in acute ischemic stroke: An update. *Therapeutic Advances in Chronic Disease*, 2(2), 119–131.

Rodwin, V. G. (2003). The health care system under French national health insurance: Lessons for health reform in the United States. *American Journal of Public Health*, 93(1), 31–37.

Rosen, B. and Samuel, H. (2009). Israel: Health system review. *Health Systems in Transition*, 11(2), 1–226.

Ruiz, F. and Breckon, J. (2014). The NICE way: Lessons for social policy and practice from the National Institute for Health and Care Excellence. London: Alliance for Useful Evidence.

Russian Federation. (1993). Foundations of the legislation of Russian Federation on the health protection of citizens (No. 5487-1). Retrieved from http://www.ilo.org/dyn/natlex/natlex4.detail?p_lang=en&p_isn=34802

Russian Federation. (2011). Basic Law on the Healthcare of Citizens of Russian Federation. (No. 323-FZ). Moscow: Russian Federation.

Saifuddin, A., Shahabuddin, S., Perveen, S., et al. (2015). Towards excellence in cardiac surgery: Experience from a developing country. *International Journal for Quality in Health Care*, 27(4), 255–259.

Sajadi, H. S. and Zaboli, R. (2016). An assessment of the positive effects of health reform plan implementation from the perspective of hospital directors. *Health Information Management*, 13(1), 55–60.

San-Kuei, H. (2014). New era of National Health Insurance in Taiwan: National Health Insurance Administration. Retrieved from https://www.pmda.go.jp/files/000152095.pdf

Sant, M., Capocaccia, R., Coleman, M. P., et al. (2001). Cancer survival increases in Europe, but international differences remain wide. *European Journal of Cancer*, 37(13), 1659–1667.

Santiano, N., Young, L., Hillman, K., et al. (2009). Analysis of medical emergency team calls comparing subjective to "objective" call criteria. *Resuscitation*, 80(1), 44–49.

Santos-Briones, S., Garrido-Solano, C., and Chavez-Chan, M. (2004). Analisis comparativo de los sistemas de salud de Cuba y Canada. *Revista Biomédica*, 15(2), 81–91.

Sari, A. B-A., Sheldon, T. A., Cracknell, A., et al. (2007). Sensitivity of routine system for reporting patient safety incidents in an NHS hospital: Retrospective patient case note review. *BMJ*, 334, 79. Retrieved from http://dx.doi.org/10.1136/bmj.39031.507153.AE

Schneider, P. and Diop, F. P. (2004). Community-based health insurance in Rwanda. In A. Preker, G. Carrin (Eds.). *Health Financing for Poor People: Resource Mobilization and Risk Sharing* (pp. 251–274). Washington, DC: World Bank.

Schnidman, A. (2012). The global effects of the brain drain on health care systems. *GU Journal of Health Sciences*, 3(1). Retrieved from https://blogs.commons.georgetown.edu/journal-of-health-sciences/issues-2/previous-volumes/vol-3-no-1-march-2006/the-global-effects-of-the-brain-drain-on-health-care-systems/

Schoen, C., Osborn, R., How, S. K., et al. (2009). In chronic condition: Experiences of patients with complex health care needs, in eight countries, 2008. *Health Affairs*, 28(1), w1–w16.

Schulte, T., Pimperl, A., Fischer, A., et al. (2014). Propensity score-matching von eingeschriebenen vs. nicht-eingeschriebenen der integrierten versorgung gesundes kinzigtal auf basis von sekun-därdaten erstellt für. Retrieved from http://optimedis.de/files/Publikationen/Studien-und-Berichte/2014/Mortalitaetsstudie-2014/Mortalitaetsstudie-2014.pdf

Scottish Executive. (2001). Patient focus and public involvement. Edinburgh, Scotland: The Stationery Office.

Scottish Executive Health Department. (2001). Scottish diabetes framework: The blueprint for diabetes care in the 21st century. Edinburgh, Scotland: Scottish Executive Health Department.

Scottish Government. (2007). Better health, better care: Action plan. Edinburgh, Scotland: The Scottish Government.

Scottish Government. (2010). Healthcare quality strategy for NHSScotland. Edinburgh, Scotland: The Scottish Government.

Scottish Government. (2011a). Achieving sustainable quality in Scotland's healthcare: A 20:20 vision. Edinburgh, Scotland: The Scottish Government.

Scottish Government. (2011b). Report of the Commission on Future Delivery of Public Services. Edinburgh, Scotland: The Scottish Government.

Scottish Government. (2012). Staff governance standard for NHSScotland employees (4th edn.). Edinburgh, Scotland: The Scottish Government.

Scottish Government. (2015). NHSScotland chief executive's annual report 2014/15. Edinburgh, Scotland: Scottish Government.

Scottish Health Council. (2014). Evaluation of Chest Heart and Stroke Scotland's Voices Scotland Programme. Edinburgh, Scotland: Scottish Health Council.

Scottish Health Council. (2015). Major service change reports. Edinburgh, Scotland: Scottish Health Council.

Scottish Health Council. (2016). Our voice: Working together to improve health and social care. Edinburgh, Scotland: Scottish Health Council.

Scottish Office. (1997). Designed to care. Edinburgh, Scotland: The Stationery Office.

Scottish Office. (1998). Acute services review report. Edinburgh, Scotland: Scottish Office.

Scottish Parliament. (2011). The Patient Rights (Scotland) Act 2011. Edinburgh, Scotland: The Stationery Office.

Sears, K., Archer, L., Irani, L., et al. (2015). The impact of private health sector policy on health systems and outcomes. Washington, DC: Futures Group, Health Policy Project.

Secretaría de Salud. (2002). Salud México 2001. Mexico City, Mexico: Secretaría de Salud.

Secretaría de Salud. (2003). Salud México 2002. Mexico City, Mexico: Secretaría de Salud.

Secretaría de Salud. (2004a). Observatorio del Desempeño Hospitalario 2003. Mexico City, Mexico: Secretaría de Salud. Retrieved from http://www.salud.gob.mx/unidades/evaluacion/publicaciones/odh/odh2003/odh2003.pdf

Secretaría de Salud. (2004b). Salud México 2003. Mexico City, Mexico: Secretaría de Salud.

Secretaría de Salud. (2005a). Observatorio del Desempeño Hospitalario 2004. Mexico City, Mexico: Secretaría de Salud.

Secretaría de Salud. (2005b). Salud México 2004. Mexico City, Mexico: Secretaría de Salud.

Secretaría de Salud. (2006a). Observatorio del Desempeño Hospitalario 2005. Mexico City, Mexico: Secretaría de Salud.

Secretaría de Salud. (2006b). Salud México 2001–2005. Mexico City, Mexico: Secretaría de Salud.

Seddon, M., Hocking, C., Mead, P., et al. (2011). Aiming for zero: Decreasing central line associated bacteraemia in the intensive care unit. *New Zealand Medical Journal*, 124(1338), 9–21.

Shahian, D. M., Edwards, F. H., Ferraris, V. A., et al. (2007). Quality measurement in adult cardiac surgery: Part 1—Conceptual framework and measure selection. *The Annals of Thoracic Surgery*, 83(4), S3–S12.

Sharek, P. J., Parry, G., Goldmann, D., et al. (2011). Performance characteristics of a methodology to quantify adverse events over time in hospitalized patients. *Health Services Research*, 46(2), 654–678.

Shishkin, S. V. and Vlassov, V. V. (2009). Russia's healthcare system: In need of modernisation. *British Medical Journal*, 338. Retrieved from http://dx.doi.org/10.1136/bmj.b2132

Shojania, K. and Marang-van de Mheen, P. (2015). Temporal trends in patient safety in the Netherlands: Reductions in preventable adverse events or the end of adverse events as a useful metric. *BMJ Quality & Safety*, 24(9), 541–544.

Silber, J. H., Rosenbaum, P. R., Trudeau, M. E., et al. (2005). Changes in prognosis after the first postoperative complication. *Medical Care*, 43(2), 122–131.

Simini, B. (2000). Tuscany doubles organ donation rates by following Spanish example. *The Lancet*, 355 (9202), 476.

Siviero, P. D. (2012). Managed-entry agreements as a way of enabling patient access to innovation. *European Journal of Oncology Pharmacy*, 6(3–4), 30–31.

Smart Card Alliance. (2005). The Taiwan health care smart card project. Retrieved from http://www.smartcardalliance.org/resources/pdf/Taiwan_Health_Card_Profile.pdf

Snow, R. C., Asabir, K., Mutumba, M., et al. (2011). Key factors leading to reduced recruitment and retention of health professionals in remote areas of Ghana: A qualitative study and proposed policy solutions. *Human Resources for Health*, 9(13). Retrieved from https://human-resources-health.biomedcentral.com/articles/10.1186/1478-4491-9-13

Sodzi-Tettey, S. (2015). Ghana. In J. Braithwaite, Y. Matsuyama, R. Mannion, et al. (Eds.). *Healthcare Reform, Quality and Safety: Perspectives, Participants, Partnerships and Prospects in 30 Countries* (pp. 10–15). Farnham, UK: Ashgate Publishing.

Solimano, G. and Valdivia, L. (2015). Chile. In J. Braithwaite, Y. Matsuyama, R. Mannion, et al. (Eds.). *Healthcare Reform, Quality and Safety: Perspectives, Participants, Partnerships and Prospects in 30 Countries* (pp. 183–192). Farnham, UK: Ashgate Publishing.

Sonneland, H. (2016). Update: Venezuela is running short of everything: Americas Society/Council of the Americas. Retrieved from http://www.as-coa.org/articles/update-venezuela-running-short-everything

Sposato, L. A. and Saposnik, G. (2012). Gross domestic product and health expenditure associated with incidence, 30-day fatality, and age at stroke onset. *Stroke*, 43, 170–177.

Steinberg, S. M., Popa, M. R., Michalek, J. A., et al. (2008). Comparison of risk adjustment methodologies in surgical quality improvement. *Surgery*, 144(4), 662–667; discussion 662–667.

St. James's Hospital. (2015a). Achieving world class patient safety and efficiency in Irish Healthcare: Whitepaper. Dublin: St. James's Hospital. Retrieved from https://www.gs1ie.org/Download_Files/Healthcare_Files/St-James-Hospital-eProcurement-Whitepaper.pdf

St. James's Hospital. (2015b). Prospectus of learning and development opportunities 2015. Dublin: St. James's Hospital. Retrieved from http://www.stjames.ie/Departments/DepartmentsA-Z/C/CentreforLearningDevelopment/DepartmentinDepth/SJH%20Prospectus2015.pdf

Stafinski, T., McCabe, C. J., and Menon, D. (2010). Funding the unfundable: Mechanisms for managing uncertainty in decisions on the introduction of new and innovative technologies into healthcare systems. *Pharmacoeconomics*, 28(2), 113–142.

Staines, A., Mattia, C., Schaad, N., et al. (2015). Impact of a Swiss adverse drug event prevention collaborative. *Journal of Evaluation in Clinical Practice*, 21(4), 717–726.

Statistics Austria. (2016). Jahrbuch der gesundheitsstatistik [Yearbook of health statistics] 2014. Vienna, Austria: Verlag Österreich.

Statistics Centre [Abu Dhabi]. (2016). Statistics. Retrieved from https://www.scad.ae/en/Pages/default.aspx

Statistics Finland. (2015). Population. Retrieved from http://www.stat.fi/tup/suoluk/suoluk_vaesto_en.html

Steiner, M. M. and Brainin, M. (2003). The quality of acute stroke units on a nationwide level: The Austrian Stroke Registry for acute stroke units. *European Journal of Neurology*, 10(4), 353–360.

Suleiman, A. B., Mathews, A., Jegasothy, R., et al. (1999). A strategy for reducing maternal mortality. *Bulletin of the World Health Organization*, 77(2), 190–193.

Sulović, M. Z. (2016). Analysis of expert teams to protect children from abuse and neglect in the health institutions of the Republic of Serbia in 2014. Belgrade, Serbia: Institute of Public Health of Serbia. Retrieved from http://www. batut.org.rs/download/publikacije/Rad%20strucnih%20timova%20zlostavljanje%20dece%202014.pdf

Supreme Council, Russian Soviet Federative Socialist Republic. (1993). On amendments to the Law of Russian Federation: "On medical insurance of citizens in RSFSR." Approved by Supreme Council RSFSR 2.4.1993. Vedom Verh Soveta RF, (17):602.

Svenska Höftprotesregistret. (n.d.). Swedish Hip Arthroplasty Register. Retrieved from http://www.shpr.se/en/

Swedish Rheumatology Quality Register [SRQ]. (n.d.). About SRQ. Retrieved from http://srq.nu/en/about-srq/

Syed-Abdul, S., Hsu, M. H., Iqbal, U., et al. (2015). Utilizing health information technology to support universal healthcare delivery: Experience of a national healthcare system. *Telemedicine and e-Health*, 21(9), 742–747.

Syrett, K. (2003). A technocratic fix to the "legitimacy problem"? The Blair government and health care rationing in the United Kingdom. *Journal of Health Politics, Policy and Law*, 28(4), 715–746.

Telesur. (2015). Barrio Adentro suma más de 704 millones de consultas gratuitas en Venezuela. Retrieved from http://www.telesurtv.net/telesuragenda/12-anos-de-Barrio-Adentro-20150415-0079.html

Teyrouz, Y. (2011). Transforming a tragedy [Video File]. Retrieved from https://www.youtube.com/watch?v=buv8e5fUOVc

Thompson, A. and Steel, D. (2015). Scotland. In J. Braithwaite, Y. Matsuyama, R. Mannion, et al. (Eds.). *Healthcare Reform, Quality and Safety: Perspectives, Participants, Partnerships and Prospects in 30 Countries* (pp. 273–284). Farnham, UK: Ashgate Publishing.

Thouvenin, D. (2011). French medical malpractice compensation since the act of March 4 2002: Liability rules combined with indemnification rules and correlated with several kinds of proceedings. *Drexel Law Review*, 4(1), 165–197. Retrieved from https://www.google.fr/#q=Kouchner+act%2C+patient+rights+in+france

Times of Malta. (2015). Brain drain reversal? UK doctor says better to work in Malta. 24 September. Retrieved from http://www.timesofmalta.com/articles/view/20150924/local/brain-drain-reversal-uk-doctor-says-better-to-work-in-malta

Towse, A. and Garrison, L. P., Jr. (2010). Can't get no satisfaction? Will pay for performance help? Toward an economic framework for understanding performance-based risk-sharing agreements for innovative medical products. *Pharmacoeconomics*, 28(2), 93–102.

Transparencia Venezuela. (2015). Misiones Transparentes Gran Misión Barrio Adentro. Retrieved from http://transparencia.org.ve/wp-content/uploads/2015/01/InformeBarrio1.pdf

Tsui, E., Au, S. Y., Wong, C. P., et al. (2015). Development of an automated model to predict the risk of elderly emergency medical admissions within a month following an index hospital visit: A Hong Kong experience. *Health Informatics Journal*, 21, 46–56.

UNICEF. (2008). State of the world's children. Retrieved from http://www.unicef.org/sowc08/docs/sowc08_table_8.pdf

UNICEF. (n.d.). Protecting children from violence in South East Europe. Retrieved from http://www.unicef.org/ceecis/EU_UNICEF_project_Protecting_children_from_violence_in_South_East_Europe.pdf

United Nations Development Programme. (2014a). Human development report. Retrieved from http://hdr.undp.org/en/2015-report

United Nations Development Programme. (2014b). Rwanda millennium development goals- Final progress report: 2013. Retrieved from http://www.undp.org/content/dam/undp/library/MDG/english/MDG%20Country%20Reports/Rwanda/Rwanda_MDGR_2015.pdf

United Nations Development Programme. (2015). Recovering from the Ebola crisis: Full report. Retrieved from http://www.undp.org/content/undp/en/home/librarypage/crisis-prevention-and-recovery/recovering-from-the-ebola-crisis---full-report.html

United Nations General Assembly. (1990). Convention on the Rights of the Child (Article 19). Retrieved from http://www.un.org/documents/ga/res/44/a44r025.htm

United Nations General Assembly. (2006). Violence against children: UN Secretary-General's study. Retrieved from http://www.unviolencestudy.org

United States Agency for International Development. (2013). Health care accreditation project: Final report. Retrieved from http://pdf.usaid.gov/pdf_docs/pdacy095.pdf

United States Agency for International Development. (2014a). Sustainable Improvement in PHC/FP Services: Jordan's Accreditation Experience. Retrieved from http://www.initiativesinc.com/resources/publications/docs/HSSII_AC_EOP_Report_Aug2015.pdf

United States Agency for International Development. (2014b). Yemen: Country Development Cooperation Strategy 2014–2016. Retrieved from https://www.usaid.gov/sites/default/files/documents/1860/CDCS_Yemen_Public%20Version.pdf

United States Department of Health and Human Services, Centers for Disease Control and Prevention, National Center for Health Statistics. (2010). National Hospital Discharge Survey, 2007. Retrieved from http://doi.org/10.3886/ICPSR28162.v1

Venezolana de Televisión. (2014). En 11 años Misión Barrio Adentro ha fortalecido la salud pública del país. Retrieved from http://www.vtv.gob.ve/articulos/2014/04/09/en-11-anos-mision-barrio-adentro-ha-fortalecido-la-salud-publica-del-pais-8474.html

Venezuela's medical crisis requires world's attention. (2015). *Boston Globe*. April 28. Retrieved from http://www.bostonglobe.com/opinion/editorials/2015/04/28/medical-crisis-venezuela-requires-world-attention/EAgdzuzc9WebDGCZ0QY8GI/story.html

Vergara, M., Bisama, L., and Moncada, P. (2012). Competencias esenciales para la gestión en red. *Revista Médica de Chile*, 140, 1606–1612.

Vest, J. R., Kern, L. M., Campion, T. R., Jr., et al. (2014). Association between use of a health information exchange system and hospital admissions. *Applied Clinical Informatics*, 5(1), 219–231.

Vetter, P. and Boecker, K. (2012). Benefits of a single payment system: Case study of Abu Dhabi health system reforms. *Health Policy*, 108(2–3), 105–114.

Vincent, C. (2007). Incident reporting and patient safety. *BMJ*, 334, 51. Retrieved from http://dx.doi.org/10.1136/bmj.39071.441609.80

Vincent, C., Burnett, S., and Carthey, J. (2014). Safety measurement and monitoring in healthcare: A framework to guide clinical teams and healthcare organisations in maintaining safety. *BMJ Quality & Safety*, 23, 670–677.

Vlassov, V. V. (2016). Russian experience and perspectives of quality assurance in healthcare through standards of care. *Health Policy and Technology*, 5(3), 307–312.

Wagner, E. H., Austin, B. T., and Von Korff, M. (1996). Organizing care for patients with chronic illness. *The Milbank Quarterly*, 74(4), 511–544.

Wang, L., Wu, Y. and Ren, L. (2008). Usage of self-service report system in laboratory medicine. *West China Medicine*, 6(1396), 1396.

Wang, Zh., He, M., Ke, Y., et al. (2013). Design and application of a digital hospital laboratory information system. *Research and Exploration in Laboratory*, 32(7), 104–106.

Welsh Government. (2015). Mid year estimates of the population, 2014. Retrieved from http://gov.wales/statistics-and-research/mid-year-estimates-population/

Welsh Government. (2016). Prudent healthcare. Retrieved from http://gov.wales/topics/health/nhswales/prudent-healthcare/?lang=en

Welsh Government. (n.d.). Organ donation Wales. Retrieved from http://organdonationwales.org/?lang=en

Wensing, M., Bal, R., and Friele, R. (2012). Knowledge implementation in healthcare practice: A view from the Netherlands. *BMJ Quality & Safety*, 21(5), 439–442.

WHO (World Health Organization). (2000). The world health report 2000: Health systems—Improving performance. Geneva, Switzerland: WHO.

WHO (World Health Organization). (2001). The World Health Report 2000: Health systems improving performance. Geneva, Switzerland: World Health Organization.

WHO (World Health Organization). (2002). *Quality of care: Patient safety*. Report by the Secretariat at the Fifty Fifth World Health Assembly (A55/13). Geneva, Switzerland. 2002.

WHO (World Health Organization). (2005a). International Health Regulations. WHO. Geneva, Switzerland.

WHO (World Health Organization). (2005b). Efforts under way to stem "brain drain" of doctors and nurses. *Bulletin of the World Health Organization*, 83(2), 5.

WHO (World Health Organization). (2006). Quality of Care: a process for making strategic choices in health systems. Retrieved from http://www.who.int/management/quality/assurance/QualityCare_B.Def.pdf

WHO (World Health Organization). (2009). Country Cooperation Strategy for WHO and the Republic of Yemen 2008–2013. Retrieved from http://www.who.int/countryfocus/cooperation_strategy/ccs_yem_en.pdf

WHO (World Health Organization). (2010a). The ICD-10 International statistical classification of diseases and health related problems. Retrieved from http://www.who.int/classifications/icd/ICD10Volume2_en_2010.pdf

WHO (World Health Organization). (2010b). A framework for national health policies, strategies and plans. Retrieved from http://www.who.int/nationalpolicies/FrameworkNHPSP_final_en.pdf

WHO (World Health Organization). (2011). Health systems strengthening: Glossary. Retrieved from http://www.who.int/healthsystems/Glossary_January2011.pdf?ua=1

WHO (World Health Organization). (2012). Management of patient information trends and challenges in member states. *WHO Global Observatory for eHealth series, 6.* Retrieved from http://apps.who.int/iris/bitstream/10665/76794/1/978924150 4645_eng.pdf

WHO (World Health Organization). (2013). United Arab Emirates, *National Expenditure on Health*. Retrieved from http://apps.who.int/nha/database

WHO (World Health Organization). (2014). Global status report on noncommunicable diseases. Retrieved from www.who.int/nmh/publications/ncd-status-report-2014/en/

WHO (World Health Organization). (2015a). Iran (Islamic Republic of): WHO Statistical profile. Retrieved from http://www.who.int/gho/countries/irn.pdf?ua=1

WHO (World Health Organization). (2015b). WHO global strategy on people-centred and integrated health services. Retrieved from http://www.who.int/servicedeliverysafety/areas/people-centred-care/global-strategy/en/

WHO (World Health Organization). (2015c). Health in 2015: From MDGs to SDGs. Retrieved from http://www.who.int/gho/publications/mdgs-sdgs/en/

WHO (World Health Organization). (2015d). Health worker Ebola infections in Guinea, Liberia and Sierra Leone: Preliminary report. Retrieved from http://www.who.int/csr/resources/publications/ebola/health-worker-infections/en/

WHO (World Health Organization). (2015e). WASH training of trainers. Retrieved from http://www.who.int/csr/disease/ebola/wash-training-2015/en/

WHO (World Health Organization). (2015f). World health statistics 2015. Retrieved from http://www.who.int/gho/publications/world_health_statistics/2015/en/

WHO (World Health Organization). (2016a). Yemen: Country profile. Retrieved from http://www.who.int/countries/yem/en/

WHO (World Health Organization). (2016b). Situation report. Retrieved from http://apps.who.int/iris/bitstream/10665/208883/1/ebolasitrep_10Jun2016_eng.pdf?ua=1

WHO (World Health Organization). (2016c). Health worker infection report. Retrieved from http://www.who.int/features/ebola/health-care-worker/en/

WHO (World Health Organization). (2016d). Health systems, international health regulations and essential public health functions: Report of the WHO Interregional Internal Working Meeting. Retrieved from http://www.who.int/servicedeliverysafety/areas/qhc/CopenhagenMeetingReport.pdf?ua=1

WHO (World Health Organization). (2016e). Recovery toolkit: Supporting countries to achieve health service resilience. Retrieved from http://www.who.int/csr/resources/publications/ebola/recovery-toolkit/en/

WHO (World Health Organization). (n.d.a). Health systems: Key expected results. *Secondary Health Systems: Key Expected Results.* Retrieved from http://www.who.int/healthsystems/about/progress-challenges/en/

WHO (World Health Organization). (n.d.b). HEN Sources of Evidence Database. Finnish Office of Health Technology Assessment (Finohta). Retrieved from http://data.euro.who.int/HEN/Search/SearchResult.aspx?SourceEvidenceId=17

WHO (World Health Organization). (n.d.c). Institutional health partnerships. Retrieved from http://www.who.int/csr/disease/ebola/health-systems-recovery/partnerships/en/

WHO (World Health Organization). (n.d.d). Quality in universal health coverage. Retrieved from http://www.who.int/servicedeliverysafety/areas/qhc/en/

WHO (World Health Organization). (n.d.e). WHO commitment: Focusing efforts. Retrieved from http://www.who.int/servicedeliverysafety/areas/qhc/commitment/en/

Wiederhold, G. (1980). Databases in healthcare. (Report No. STAN-CS-80-790). Stanford, CA: Stanford University, Computer Science Department.

Wildridge, V., Childs, S., Cawthra, L., et al. (2004). How to create successful partnerships: A review of the literature. *Health Information and Libraries Journal*, 21, 3–19.

Williams, I. (2016). The governance of coverage in health systems: England's National Institute for Health and Care Excellence (NICE). In S. L. Greer, M. Wismar and J. Figueras (Eds.). *Strengthening Health System Governance: Better Policies, Stronger Performance*. Berkshire, UK: Open University Press.

Wilson, P. (2015). The collapse of Chávezcare. *Foreign Policy*. Retrieved from http://foreignpolicy.com/2015/04/27/chavez-maduro-healthcare-venezuela-cuba/

Winters, B. and DeVita, M. (2011). Rapid response systems: History and terminology. In M. DeVita, K. Hillman, and R. Bellomo (Eds.). *Textbook of Rapid Response Systems: Concept and Implementation* (pp. 3–12). New York, NY: Springer.

Woodall, J., Raine, G., South, J., et al. (2010). Empowerment and health & well-being: Evidence review. Leeds, UK: Center for Health Promotion Research, Leeds Metropolitan University.

World Bank. (1998). Pakistan: Towards a health sector strategy. World Bank. Retrieved from http://www-wds.worldbank.org/external/default/WDSContentServer/WDSP/IB/1998/04/22/000009265_3980625101315/Rendered/PDF/multi0page.pdf

World Bank. (2000). Republic of Yemen: Health sector strategy note. Retrieved from https://openknowledge.worldbank.org/bitstream/handle/10986/14953/444950replacem1s0file0to0catalogue1.pdf;sequence=1

World Bank. (2003). Papua New Guinea public expenditure review and rationalization. Overview of discussion paper. Retrieved from http://documents.worldbank.org/curated/en/546441468287094426/Papua-New-Guinea-Public-expenditure-review-and-rationalization-overview-of-discussion-paper

World Bank. (2009). Rwanda: Country status report. Washington, DC: World Bank.

World Bank. (2015). The state of health care integration in Estonia: A review of Estonia's quality assurance system for health care. Retrieved from https://www.haigekassa.ee/sites/default/files/Maailmapanga-uuring/estonia_quality_assurance_analysiswb_20150226.pdf

World Bank. (2016a). Iran: Country overview. Retrieved from http://www.worldbank.org/en/country/iran/overview

World Bank. (2016b). Jordan: Data. Retrieved from http://data.worldbank.org/country/jordan

World Bank. (2016c). Nigeria: Data. Retrieved from http://data.worldbank.org/country/nigeria

World Bank. (n.d.). Indicators. Retrieved from http://data.worldbank.org/indicator/SP.POP.65UP.TO.ZS

World Federation of Hemophilia. (2012). About bleeding disorders. Retrieved from http://www.wfh.org/en/page.aspx?pid=637#Life_expectancy

Work Group Report. (1995). Sosiaali-ja terveydenhuollon tietoteknologian hyödyntämisstrategia [The Strategy for Utilisation of Information and Communication Technologies in Welfare and Health], Work Group Report. Helsinki: Ministry of

Social Affairs and Health. Retrieved from https://julkaisut.valtioneuvosto.fi/bitstream/handle/10024/74034/TRM199527.pdf?sequence=2

World Health Organization Regional Office for the Eastern Mediterranean. (n.d.). National Health Strategy for Yemen 2011–2025. Retrieved from http://www.emro.who.int/yem/programmes/health-systems-development.html

Xiao, F., Huang, Z., Zhang, W., et al. (2012). Design and application of laboratory self-service report system for outpatients. *Military Medical Journal of South China*, 26(1), 63–73.

Yen, J. C., Chiu, W. T., Chu, S. F., et al. (2016). Secondary use of health data. *Journal of the Formosan Medical Association*, 115(3), 137–138.

Yiu, R., Fung, V., Szeto, K., et al. (2013). Building electronic forms for elderly program: Integrated care model for high risk elders in Hong Kong. *Studies in Health Technology and Informatics*, 192, 1016.

Yuan, W. (2013). Establishment of hospital information system. *World of Electronics*, 23, 102.

Zhang, Y. (2012). Establishment and application of hospital internet system. *Modern Economic Information*, 10(234).

Zhao, M., Liang, M., Yu, R., et al. (2009). China Healthcare Quality Indicators System (CHQIS). *Chinese Hospitals*, 13(4), 2–4.

Zimlichman, E. (2015). Israel. In J. Braithwaite, Y. Matsuyama, R. Mannion, et al. (Eds.). *Healthcare Reform, Quality and Safety: Perspectives, Participants, Partnerships and Prospects in 30 Countries* (pp. 35–44). Farnham, UK: Ashgate Publishing.

Index

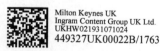

Milton Keynes UK
Ingram Content Group UK Ltd.
UKHW021931071024
449327UK00022B/1763